Giving Bodies Back to Data

Leonardo

Roger F. Malina, Executive Editor
Sean Cubitt, Editor-in-Chief

Synthetics: Aspects of Art & Technology in Australia, 1956–1975, Stephen Jones, 2011

Hybrid Cultures: Japanese Media Arts in Dialogue with the West, Yvonne Spielmann, 2012

Walking and Mapping: Artists as Cartographers, Karen O'Rourke, 2013

The Fourth Dimension and Non-Euclidean Geometry in Modern Art, revised edition, Linda Dalrymple Henderson, 2013

Illusions in Motion: Media Archaeology of the Moving Panorama and Related Spectacles, Erkki Huhtamo, 2013

Relive: Media Art Histories, edited by Sean Cubitt and Paul Thomas, 2013

Re-collection: Art, New Media, and Social Memory, Richard Rinehart and Jon Ippolito, 2014

Biopolitical Screens: Image, Power, and the Neoliberal Brain, Pasi Väliaho, 2014

The Practice of Light: A Genealogy of Visual Technologies from Prints to Pixels, Sean Cubitt, 2014

The Tone of Our Times: Sound, Sense, Economy, and Ecology, Frances Dyson, 2014

The Experience Machine: Stan VanDerBeek's Movie-Drome and Expanded Cinema, Gloria Sutton, 2014

Hanan al-Cinema: Affections for the Moving Image, Laura U. Marks, 2015

Writing and Unwriting (Media) Art History: Erkki Kurenniemi in 2048, edited by Joasia Krysa and Jussi Parikka, 2015

Control: Digitality as Cultural Logic, Seb Franklin, 2015

New Tendencies: Art at the Threshold of the Information Revolution (1961–1978), Armin Medosch, 2016

Screen Ecologies: Art, Media, and the Environment in the Asia-Pacific Region, Larissa Hjorth, Sarah Pink, Kristen Sharp, and Linda Williams, 2016

Pirate Philosophy: For a Digital Posthumanities, Gary Hall, 2016

Social Media Archeology and Poetics, edited by Judy Malloy, 2016

Practicable: From Participation to Interaction in Contemporary Art, edited by Samuel Bianchini and Erik Verhagen, 2016

Machine Art in the Twentieth Century, Andreas Broeckmann, 2016

Here/There: Telepresence, Touch, and Art at the Interface, Kris Paulsen, 2017

Voicetracks: Attuning to Voice in Media and the Arts, Norie Neumark, 2017

Ecstatic Worlds: Media, Utopias, Ecologies, Janine Marchessault, 2017

Interface as Utopia: The Media Art and Activism of Fred Forest, Michael F. Leruth, 2017

Making Sense: Art, Computing, Cognition, and Embodiment, Simon Penny, 2017

Weather as Medium: Towards a Meteorological Art, Janine Randerson, 2018

Laboratory Lifestyles: The Construction of Scientific Fictions, edited by Sandra Kaji-O'Grady, Chris L. Smith, and Russell Hughes, 2018

Invisible Colors: The Arts of the Atomic Age, Gabrielle Decamous, 2018

Virtual Menageries: Animals as Mediators in Network Cultures, Jody Berland, 2019

From Fingers to Digits: An Artificial Aesthetic, Ernest Edmonds and Margaret A. Boden, 2019

MATERIAL WITNESS: Media, Forensics, Evidence, Susan Schuppli, 2020

Tactics of Interfacing: Encoding Affect in Art and Technology, Ksenia Fedorova, 2020

Giving Bodies Back to Data: Image Makers, Bricolage, and Reinvention in Magnetic Resonance Technology, Silvia Casini, 2021

See <https://mitpress.mit.edu> for a complete list of titles in this series.

Giving Bodies Back to Data

Image Makers, Bricolage, and Reinvention in Magnetic Resonance Technology

Silvia Casini

The MIT Press
Cambridge, Massachusetts
London, England

This book was made possible by generous funding from the Leverhulme Trust.

LEVERHULME
TRUST

This book was set in Stone Serif and Stone Sans by Westchester Publishing Services. Printed and bound in the United States of America.

Library of Congress Cataloging-in-Publication Data

Names: Casini, Silvia, 1977- author.
Title: Giving bodies back to data : image makers, bricolage, and reinvention in magnetic resonance technology / Silvia Casini.
Other titles: Leonardo (Series) (Cambridge, Mass.)
Description: Cambridge : The MIT Press, [2021] | Series: Leonardo | Includes bibliographical references and index.
Identifiers: LCCN 2020032364 | ISBN 9780262045292 (hardcover)
Subjects: MESH: Magnetic Resonance Imaging--History | Data Visualization
Classification: LCC RC386.6.M34 | NLM WN 11.1 | DDC 616.07/548--dc23
LC record available at https://lccn.loc.gov/2020032364

10 9 8 7 6 5 4 3 2 1

To Margaret Foster Hutchison

Contents

Series Foreword: Leonardo/International Society for the Arts, Sciences, and Technology (ISAST)

Leonardo, the International Society for the Arts, Sciences, and Technology, and the affiliated French organization Association Leonardo, have some very simple goals:

1. To advocate, document, and make known the work of artists, researchers, and scholars developing the new ways in which the contemporary arts interact with science, technology, and society.
2. To create a forum and meeting places where artists, scientists, and engineers can meet, exchange ideas, and, when appropriate, collaborate.
3. To contribute, through the interaction of the arts and sciences, to the creation of the new culture that will be needed to transition to a sustainable planetary society.

When the journal *Leonardo* was started some fifty years ago, these creative disciplines usually existed in segregated institutional and social networks, a situation dramatized at that time by the "Two Cultures" debates initiated by C. P. Snow. Today we live in a different time of cross-disciplinary ferment, collaboration, and intellectual confrontation enabled by new hybrid organizations, new funding sponsors, and the shared tools of computers and the internet. Sometimes captured in the "STEM to STEAM" movement, new forms of collaboration seem to integrate the arts, humanities, and design with science and engineering practices. Above all, new generations of artist-researchers and researcher-artists are now at work individually and collaboratively bridging the art, science, and technology disciplines. For some of the hard problems in our society, we have no choice but to find new ways to couple the arts and sciences. Perhaps in our lifetime we will see the emergence of "new Leonardos," hybrid creative individuals or teams that will not only develop a meaningful art for our times but also drive new agendas in science and stimulate technological innovation that addresses today's human needs.

For more information on the activities of the Leonardo organizations and networks, please visit our websites at https://www.leonardo.info/ and http://www.olats.org/. The Arizona State University–Leonardo knowledge enterprise provides leadership to advance ASU's transdisciplinary art-science research, creative practice, and international profile in the field: https://leonardo.asu.edu/.

Roger F. Malina

Advising Editor, Leonardo Publications

Acknowledgments

Over the lifetime of this book, I have been inspired, encouraged, and challenged by the company and intellectual exchange of many scholars, artists, and friends. I am most grateful for the intellectual generosity of people who read portions of this manuscript, provided me with invaluable feedback at conferences, and otherwise helped it along, including Amit Prasad, Katherine Groo, Peter Weibel, Suzannah Biernoff, Ben Marsden, Frances Robertson, Ella Chiemlevska, Matteo Valleriani, Michael Sappol, Leeanne Bodkin, Joseph Dumit, Paolo Maccagno, Roberta Buiani, Eleonora Montuschi, Angela Vettese, and Neil Curtis. With her positive attitude, my colleague Amy Bryzgel cheered me up on several occasions. Des O'Rawe has offered his advice whenever I needed it. It has been a pleasure to collaborate with all staff at the Suttie Arts Space. Ralph O'Connor, my mentor during the probation period, has encouraged me to trust my project when it was at an embryionic stage. Thanks to Nicola Miller and our inspiring conversations over coffee and cake. Michael Reinsborough read parts of the final manuscript with intellectual curiosity and kept asking the right questions even when I did not want to hear them.

The book *Atlante Occidentale*, conceived in the early 1980s by the Venice-based writer Daniele Del Giudice while doing a fieldwork visit at the CERN laboratory, has become a north star during my own writing. The dialogues and encounters between the two protagonists, the young particle physicist Pietro Brahe and the old writer Ira Epstein, showed me how the solid world of magnets, cables, and electronic circuits can suddenly reveal an elusive world of impalpable and invisible phenomena to which artists can give a form.

Like many others, I spent years both inside and outside the Italian academia, juggling multiple jobs to make ends meet. Albeit so different, the communities of artists/curators and start-uppers to whom I belonged showed me the importance of dreaming big while carrying out every job, even the modest ones, with care and attention to the wider community. After years of precarious employment, I was grateful to the University of Aberdeen for taking the risk and trusting my individual research trajectory.

The School of Languages, Literature, Music and Visual Culture offered me many opportunities to thrive. My biggest debt of gratitude, though, goes to the biomedical physics department of the University of Aberdeen and, in particular, to David Lurie,

Lionel Broche, and James Ross for taking seriously the questions of a humanities scholar. I owe a debt of gratitude to my students who pushed me to think out of the box. While this book existed only in my imagination, I benefited from the stimulating meetings of the Picturing Science reading group that I ran in Aberdeen. Thank you also to the guidance of the wonderful professionals of the Special Collections of the University of Aberdeen and of the University of Nottingham.

My unbounded thanks go to my editors Sean Cubitt, Doug Sery, and Roger Malina for believing in this project when it was still at an early stage. Three anonymous reviewers offered invaluable suggestions and constructive criticism. A small grant from the Carnegie Trust helped me to undertake the initial pilot research project necessary to shape this study. A generous yearlong fellowship by the Leverhulme Trust allowed me to be released from teaching and administrative duties in order to carry out the research and complete the writing of this book. Although the ideas and concepts discussed in this book originated from conversations I had with many people, any remaining error is mine.

My gratitude goes to my parents for their encouragement and to Ilaria Casini for being a true sister. My friends across countries and continents make me feel at home regardless of where I am. In our ongoing lifelong adventure together, my beloved Nicola trusted me enough to let me pursue my goals. He read the book from the first to the last page. He has accompanied me with his strength of spirit, smiles, and wisdom.

This book is dedicated to Margaret Foster Hutchison—woman, biologist, and lifelong partner of James Hutchison.

Introduction

> Once the subject of making visible in science leaves the domain of mere illustration or mere technology and becomes a matter of making knowledge, then the making acquires much higher status. Makers of images, along with their materials and techniques, must then appear in the same space with writers and readers of verbal ideas. The dichotomies of doing versus thinking, craftsperson versus creator of ideas, and body versus mind (or the senses versus the intellect) must then be transformed into overlapping actions, or intersections, where the "and" of collaboration replaces the "either/or" of intellectual conceit.
>
> —Norton Wise, "Making Visible"

Scene I

Sitting at his laboratory desk in Madrid in 1882, surrounded by the microtomes he uses to cut brains into thin slices, Santiago Ramón y Cajal peers through a light microscope at silver-stained cerebral tissues. Accustomed to looking at brains of humans and animals, and with an exceptional talent for drawing, Cajal sketches countless pen-and-ink diagrams. More than merely beautiful creations, though, these drawings are scientific data—accurate representations of the structures of the nervous system. With a keen eye for discerning form and function in the midst of a tangle of grey matter, Cajal sees separate cells—neurons, or, as he calls them, "the mysterious butterflies of the soul."[1]

Scientific and artistic practices are often about creating new worlds and new objects (so that they become visible) or about throwing new light onto familiar things (so that the way we look at them changes).[2] Well-known examples from different historical periods across art–science are Leonardo da Vinci's anatomical drawings, Galileo Galilei's observations of the moon's surface, Santiago Ramón y Cajal's drawings of neurons, and today's brain scans that purport to show us neural functions in full color. These images and data visualizations use aesthetics and craftsmanship to interrogate, rather than simply represent, the object made visible. They work as a "question-generating machine."[3]

Cajal (1852–1934) is now regarded as the father of modern neuroscience. His drawings, in their graphic and chromatic fragility and coupled with his cognition and vision, managed to solve the most complex maze that exists: the headquarters of intelligence

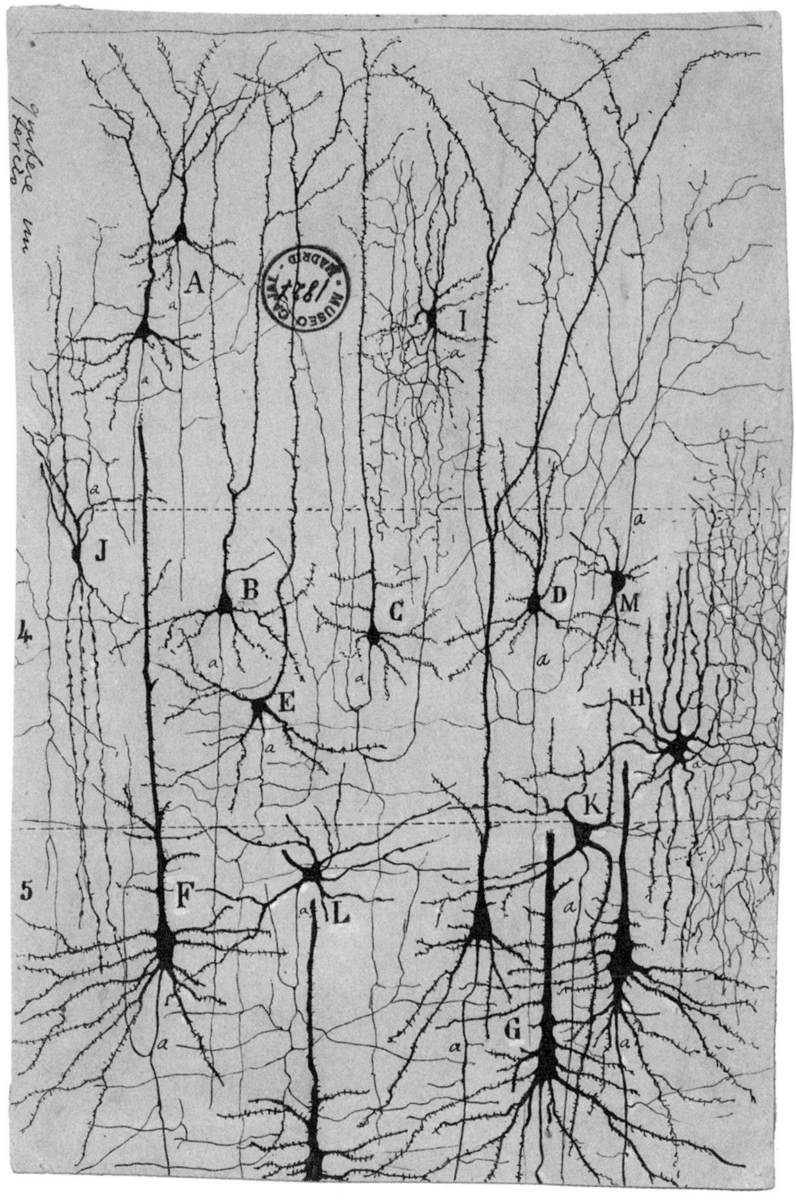

Figure 0.1

Santiago Ramón y Cajal, M1827 Diversos tipos celulares de la corteza esfenoidal del gato de 24 días, 1899.

Source: Courtesy of the Cajal Institute, Cajal Legacy, Spanish National Research Council (CSIC), Madrid, Spain.

located in the cortex (see figure 0.1).[4] Aesthetics acted as an instrument of both perception and knowledge production.

Cajal conducted his observation using his eyes (physiological vision), technology (the light microscope and the staining technique), previous knowledge (Camillo Golgi's seminal studies on neurons), and his hand (the drawings).[5] The object observed (the neuron) was known, but its precise configuration was not. Cajal postulated that neurons were individual contiguous cells in the brain capable of sending and receiving information. He drew how information flew through the brain, how neurons communicated with one another by sending information along axons to dendrites, and thus established a new framework for understanding the brain as a circuit.[6] He intuited that our thinking, learning, and memory were most likely to occur in the gaps between neurons, which he called synapses. Although it would take another half century until the electron microscope could confirm what Cajal had seen in his mind's eye, Cajal was able to persuade his fellow scientists of the value of his observations by showing them his diagrammatic drawings. With its synthetic and accurate character, Cajal's method of visualizing data gave the onlooker a direct and intuitive awareness of the brain's functions.[7]

Scene II

March 1974: a biomedical physics laboratory in Scotland. The experimental subject, a mouse, must remain completely still during the long image acquisition time. The biologist, Margaret Foster, breaks its neck. The experiment can begin.

Data are slowly acquired. James Hutchison, a physicist working in the same laboratory, meticulously hand-paints a map offering a dorsal view of the mouse. He uses Margaret's crayons, color-coding the map from data obtained using a small but powerful magnetic system. As he colors, square by square, patterns begin to form. When he reaches the area of the map corresponding to the neck of the mouse, the color code dictates a striking black. The magnetic system could "see" the edema in the mouse's broken neck, and the color-coded data revealed, in plain sight, this difference between healthy and injured tissue.

At a time when computers were not yet that powerful, the manual labor put into the creation and display of the mouse image was part of its visual performance. The mouse map (figure 0.2) enabled the immediate visualization of information related to the health status of soft tissues. It thus became the first clinically useful magnetic resonance imaging (MRI) image obtained by the team in the University of Aberdeen biomedical physics laboratory led by the physicist John R. Mallard. The striking copresence of numbers and pictorial elements on the map shows how scientists combine physics, mathematics, and aesthetic choices. The colors increased the visual appeal of the map and conveyed its information more clearly and directly. The magnetic system used to create it was the predecessor of the world's first whole-body MRI scanner, which would become one of the most widely used clinical image-generating technologies in the field of biomedicine and neuroscience.

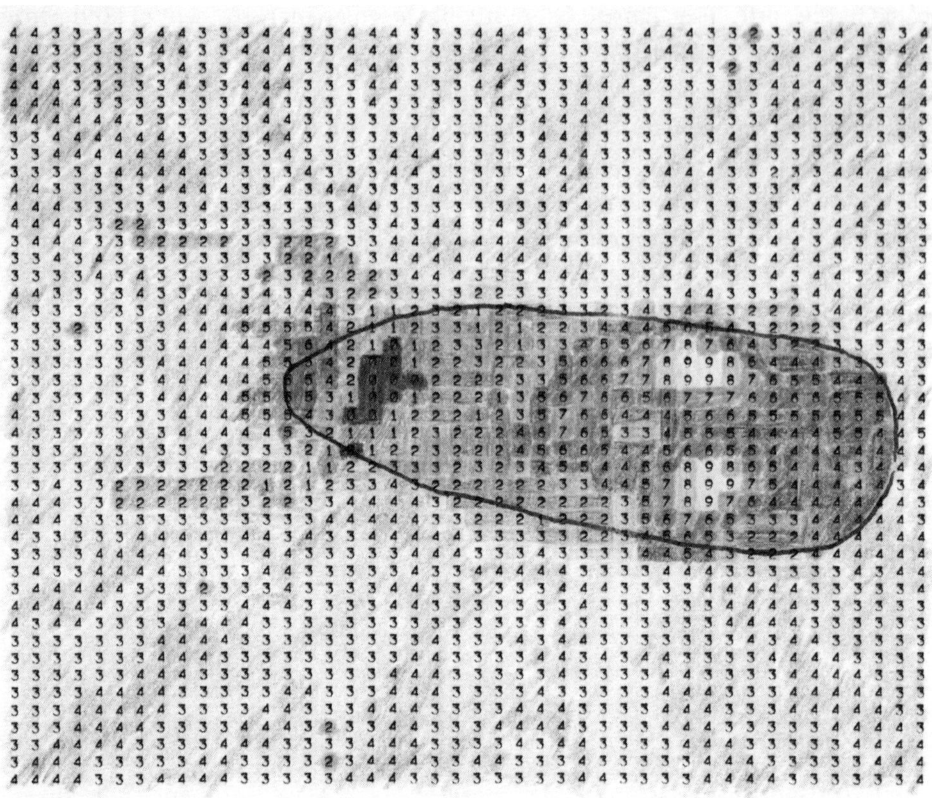

Figure 0.2
Map 2 of mouse produced in 1974.
Source: Courtesy of Professor David J. Lurie, University of Aberdeen. See plate 1.

Visual perception (seeing) is fast and requires little effort. Cognition (thinking) is much slower and less efficient. Traditional data sensemaking and presentation methods privilege thinking over seeing, but modern methods of data visualization take advantage of vision whenever possible, resulting in more immediate assimilation of information.

Direct apprehension through vision becomes difficult when the phenomenon under investigation is ambiguous. In the same laboratory where Hutchison used to work, scientists are now developing a new biomedical imaging technique called fast field-cycling MRI (FFC-MRI), which reveals biochemical information at the molecular level by exploring a range of magnetic field strengths during the scanning procedure.[8]

Data-visualization conventions tend to work against ambiguity because their aim is to convey the idea that the visual output is true. Clean lines, easy-to-read patterns, and simplified representational strategies are all ways of reducing complexity and disciplining the object represented. However, the visual output is not always easy to interpret or communicate. For example, FFC-MRI produces a graph as its initial visual output—the T_1 dispersion curve (figure 0.3; see also chapter 1). Rather than the image being

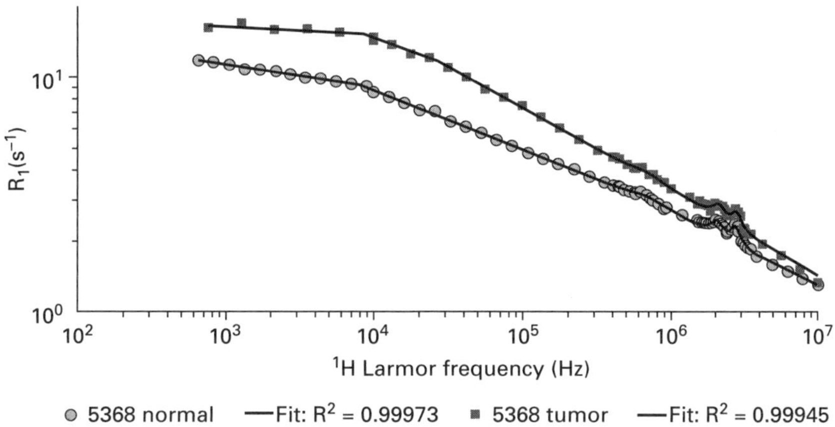

Figure 0.3
Dr. Lionel Broche, Dispersion curves from colorectal tissues (light gray) and colorectal cancer (dark gray). Large differences are observed at low magnetic fields, whereas almost no contrast appears in the high-field end of the spectrum.
Source: Courtesy of University of Aberdeen.

an object with defined borders and surfaces that stands against a background, it is an epistemic thing—that which one does not yet know.[9]

After a long period in which experts and nonexperts became accustomed to almost photographic biomedical images of the inner structure and workings of the body, the FFC-MRI graphs leave us baffled. What exactly are we looking at?

FFC-MRI lacks the immediacy and realism of Cajal's drawings or the mouse map. The T_1 dispersion graph represents "becoming" (tracking how the behavior of water changes in diseased tissues) rather than "being" (a mouse with a broken neck). The "becoming" is solidified in the visual framework of the graph, but there is no one-to-one relationship between the observer and the observed.

Scene III

The blackened gallery unfolds like a film strip marked by three illuminated poses: three sculptures lined up on the floor. These constitute a whole—a unique sculpture—despite their difference in form, material, and mode of installation. I walk around one of them, Marc Didou's *Skull I*. It is a white marble monolith of no discernible shape, set on a black marble and pinewood pedestal. The contour of the layers is accurate and clear-cut, a result of water used in the production process. The marble surface becomes light, dissolving the boundary between the material and immaterial—the artwork and its environment, contours and background. I raise my gaze to the ceiling, where a black marble mirror hangs. I stand still, eyes immobile. A white, lucent skull appears in the mirror.[10]

First created by Leonardo da Vinci, who included anamorphic drawings of a child's head in his *Codex Atlanticus* (1483–1518), anamorphosis became popular in the sixteenth

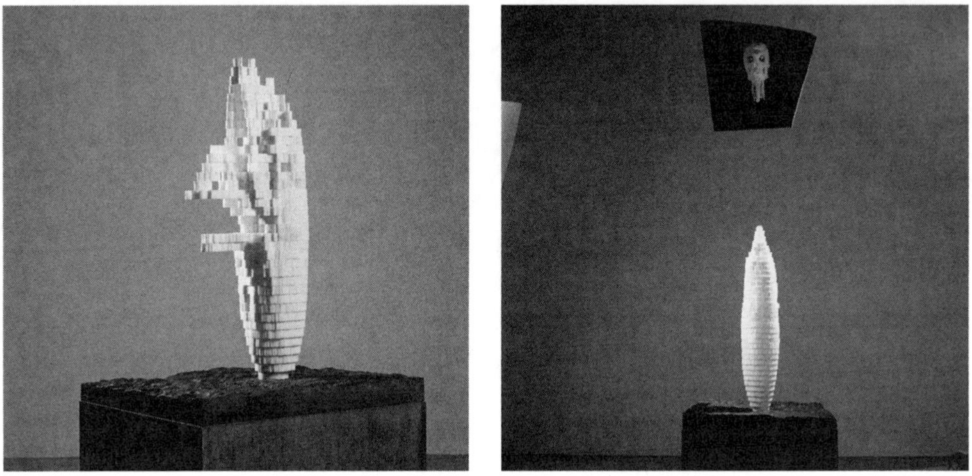

(a) (b)

Figure 0.4
Marc Didou, *Skull I*. Three elements: white marble, black marble pedestal, black marble mirror, 2007.
Source: Photograph by Alain Le Nouail. Courtesy of the artist.

and seventeenth centuries and has recently been rediscovered by artists and critical theorists. The technique is a method for producing a distorted image of an object, which is revealed in its proper form when viewed at certain angles or reflected in a curved mirror. With anamorphosis, the world as represented by classical perspective came under pressure from dark forces of desire, irrational imagination, images feeding upon themselves instead of upon a reference.[11]

Skull I (figure 0.4) embodies the sculptural gesture that begins within the MRI scanner and continues in Didou's atelier with the creation of casts from the MRI image data. The artist rematerializes the MRI data-visualization process, giving a body back to data. The mirror placed within the MRI scanner above the head of the patient is the getaway point that allows the gaze to escape outside the scanner. In *Skull I*, the getaway point is an anamorphic mirror, a widening of space and time through which the sculpture migrates from the physical space to an imaginary but no less real one—that of the mirror. *Skull I* loses its attributes of weight, substance, and materiality. The mirror functions as a centripetal black hole where time as a linear succession collapses. Thanks to the curved mirror, viewers walk through the sculpture backward, facing what had been its starting point: the physical body of the artist inside the MRI scanner.

* * *

Today, almost forty years after the world's first clinical full-body MRI scanner was developed in John R. Mallard's Aberdeen physics laboratory, MRI images help clinicians interpret the significance of biodata for patients all around the world. But what is it that the image makers in Mallard's lab first saw before a protocol solidified for generating images out of data, data from signal/noise, and interpretation of the data from the data-generated image? How do scientists visualize data when an image-generating technique is still under development, when the protocol for image generation/data interpretation has not yet crystallized into a visual output? What do they see? And how can what they see be reinvented by artists? What visual practices and theories do visual artists adopt when they use biomedical imaging techniques to engage with and reconfigure the neurosciences and other biomedical imaging fields?

I give bodies back to data. My aim is to reframe and reorient existing narratives of biomedical imaging innovation, which have tended to neglect the submerged but important role played by aesthetics, affectivity, and craft practice. To do that, I historicize and denaturalize visualization tropes and practices around the development of MRI technology, thanks to a methodology that combines laboratory ethnography, archival research, and collaborative art–science work.[12] In this book, I uncover archival sources (sketches, photographs, papers, drawings) to assess how methods and theories from the arts and humanities, usually considered peripheral to science, feed into past and present MRI innovation networks. *Giving Bodies Back to Data* analyzes some of the patterns and assumptions made by scientists and artists in visualizing, interpreting, and displaying data that underlie the dominant approaches to studying the body and brain. By doing so, I respond to the historian of science Mario Biagioli's call to improve the interface between the sciences, the arts, and the humanities, encompassing a wider range of contemporary imaging techniques and visualization practices across these disciplines.[13]

I make use of theories, methods, and concepts from different theoretical traditions, borrowing from science and technology studies (STS) through to medical anthropology and historical epistemology, to history and philosophy of technology and art–science studies. The glue holding together all these approaches is the focus on the physical-material dimension of reality that can be called "epistemology of the concrete" (Hans-Jörg Rheinberger), "mangle of practice" (Andrew Pickering), or, more recently, "multiple ontologies" (Annemarie Mol), "vibrant materialism" (Jane Bennett), and "agential realism" (Karen Barad).[14]

Through laboratory ethnography and archival research, I retrieve the multiple presences and agencies of bodies. Bodies of the image and technology makers; human and non-human subjects of experiments (patients, researchers, animals); the artifacts through which both scientists and artists create new body-worlds. In the process of technological development, these bodies are often left behind in the ensuing object or data visualization. Bodies are present as ghosts—traces that witness scientists' bodywork and embodied imagination with data collection, interpretation, and transmission. The body is the "body multiple" that philosopher of health care and medicine Annemarie Mol describes as "The body, the patient, the disease, the doctor, the technician, the technology: all of these are more than one.... No body is singular because it attends to the multiplicity of reality that sustains it."[15]

The bodies are those involved in the image production (patients/experimental subjects, not just human but also non-human), physicists, biologists, technicians, artists.

I never separate these bodies from the practices and the instruments through which bodies are sliced (digitally), reassembled, peered into, quantified, and visualized from and as data. I explore how bodies are enacted both in the laboratory and in the context of art–science collaborative projects.

Data visualization is a form of critical practice that opens a discursive *space*. It is not only a practice to make visible that which is not in sight, but a vital process capable of producing cognitive and affective relationships between concepts, spaces, and people.[16] Looking at how scientific knowledge is produced, rather than innocently discovered, is akin to looking *under* data visualization to consider its assumptions and conventions.[17] What does "looking under" data visualization mean? There is nothing natural or predetermined when it comes to data visualization. *Data* (literally, "the givens") is a taken-for-granted word across all the sciences: short and down to earth, it seems to encompass the simplest elements of empirical research.

Whether inscribed as magnetic signals, digital information, scribbles on envelopes, or meticulous entries in lab notebooks, data supply the essential materials for all scientific activity, from observing to theorizing. Data are not given; they are made. Philosopher of data science Sabina Leonelli says, "They are the results of complex processes of interaction between researchers and the world, which happen with the help of interfaces."[18] If one brings to the foreground the role of human agency in producing, interpreting, and displaying data, then it emerges that data are already aesthetic-laden and affective inside the laboratory. Aesthetics, bricolage, and affective investment are part of the situated, material conditions of knowledge production that have been considered peripheral to science and that scholars and artists alike can bring to the foreground.

I argue that experimentation, the use of aesthetics, and bricolage can help establish a common ground for collaboration between art and science. Science and art are both skilled pursuits involving a synergy between the body, the tools, the raw material, and the environment.[19] Since the Scientific Revolution, science has been considered a cultural activity characterized by a set of procedures that are carried out in view of changing nature and/or creating other worlds.[20] Attention to the role of aesthetics and craftsmanship in science can nurture language for starting a mute conversation from material practice and objects rather than from concepts.

I approach art–science collaboration from the perspective of data visualization, which has always been an important scholarly topic at the crossroads of the two disciplines. The point of departure of artists' work is also data in the broadest sense: data obtained by automated algorithms; data from human exchanges; and physiological or phenomenological data, such as the sensory experience inside the MRI scanner. The dichotomy between data and visualization, between what becomes visible and what remains hidden from view, becomes a space of creative possibility.

If artists and scientists want to collaborate, they each need to understand some of the methods, tools, and metaphors used by the other. Scientists need to become aware of the role played by aesthetics and sociocultural histories/practices embedded in the data-visualization pipeline. Artists need to pay attention to the materiality and craftsmanship of the image-making process (turning data into a visual output; making aesthetic decisions) as a reference to what happens in the body. This is not always doable due to the specialization and technical knowledge required just to grasp the basics of a scientific discipline or the workings of a technology. The epistemic gap between art and science is, therefore, the reality of many art–science projects. It is only by inhabiting this gap, rather than by seeking to close it, that an opportunity can arise for an art–science collaboration on equal terms. If artists limit themselves to the task of engaging with science, their final works might fail to be more than a demonstration of some measurable or sensible phenomena rather than transcending this to manifest truly as art.

Visualizing the Body in the Digital Age: A Brief Historical and Conceptual Background

From early modernity with Leonardo da Vinci's anatomical sketches and drawings and Vesalius's engraved atlas of the human body (*De Humani Corporis Fabrica*, 1543), through to Roentgen's discovery of X-rays in 1895, to the digital biomedical body constructed with modern imaging techniques, medical imaging technologies and their images have redefined the cultural history of the body, catalyzing new ways of seeing. The category of transparency functions both as an ideal to pursue and as an ideology by which to navigate our anxieties related to our bodies.[21] Although the anatomical body seems to have dissolved, first, in a digital data set of cross-sectional photographs with the Visible Human Project (1994–1995) and, then, into a map of genes and molecules with the advent of the Human Genome Project (1990–2003), the Medusa myth—the curiosity and fear of looking at our own interiority—still survives.[22] Modern medicine, despite its evident ability to unveil and map the body's interior landscape, makes this interior accessible only through representative images. The difference between information and flesh, made possible by the Human Genome Project with its extraction of data from bodies, has been questioned by biomedia artists working with biological material to create novel life forms.[23]

Research in biomedicine and genetics after the Second World War was boosted by the advent of digital techniques of visualization and computer-assisted imaging technology. It opened up a new era in the investigation of the interiors of the body and brain, from the anatomic to the molecular body, with increased attention on the brain as a cultural, aesthetic, and scientific object.[24] Thanks to the computerization of medical observation, imaging has gained a primacy in medicine and health care that it never had before. Imaging is a central feature of diagnostic and treatment procedures, and of the patient experience. It is also a field in transition, tied to cycles of innovation in biomedicine and to a transformation of the relationship between the patient's body and the medical image. Noninvasive imaging procedures put the living body of the patient at the center of their investigation, but often in the guise of a medical image with the actual body remaining absent.

A technology is made not just with engineering but also with a leap of the imagination. For example, in the early days of MRI development, scientists acted as guinea pigs, putting their own bodies through scans to provide the normative references for patients' bodies. When clinical trials started, components of the scanner (such as the bed) needed adjusting because the prototype scanner had not been designed with the patient's body in mind. Changing this process, which frequently occurs in the early phases of technological development, is not just a matter of small tweaks but requires a big shift in mindset. A failure in the technology is largely a failure of the imagination.

The history of MRI development must be framed within this broader tendency to grasp and represent the body in techno-visual terms.[25] This book is not a comprehensive historical study of biomedical imaging technologies but an in-depth analysis of one trajectory of the cluster of actions, decisions, and challenges undertaken by the biomedical physics laboratory at the University of Aberdeen. It begins in the early days of clinical MRI development, from the late 1960s to the early 1980s, then fast-forwards to the present day as the same laboratory is now working on developing FFC-MRI.

While the first MRI scanner was in development, the cross-disciplinary field of neuroscience was also being established. Interestingly, the close relationship between physics and medicine in the laboratory has always shaped brain research since it began (in earnest) at the start of the nineteenth century, thanks to newly available instruments (e.g., microscopes) for observing life phenomena.[26] In this book, I show a preference for those artists and practices that focus on the body–brain system rather than on the brain as a monolithic object whose study can be undertaken by a single discipline called neuroscience. Failing to do so, as the historian of science and technology Cornelius Borck states, turns the brain into "an almost fictional object, created when the public and the media ... use the singular 'brain' for summarizing complex lines of research."[27]

Challenging Techno-Fetishism

Paradoxical though it might sound, a sustained attention to the technicalities of the data-visualization pipeline is crucial to avoid the fetishism of technology, which is specular to ahistorical art–scientism.[28] Combining the medium of drawing with new technologies such as MRI and movement-simulation techniques in her studies on human locomotion, the artist and researcher Jeanine Breaker recommends that fellow artists test the quality of the claims and visual outputs made possible by cutting-edge technologies against previous techniques for studying movement and anatomy such as drawing: "It becomes increasingly critical that we monitor and enhance the quality of these new tools upon which we have come to rely. The nuanced movement-analysis learned from past methodology can help us to monitor the quality of the technology that we are so eager to embrace."[29]

Although I refuse to endow MRI with powers it does not have, I have chosen to focus on it over other biomedical imaging techniques to tackle data-visualization challenges. First, MRI is constantly evolving. It keeps being reinvented; its multiple origin forces the scholar to reject any technological determinism and linear approach to innovation trajectory that goes from research and design to development and implementation, and finally to diffusion. Second, MRI, along with other research tools, technologies, methods, and media, participated not only in shaping the brain as a scientific object but also in unveiling the richness of the wider cultural context of brain research.[30]

By looking at the early stages in which MRI was developed for clinical purposes in the Aberdonian biomedical physics laboratory, I accept the invitation made to scholars by sociologist Kelly Joyce to engage with emergent narrative practices related to MRI technology beyond 1999–2006, the time frame she focused on.[31] Orit Halpern, one of the key theorists of the intertwined history of vision, data, and cognition, argues that "our current focus on built or existing technologies ignores questions of desire, aspiration, epistemology, and imagination that exist before and often outside of specific material instantiations in built objects."[32] These discourses might never become visible in the final technology. Yet they can be made to surface again in artistic interventions and impact the way in which we integrate visualization technologies into our media systems. They can provide new ways of thinking about man–machine relationships, which we produce inside and then outside the laboratory.

The fictive point of origin of MRI development at the University of Aberdeen is the hardware rather than in the visual output. My choice is not neutral. It means taking off from the material history and practice that lie beneath the final image visualized on the computer screen, to highlight the material labor of professionals who decided to control the process of visualizing data from the very first cable laid on the ground and even from the imagination that set this task. As the literary historian Sander Gilman says, "To study 'medical technology,' without understanding how its generation of representations is the key to its understanding, is limited…; to study the representations without understanding the technology and the knowledge it generates is equally one-sided."[33] Therefore, in examining the process and challenges of data visualization in MRI, I keep side by side the technology and its representational output.

In this book on data visualization, I often give space to the dimension of noise. Image makers need to distinguish between signal and noise. In physics, being able to discern noise from signal in the data-visualization pipeline is paramount to creating meaningful visualizations that can convey information. Noise is not just a technical disturbance, however, but an epistemological element. Noise is crucial for contextualizing the signal, for understanding its origin and relationship to other elements inside and outside the laboratory. Noise is what gives data their relational character, their bodies, back.[34]

Laboratory Microhistories and Encounters within Archives

Although this is not a book on the history of technology, I have been inspired by the microhistorical approach of the historian Carlo Ginzburg. The "micro" dimension of doing history, as Ginzburg understands it, is not related to the symbolic or actual dimension of the topic/object being studied.[35] The approach is analytical, as if carried out using a microscope. For example, I use an analytical approach to study the data-visualization maps (such as the mouse series) created by scientists. The detailed examination of local data-visualization methods does not imply the attempt to build upon them as if they were "case studies" enabling generalizations. The study of local practices and microhistories related to a specific laboratory can inform discussion on wider conceptual key threads and questions that concern the participation of a certain imaging technology to the history of biomedicine and neurosciences development in the twentieth century.

My approach seeks to subvert existing hierarchies such as those between theory and practice, rationality and affectivity, invention and development. Where and when does one locate innovation materially and at a conceptual level in MRI history and ongoing development? Which were/are the most salient forces driving innovation in the development of a new technology? What is the role played by aesthetics and epistemologies coming from the humanities and the arts in the innovation trajectory of a specific image-generating technique such as MRI? Things perceived as peripheral to the science are in fact central to it.

Although the Aberdonian case study is an underexplored thread within the broader transnational history of MRI technology, it offers the opportunity to engage with the early developmental stages of a technology using a combined methodology. The approach is both diachronic (from the early stage until its recent "reinvention" with a new type of MRI technology, plus the wider cultural-historical and philosophical context) and synchronic (internal analysis of archive material and fieldwork).

In *Giving Bodies Back to Data*, I give space to my encounters with archival materials, people, and bits and pieces of technologies—in short, "the mangle" of scientific practice.[36] I conduct a detailed ethnographic account of scientific practice as it unfolds, conceptually and materially, at the laboratory bench. I weave together maps, objects, laboratory experiments, scientists' academic papers, anecdotes and memories, and detailed explanations of scientific concepts and technologies. I combine laboratory ethnography with archival research in both institutional and private repositories.

The use of hitherto unavailable archival holdings (research notes contained in private journals or laboratory notebooks by scientists, work-in-progress images and sketches, poems, photographs) and laboratory ethnography enables the researcher to study how science practice unfolds in the everyday laboratory life and activities performed by scientists. The aforementioned elements can contribute to unveil the humanities aspect of biomedical imaging, foregrounding the bodily, situated aspects of data-visualization work. Furthermore, sketches of experiments and pieces of technology related to the early stages of MRI development could be potentially repurposed as both art and research, for example, to construct or improve existing technologies for users that are currently excluded from taking advantage of them due to the high costs of high-field MRI scanners.

I triangulate historical epistemology with archival research and art–science collaboration. The archive can become the repository of sociotechnical and affective imaginaries rather than of dead documents and objects waiting to be brought back to life.[37]

The role of archival research in art–science collaboration, furthermore, places history as the often-neglected root of contemporary collaborative art–science projects. The role of history becomes central because it generates images and visions of the world, offering us the key to understanding our present time and the images we create. A detail-rich archival (and, when possible, laboratory ethnographic) study focusing on the intimate process of developing a technology can raise questions that are usually neglected by typical discussions of existing technologies and by many art–science projects.

Book Structure

This book is written for both scholars and practitioners with aesthetic, historical, and philosophical interests in art–science collaboration. Artists, scientists, and humanities/social sciences researchers (in visual studies, medical humanities, history of technology, and media arts) will find here a methodology and a set of conceptual questions to guide their thinking and practice. Several valuable books have been published on the topic of art–science collaboration.[38] Although exhaustive in the range of examples discussed and in highlighting some of the major concerns of collaborative projects, these studies run the risk of adopting a surveylike approach, failing to engage in a sustained critical examination of an intimate collaborative process.

My aim is not to provide yet another study of how successful a collaborative project has been, nor to prescribe a series of "dos and don'ts." Rather, I offer a method that shows how to set up and implement a collaborative art–science project without huge infrastructure capacities and funding, combining laboratory fieldwork and archival research. This is the first step in nurturing the culture required to push forward from the integration of science, technology, engineering, and math (STEM) with the arts (STEAM) across the wider curriculum.[39]

I do not engage with art–science *sub specie aeternitatis*. My own thinking stems from a sustained experience of collaborative art–science projects. The choice of using a first-person essayistic style ought to remind the reader of my own situated position inside the laboratory, that of a participant-observer able to trigger dialogues and collaborative work.[40] My chosen critical method is conceptual rather than chronological, inclined toward a speculative and creative form of thinking through images—one that I believe needs to be encouraged by researchers and teachers working in visual culture and media arts.

Giving Bodies Back to Data is organized in two parts: the first part (chapters 2–4) is a close-up examination of laboratory practices; the second part (chapters 5–7) gradually zooms out from the curatorship of an art–science project to broadening the conceptual framework and the range of artists' practices beyond the focus on MRI. As I demonstrate in parts I and II, archival research and laboratory ethnography are two ways of opening up the data-visualization material process, giving bodies back to data.

Chapter 1 lays the groundwork for understanding the material culture and history of data visualization in science and art, with a focus on the transnational history of MRI invention and development. The chapter is organized around the center–periphery pair, offering the conceptual framework for appreciating the role of aesthetics and bricolage in scientific practice that I use throughout the book. To support my relational view of data, I introduce concepts and approaches from disciplines such as history of science, visual studies, philosophy of science, and STS, referring to the scholarly works of Hans-Jörg Rheinberger, Peter Galison, Sabina Leonelli, Bruno Latour, Orit Halpern, and Annemarie Mol.[41]

Chapters 2–4 (part I) are an in-depth ethnographic study of MRI development at the University of Aberdeen's biomedical physics laboratory in two different periods. Chapter 2 uses the tools of STS and historical epistemology to focus on data-visualization challenges between the late 1960s and early 1980s, when the first whole-body clinical scanner was constructed. An analysis of the data-visualization pipeline and archival material demonstrates how the transformation of data into an image was never taken for granted in the initial development of MRI. When the procedure for transforming data into images was black boxed and became standardized, it was no longer subject to further examination or questioning.

Chapter 3 continues the ethnographic investigation on the features and limits of data visualization in the ongoing development of FFC-MRI. I focus on two aspects. First, I critically examine the conventions, aesthetic decisions, and theoretical and practical knowledge used by physicists to help or hinder their attempt to put the patient's body at the center of exchanges between scientists, technologies, and data. Second, I discuss how image quality in biomedical data visualization is differently understood by those engaged in the process of stabilizing the data-visualization pipeline.

Is anything unrepresentable in today's biomedical imaging and neuroscientific research, which is saturated by data, information, and visualization? To address the limits of data visualization in FFC-MRI, in chapter 4 I analyze selected passages of a short book in which the philosopher Giorgio Agamben engages with the implications of the new regime in physics characterized by the introduction of statistics, probability, and potentiality in the study of phenomena. I place FFC-MRI within the broader discourse, imagery, and practice of personalized/predictive medicine, which rests upon the move from the transparent, molar body to the potential, molecular body that was undertaken at the beginning of the twenty-first century.[42] What do the strange profiles of FFC-MRI hope to reveal? Not just the present reality but the probability of a given condition developing.

A short intermezzo connects the first and second parts of the book by discussing the role of the grid both in art and in the sciences—the grid being the matrix of Cartesian coordinates used to organize data and turn them into a visual output. We live in a regime populated by algorithms, machine-learning techniques, and data-visualization technologies used in the military, medicine, and security, all critically based on the grid. Applying Louise Amoore's work on risks and prediction to the analysis of the grid's role in the data-visualization pipeline, I discuss how the grid contributes to transforming how we perceive our bodies and make decisions related to them.[43]

In chapter 5 I analyze a selection of neuroscience/biomedicine-based or inspired artistic interventions from the 1990s onward by artists working in different media from sculpture and drawing to virtual reality and bio art. The chapter focuses on the visual component of the neurorealism fallacy discussed by the anthropologist Joseph Dumit in his examination of brain imaging.[44] Neurorealism is the belief that brain scans are the visual evidence of brain activity, despite the complexity inherent in data acquisition and image creation. I argue that artists run the risk of reproducing the neurorealism fallacy at the visual level simply by carrying the laboratory-stabilized image interpretations out into the world. To avoid this, artists have two pathways. They can either work with the artisanship of image making in the laboratory, or they can reappraise the systems-thinking approach of second-order cybernetics with its holistic view of the body–brain system.

Chapter 6 shows how to design and carry out a small-scale art–science project. I demonstrate this by providing a methodology that combines laboratory ethnography with archival research, including newly uncovered private notebooks by James Hutchison that become a space for literary trails and experimentation on paper. The chapter critically describes the collaboration I set up between the biomedical physics laboratory, the artist Beverley Hood, the Suttie Arts Space gallery, and myself, with the goal of highlighting the relational and aesthetic-laden character of data that are the product of craftsmanship and affective labor at the laboratory bench.

The concluding chapter 7 moves beyond the specific laboratory and collaboration discussed in the previous chapters. It expands the body–brain ensemble beyond data visualization by conceptualizing it in relation to material and immaterial infrastructures and media systems, opening the discourse to operational images and neural networks. I problematize the question of what space humans can claim back in the era of operational images. Machine learning and artificial intelligence (AI) remind us how easily the world seems never to be completely human centered. However, the works of art I critically examine here (focusing, in particular, on artists such as Liz Orton, Ilona Sagar, and Thomas Feuerstein) ask us not to give up our responsibility as humans in the process of analyzing, interpreting, and displaying information from operational images, giving bodies back to data.

1 Center–Periphery in Data Visualization: Concepts and Methods

> All my life, all my work has been nothing more than connecting people to objects, and objects to experience and feelings, to self-perception, to ideas. Perhaps what I have invented so far is nothing more than a special lens, which allows you to see the background and the figure in their relationship, with equal dignity. As a boy you will have been brought up for math, or science. I had an aptitude for people.
>
> —Writer Ira Epstein to physicist Pietro Brahe in Daniele Del Giudice, *Atlante Occidentale* (author's translation)

The Relational View of Data

Historian of science and biologist Hans-Jörg Rheinberger argues that the foundational gesture of science is to make things visible in the broader context of laboratory experimentation.[1] Instruments produce marks (traces, signals), which become data only after further manipulations from observation or experiments. Once marks become data, they can be stored and made available to others.

Data are relational entities, rather than straightforward representations of the phenomenon under investigation. Building on Rheinberger's work and using case studies from molecular biology, the philosopher of social sciences Sabina Leonelli is one of the first scholars to pay attention to the relational character of data and to their multiple journeys in two ways. First, she highlights how data are an "embarrassing dent in scientific legitimacy.… How can intrinsically located, situated, idiosyncratic, theory-laden results serve as confirmation for universal truths about nature?"[2] Data are not "given," in the sense that they do not express incontrovertible facts on a given entity or process. They are assembled. They are a context-dependent expression of tacit skills and embodied knowledge.[3] Second, part of the definition of data, Leonelli explains, is their portability.[4] In fact, data acquire value as evidence not by virtue of an intrinsic representational power but because they can travel after being collected and stored.[5] In order to understand how data are generated, how they circulate, and how they contribute to knowledge, Leonelli explores the journeys undertaken by data from the sites in which data are created (laboratories, clinical studies, and so forth) to the sites of data mobilization (databases, archives, data banks, publications) and interpretation (laboratories, journalism, social media).[6]

In this book I ask the following questions: What counts as data in the scientific laboratory and, more specifically, in the early development of a technology such as MRI? What is the role played by aesthetics and craftmanship in the construction, interpretation, and display of data within the laboratory? What do data become when they are remediated in artists' practices? The answers to these questions are key to laying out the possibility of a trading zone between scientists and artists. When data are recontextualized and remediated, they might become something else—noise, waste, or facts.[7] This material process of creating "data after data" is often the springboard for collaborative work between scientists and artists. Remediated data can feed back into laboratory research.

Leonelli's relational view of data-driven science can be used as a springboard for studying data visualization across sciences and the arts. The act of visualizing reinforces and expands the relational view of data. Visualization plays a key role in how data are formed, contextualized, and made to travel not only across laboratories but also from the laboratory to the wider cultural arena. Understanding how data visualization works is important for developing a micropolitics of the visual field, as emphasized by artist and researcher Susan Schuppli:

> Politics enters into the visual field not simply at the level of representation—the content displayed in the image—but at the structural level of its information acquisition, processing, and transmission; at the moment when pure data is captured by sensors, transformed into binary code, assigned pixel values, algorithmically adjusted, composited to produce a digital image, saved in a standardised file format, and transmitted to recombine with others circuits of technical and social assembly. This is what I am calling the micro-politics of [image] processing.[8]

To study the micropolitics of data visualization, Leonelli's conceptual relational view of data needs to be integrated with concepts and methods from science and technology studies (STS) and ethnographic laboratory studies. Research on the role of images and visualization in the production and diffusion of knowledge must be studied as part of the wider discursive and social context in which they are embedded.[9]

The Epistemic Functions of Images and Visualization in Science

The focus of my analysis is on the material form and iconology of technical images.[10] The technical image, which originates primarily in science and medicine and from the German tradition of image science (*Bildwissenschaft*), is created using instruments, technologies, or imaging procedures. Technical images come into being as ways of thinking through, presenting, and mediating constellations of material artifacts, bodies, or data by the image makers—scientists or artists.

The historian of physics Peter Galison offers a conceptual framework to describe two traditions present in technical images produced within twentieth-century microphysics. The first, called the *image tradition*, describes images as natural, illusionary, or mimetic. The second, the *logic tradition*, replaces images with the notion of statistical projections of data and digital information.[11] These two traditions use different forms of experimentation. The first seeks to base its demonstrations not on statistics but on single "golden" events, such as those proving the forms of the subatomic world. The second tradition uses statistical demonstrations and is based on the aggregation of data. The images belonging to this second tradition tend to be pixelated or statistical graphs, which are averages, rather than a direct visualization. Galison argues that these two traditions have merged into a hybrid one characterized by the co-presence of numbers (data) and pictorial values (image). Being able to move between these two traditions and to produce good quality image data is paramount to enabling physicists to reach out to different communities—radiologists, clinicians, patients, and the lay public. To give an example, for brain data to travel successfully from the physicist's laboratory to the radiologist's console to the patient, they need to take the form of an image.

Pictures and images belong to a different conceptual tradition than visualizations of data, but the terminological ambiguity used to describe the visual output of the latter (images, image data, scans, maps, visualizations, graphs) mirrors the reality of the attitude that scientists have toward images, moving between the iconophile and the iconoclastic stance.[12] In biomedical imaging, for instance, physicists refer to the visual output obtained using imaging apparatus either as data visualization or as an image, with the implicit understanding that, in the latter case, what they really mean is "image data."

Visualizing differs from observing and imaging. The act of observing a phenomenon involves seeing and is a learned practice helped by instruments. The act of visualizing is akin to a mental act, a type of inner seeing. Imaging, used in the medical context, is the technique or practice of creating images of otherwise invisible aspects of an object, for instance, a body part. The final visual output of an imaging procedure is called a "visualization" rather than a "picture." A picture is a representation of something (a person, a landscape, an object) obtained by drawing, painting, photography, and so forth. Visualization incorporates features of the phenomenon under study as well as the properties of the technique used to visualize the phenomenon.

Contemporary forms of observation are not linked to single bodies or unified subjectivities, for they comprise all kinds of human and machinic interfaces. Similarly, computerized technologies and visualization techniques in contemporary neuroscience and biomedicine coexist with analog forms of representation (e.g., drawing and writing on paper, modeling).[13] Furthermore, data visualization is not just about observing, organizing, and making available information as an image in the present, but can expand to future scenarios that incorporate other aspects, including imagination."[14]

Visualization is often how science creates its objects, conducts its inquiries, advances its arguments among peers, and communicates its results to the lay public, thus covering three epistemic functions: the exploration, transformation, and transmission of knowledge. The use of images and data visualization in scientific practice has raised the interest of historians, philosophers, and sociologists of science since Martin Rudwick's seminal paper on the emergence of a "visual language" for geologists in the eighteenth and nineteenth centuries.[15] The historical study of images and their context of production can trigger wider questions related to the cultural representation of science among its different publics.[16] Sociologists and STS scholars treat visual representation as an integral part of scientific practice. The philosopher and sociologist Bruno Latour highlights the relationship between visualization and embodied cognition at a time when the introduction of digital imaging, automated measurement, and statistics in science have partaken in the withdrawal of the hand and the eye.[17] Michael Lynch argues that the process of establishing scientific results involves making something "visible" and "analyzable," also thanks to the daily struggle with materials that need to be disciplined to achieve experimental results.[18] A philosophical approach to images tends also to focus on the epistemological function of visual modes of representation but without necessarily analyzing laboratory practices.[19]

The philosopher of science Henk W. de Regt points out that when something is visualized it can be understood.[20] Scientists define as *observable* even those phenomena that register on laboratory equipment but not on the human sensorial apparatus. With structural and functional images of the brain obtained with functional MRI (fMRI), for example, it is hard to say what becomes "observable": radio signals, neural activity, blood oxygenation? The senses, vision included, are required only for a limited number of tasks, such as testing the hardware, interacting with the interface at the console, checking the subject/patient, reading the numbers, and discriminating the colors assigned to the final image. This illustrates how much science practice involves the production and visualization of data from measurements and statistics. These data produce a nonperceptual type of evidence.

Furthermore, scientists use visualization to share their data, findings, and methods with their peers and the general public without having to reproduce the experiment. Latour explains that scientific images are inscriptions that enable scientists to work with two-dimensional objects rather than with the full subject in all its complexity. He highlights that a map (not the land it represents) is a type of inscription that can be moved to different contexts and even combined with other objects without losing its function. These inscriptions act as "immutable mobiles"—things that do not lose their meaning in transmission and that enable the standardization and repetition of a procedure.[21] An immutable mobile can move around without distortion, corruption, or decay. It maintains its shape in a physical/geographical sense and in a relational/functional one. It enables researchers and the lay public to think about the work that goes into moving scientific facts around and so producing their apparent universality.

Epistemic Cultures and Their Trading Zone

How do scientists and artists come to know what they know? What are the technical, cultural, historical, and social conditions under which the process of knowledge creation takes place? Rather than looking at knowing subjects and knowable objects as two separate entities, one can examine the space between them.[22] This in-between space, in the case of collaborative work, is connected to experimentation rather than just creativity. The anthropologist and science studies scholar Karin Knorr-Cetina introduces the concept of epistemic cultures to foster a discussion around the nature of knowledge processes within the communities and practices of molecular biologists and high-energy physicists. Epistemic cultures are communities of practice not bound to disciplines but rather to the construction of "the machineries of knowing composed of practices," both technical (e.g., how scientific instruments are used) and social (e.g., how decisions are made).[23]

What does it mean to experiment? Experimentation can follow a route independent from theory.[24] Rheinberger describes the experiment as an activity characterized by the interplay between "epistemic things" (the objects of inquiry, not yet solved) and "technical objects" (the ensemble of instruments and techniques used to tackle epistemic things).[25] Furthermore, for Rheinberger, an experimental system is set up by two different drives working together. The first is the drive toward analysis, which is about examining the constitutive elements of the phenomenon under study (molecules, chemical elements, and physical forces). The second is the drive toward synthesis—the effort to create new things.[26] What is at stake in experimental laboratory practice is not a hypothesis-testing exercise but an open-ended process, characterized by unexpected outcomes. Scientific and artistic work are both driven by the dimension of unpredictability and bricolage as epistemic and aesthetic concepts.

Bricolage comprises both improvisation and a do-it-yourself endeavor. It is the skill of using whatever is at hand and recombining it to create something new. The term has been used in a variety of fields from anthropology to cultural theory, literary studies, and the arts. The anthropologist Claude Lévi-Strauss used *bricolage* to describe mythological thinking in opposition to the goal-means-oriented thinking typical of engineers.[27] Mythical thought, according to Lévi-Strauss, reuses available materials in order to solve new problems. In contrast with the bricoleur who works with everything at hand, the specialism of the engineer requires the availability of certain materials and tools to carry out a project set out according to a specific plan. Even when not completing a project, the bricoleur, says Lévi-Strauss, "always put something of himself into it."[28] With the term *bricolage* I want to capture the craft labor and affective engagement of scientific work, moving beyond Lévi-Strauss's distinction between the engineer and the bricoleur.[29]

The Black Box of Science and Technology

In science, computing, and engineering, the black box is an object or a system that can be perceived and investigated *by looking at* its input (stimulus) and output (response) exclusively, without acknowledging its internal workings (see figure 1.1).

In science studies, Latour defines *black boxing* as the way scientific, technical, and social work is made invisible by its own success. Thus, paradoxically, the more science and technology succeed, the more opaque and obscure they become.[30] Latour argues that facts and machines are always undetermined if one pays attention to science in the making, but once they solidify and become accepted, they are referred to as *black boxes*. It is therefore important to pay attention to the process of turning phenomena, objects, and concepts into black boxes.

Latour takes the black box as a metaphor to describe scientific practice: to conduct science is to construct and close a black box. For example, it is through images of the

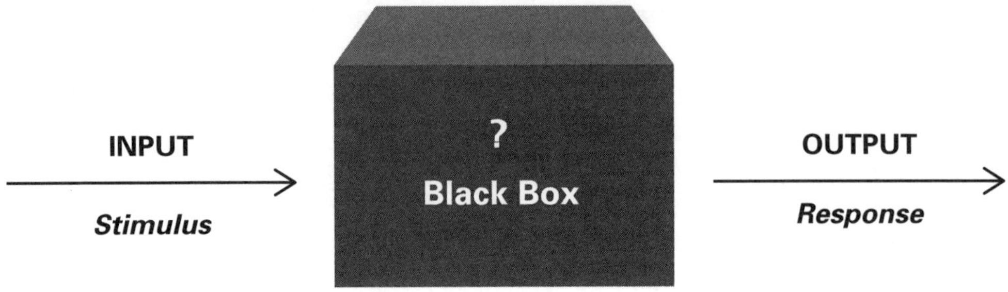

Figure 1.1
Black box diagrammatic representation.

brain that the culture and politics of neuroscience become visible, solidify, and spread across a wider public arena beyond the closed circuit of neuroscientific discourse. In spite of the highly mediated procedure for generating a brain scan, and the enormous complexity of data acquisition and image processing, these images are often presented in the mass media as if they were the photorealistic visual proof of brain activity.[31]

Reopening the black box enables a better grasp of how data are made rather than given to us. I emphasize the reopening of the black-boxed scientific process in several ways. First, when a controversy arises, the assumptions made up to that point must be reexamined. Second, a black box can be opened by looking at the early stages of development of a technology, for example, before the data-visualization protocol becomes standardized. Third, artists can open a black box by challenging the assumptions made in the laboratory or intervening in any given pipeline within the laboratory to examine what is inside the box. To do so, both researchers and artists can recur to laboratory ethnography and archival research.

The concept of the black box helps us to think about transactions between the worlds of art and science. In the laboratory, the artist examines the interior of the black box with her own set of questions, methods, and interests engaging in an exchange (a transaction) with the scientist, who can add questions, explanations, and so forth. Through this endeavor the black box can be passed back and forth between the artist and the scientist and rearranged in such a way that a shared ground is created. One can create and support such transactions by enabling a trading zone between the two epistemic cultures of art and science.

I adapt the concept of the trading zone, which stems from the history of physics, to the worlds of art and science. Galison, who has collaborated with artists including William Kentridge, defines the *trading zone* as "a social, material, and intellectual mortar binding together the disunified traditions of experimenting, theorizing, and instrument building."[32] He argues that scientists in different disciplines and belonging to different epistemic cultures (for instance, quantum physicists and molecular biologists) manage to talk to each other about a specific problem because they speak jargons, pidgins, and creoles.[33] Jargons are restricted terminologies that allow for interchange within fields. Pidgins are work languages that enable their users to trade and work across linguistic barriers. Creoles are fully fledged, rich interlanguages that emerge at borders between places in the physical/linguistic world.

These worlds intersect at the trading zones, coordinative places where exchanges and frictions can happen and be dealt with. Communication challenges can also occur within the same research community: in physics, for instance, the three subcultures of theory, experimentation, and instrument making each have their own distinctive form of reasoning and practice. Aesthetics and bricolage are something both artists and experimenters/instrument makers (and possibly theorists) do even if they might define or balance the relative importance of each term differently. Aesthetics and bricolage are found by opening up the black box—the trading zone being the place of experiment that can be accessed in the process of opening the black box.

The Collaborative Art–Science Project (and Its Discontents)

Creating a trading zone between art and science is not straightforward. The art–science divide dates back to the 1830s, when the term *scientist* was coined in analogy with the term *artist*, and the two replaced the early modern Renaissance Man, whose knowledge was universal rather than discipline specific.[34] Although art–science cross-fertilization is nothing new,[35] recent decades have seen an increase in artists challenging the split between the two cultures of science and humanities, creating works that, in some cases, are experiments conducted using the tools, methods, and aesthetics associated with scientific practice.[36]

The art historian Jean Clair, who curated the exhibition *L'âme au corps: Arts et sciences 1793–1993* (Galeries nationales du Grand Palais, Paris, October 1993 to January 1994), laments that the divorce of art and science is caused by two circumstances: art, since Romanticism, has given away the monopoly of objectivity to the sciences, keeping for itself only the soft hypertrophy of the ego that characterizes the self-styled genius of the artist; science, conversely, is lost in its graphs and fragmented specialties, cut off from the real world. "[O]nce the sciences have occupied the various fields of knowledge with their authority, the artist, kicked out from a kingdom he once shared on equal terms and sent back to the empiricism of the craftsman ('as stupid as a painter'), the artist cannot help but give himself to soliloquy or prophecy, in search of a status but also of a lost profession."[37]

The fact that collaborative art and science projects are increasingly popular softens Clair's pessimism in relation to the possibility of art regaining a status and even returning as a profession granted equal respect to medicine or law. The arts, however, seem to be too often confined to the ancillary role of being an echo chamber to scientific findings, or continuously following, when they could be leading by sketching new directions and solutions for confronting the most urgent issues of our times.[38]

In the extensive literature on collaborative art–science work, one encounters both the locutions "SciArt" and "art–science."[39] The artist and curator Nicola Triscott, founder of Arts Catalyst, one of the best-known UK programs of art–science collaboration, describes art–science as "initiatives that bring art and science into some form of interaction, exchange or conversation.... Features of this art-science include art that incorporates scientific imagery or uses scientific techniques, art that explores scientific ideas, collaborations between artists and research scientists, and artist residencies in scientific laboratories and field stations. It is also used in the context of applying artistic creativity to further scientific innovation."[40]

If the emerging quality of art–science could be valid for the 1990s, this is not the case anymore, at least for the industrialized, economically stronger part of the world.[41] Prestigious research institutions, foundations, and universities (the Wellcome Trust, CERN, the MIT Media Lab, Le Laboratoire Cambridge, Symbiotica, Laboratoria Art&Science Space, the Science Gallery Network) have been actively supporting art–science programs and initiatives aimed at communicating and engaging the lay public with scientific research and science advocacy.

My take on art–science is grounded in extensive work I have conducted as a researcher and curator. For more than a decade, I have been working on the epistemological, aesthetic, and historical role played by data-visualization practices across contemporary biomedicine, neuroscience, and the arts. For example, I set up the cross-disciplinary project *Arscientia*, a privately funded, yearlong series of art–science–entrepreneurship dialogues and pop-up events/exhibitions, which became the seed for establishing Science Gallery Venice.[42] More recently, my ethnographic study of data-visualization practices in the University of Aberdeen biomedical physics laboratory and the related archival research have become the springboard for the collaborative project comprising the exhibition *Immobile Choreography* by the artist Beverley Hood, and my archive-based exhibition *From Where Do We See?*

But art–science collaboration has a dark side. First, it runs the risk of producing bad science and bad art. On the one hand, what many art–science projects present as "scientific content" is, in fact, a surrogate of it or, as the art historian James Elkins puts it, "a remnant of scientific forms stripped of their content."[43] On the other hand, the final output of the collaboration can be of poor artistic quality, merely making science education more appealing.[44] Second, art–science programs are increasingly institutionalized and regulated by public engagement frameworks, with the artist being secluded to an ancillary role—the problem highlighted by Clair in the 1990s, which is still present. Research institutions often use art–science to strengthen the ties with industry and society at large (the so-called third mission of universities, for which the International Science Gallery Network has become an ideal vehicle). Although this is clearly not a bad thing, the risk is to objectify art.

What science discovers about the world cannot be separated from the questions of how science impacts the world and who is affected by science.[45] The dimension of responsibility in research comes to the foreground in Responsible Research and Innovation (RRI), a European Union framework used in big science projects to describe an integrated approach toward scientific research and technological development.[46]

Some RRI projects have started to use the arts and design to engage with stakeholders such as citizens, policy makers, business, third sector organizations, among others, encouraging them to work together during the whole research and innovation process in order to better align both the process and its outcomes with the values, needs, and expectations of society.[47] An RRI-informed approach to art–science collaboration can enable scientists to become more self-reflexive about their work. The risk, however, is to reproduce the unbalance of art and science power relationships, with each of them embracing a form of parasitism: the arts interested in the funding, which is greater within the sciences, and the sciences interested in art as a way to add aesthetic flavor to their own research findings.[48]

Arts at CERN (the Geneva-based European Organization for Nuclear Research), which houses the Large Hadron Collider, has become a reference point for organizations, curators, and cultural entrepreneurs interested in setting up collaborative art–science projects and residencies.[49] This and other programs, such as SciArt at the Wellcome Trust and the art program at NASA, have the merit of widening public engagement with science and, at the same time, they offer a model that can serve those willing to set up art–science projects at large institutions. The problem is that institution-sponsored art–science projects can unintentionally set the bar too high for any individuals or groups willing to set up collaborative projects without big funding schemes or substantial infrastructure.

Scholars and practitioners willing to venture in art–science collaboration should start reading those pages that never get listed in any institutional "art–science" literature. A good example is the book conceived by Daniele Del Giudice during a week-long residency at CERN in 1984. An accidental collision between two small airplanes kicks off the encounter and then friendship between the young CERN physicist Pietro Brahe and the old enigmatic writer Ira Epstein, the two protagonists of Del Giudice's laboratory-like book *Atlante Occidentale*, inspired by fieldwork he undertook at CERN and described in his handwritten notes. The two characters could not be more different. Yet, they have a common obsession: describing the world. Pietro tries it out by exploring subatomic particles inside a huge underground ring dug under the Jura mountains; Ira abdicates his profession as an analytic weaver of stories. Both are seeking to create new tools (machines) for understanding reality—Pietro a particle collider, Ira the written word.

Therefore, another scale and syntax for art–science projects can emerge from the less structured, more tentative, slower-paced grassroots approaches to setting up collaborative projects.[50] This type of art–science collaboration would benefit science research communities in a way quite different from the public engagement activities and scientific literacy that have been the more celebrated product of mainstream art–science projects. Paying attention to aesthetics and bricolage in science practice would help cultivate a community of science "amateurs" and "connoisseurs" for whom matters of concern are as important as matters of fact.[51]

Reorienting the Center–Periphery in MRI Innovation

The Multiple Origins of MRI

To tackle data-visualization challenges in biomedical imaging and the arts, I focus on MRI, a noninvasive technique that uses strong magnetic fields, radio waves, and field gradients to visualize the anatomy and the physiological processes of the body in health and disease.[52]

The patient lies inside a tube-shaped magnet and is exposed to a strong magnetic field. MRI technology is based on the principle that atomic nuclei absorb external radio-frequency waves and reemit them in a magnetic environment. Water molecules in the patient's body contain hydrogen atoms, which usually spin in random directions, but in the MRI scanner they become temporarily aligned with the direction of the applied magnetic field. A radio-frequency pulse is then applied, which excites the atoms and forces them out of equilibrium with the magnetic field. When the pulse ends, the atoms realign with the magnetic field—the time it takes for them to realign is called the "relaxation time" (abbreviated "T_1"). It is during these readjustments, which typically take just a few hundred milliseconds, that the atoms emit very faint signals that can be analyzed by the scanner to indicate whether they came from normal or diseased tissue. After being collected by the scanner, these signals are used to create cross-sectional images of the patient's tissues and organs.

MRI images are maps of tissue-specific relaxation rates of the protons of water in different tissues. The clinical usefulness of MRI derives from the fact that pathological tissues have different relaxation characteristics than healthy tissues.[53]

Like most scientific breakthroughs and discoveries, the development of MRI, involving different scientific laboratories and research teams across the world and particularly the United Kingdom, has not been linear. As with the discovery of X-rays in 1895, multiple steps led to the scientific, technological, and diagnostic breakthroughs of MRI.[54] The history of MRI might be visualized as a map with multiple centers across continents (North America, Europe, Asia) and multiple temporalities. To single out an inventor—the first to discover the principle of magnetism, the chemistry of MRI, its clinical application, the first image ever obtained, and so forth—gives the illusion of a linearity in a clustered and distributed history.

Nevertheless, it is useful to know the key milestones that led to the invention and clinical application of MRI (initially called zeugmatography, then nuclear magnetic resonance [NMR]).[55] One element that comes to the foreground in this history is the role played by visualization. Physics and chemistry were more significant in the early development of the technology; the measurement context in which MRI first appeared was one of numerical values rather than visual culture.[56] The attempt to produce a visual output came from the will to transform the technology into a diagnostic tool—a transfer from physics and chemistry to medicine. The process took twenty years, and the historical details are still a matter of debate.[57]

With a background in radar research and a familiarity with electromagnetic technology, Felix Bloch and Edward Mills Purcell applied NMR technique to experiments with liquids and solids in 1946 (which earned them the Nobel Prize in Physics in 1952).[58] In 1970, Raymond Damadian, a US-based doctor, noticed that samples from diseased tissues had longer relaxation times than normal tissues. He realized that this would open NMR to medical diagnostics. In 1971, Paul Lauterbur, who was already known for his NMR studies in the field of chemistry and was aware of Damadian's claim that NMR could be used to distinguish cancerous tissues from normal ones, thought that pictures could be made using a technique called zeugmatography. Lauterbur escaped the classic relationship between wavelength and spatial resolution by using the magnetic field gradient to encode spatial information and reconverting the frequency back into an image.[59]

In the United Kingdom, the physicist Peter Mansfield (Nottingham University), who shared the 2003 Nobel Prize in Physiology or Medicine with Lauterbur for their work on MRI, was also instrumental in discovering a better method for turning radio signals from NMR into clinical images. Test-tube small samples like the okra seed pod shown in figure 1.2 were imaged and colored in naturalistic ways.

The first NMR image showing "live human anatomy" of a finger was made in 1977 by Mansfield's group.[60] The first cross-section NMR image of a human chest, which was obtained by Damadian on July 3, 1977, was a matrix of columns and rows filled with

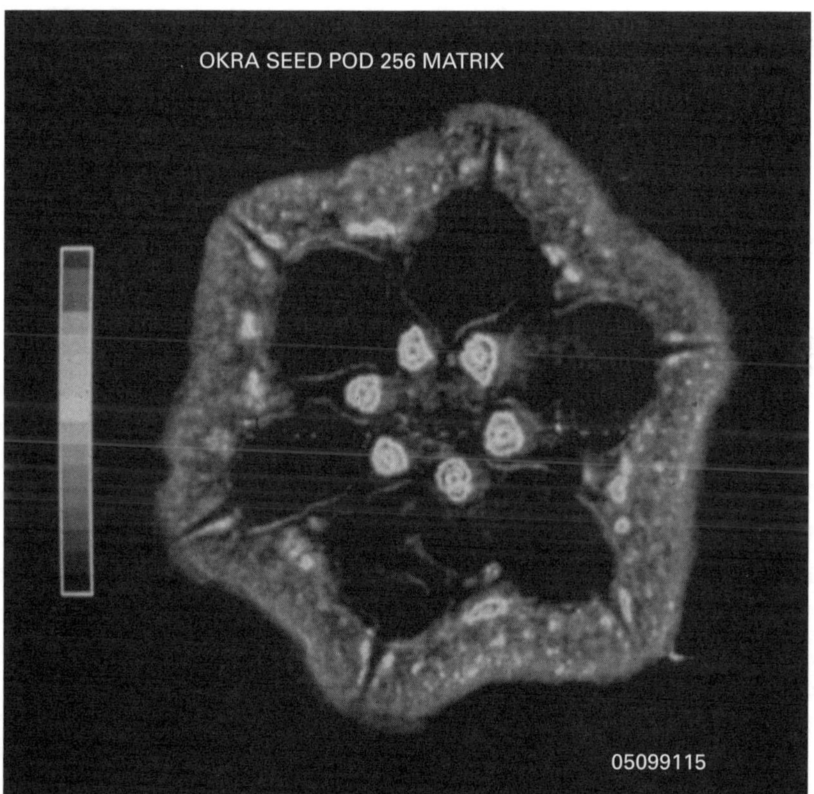

Figure 1.2
Sir Peter Mansfield, Okra seed pod 256 matrix. PPM/15/5/15.
Source: Courtesy of the University of Nottingham, Manuscripts and Special Collections.

numbers representing T_1 measurements. Rather than being a passive recording of numbers, this diagram was carefully constructed following conventions according to which a gray or color value was assigned to an NMR parameter range.[61]

There was no straightforward translation from an idea to a machine to a diagnostic aid. The passage from the theory to the early clinical use of MRI in the first half of the 1980s required more than a decade of laborious work.[62] The Aberdonian case study witnesses this complexity.

Aberdeen occupies a peripheral place within the historiographical accounts of the invention and development of MRI. Research carried out by the Aberdonian group headed MRI research until 1981, when it was superseded by research centers that could count on cutting-edge scanners manufactured by big companies. The biomedical physics laboratory in Aberdeen developed MRI in two periods. The first occurred between the late 1960s and early 1980s. The research group led by physicist James Hutchison (with John R. Mallard as head of the department) constructed *Mark I*, the world's first whole-body MRI scanner for clinical use, and invented the spin-warp method, a nuclear magnetic image-resolution technique that became the global standard for data–image conversion. Not only is this a Scottish case study of global importance, it is also relevant to a second ongoing period of Aberdonian innovation from 2014 (which I document in this book). Fast field-cycling MRI is a new noninvasive, low-cost biomedical imaging technique that enables the visualization of biochemical information at a molecular level not detectable by conventional MRI and potentially suitable for predictive medicine.

Challenging the classical narrative in innovation studies, which presumes that within an emerging global economy innovation occurs within the Western advanced metropolitan centers, the focus on the development of MRI at the University of Aberdeen reorients how researchers and practitioners theorize and foster innovation. Anthropologist Paul Rabinow highlights how simple it is to name an individual as the inventor of a technique or concept when other scientists and technicians were instrumental in bringing together what it took to make it work.[63] Rabinow's observation is valid for MRI too.

Innovation scholar Nathan Rosenberg argues that improvements to an invention after its first introduction may be vastly more important economically than the initial availability of the invention in its original form.[64] Innovation is a combination of material things and conceptual leaps from different locations and temporalities, brought together and put into a new place. The chapters related to the Aberdonian case study trace the topography through which scientific practice moves. The nodes of this topography are research centers, institutions, academic journals; different expertise from physics, design, clinical practice, engineering; as well as memories, affective investment, and bricolage. These nodes become the cartography that embodies the dynamics of the center–periphery relationship in the history of MRI innovation.

Moving Craftsmanship and Affectivity from the Periphery to the Center of Science Practice

This study of scientific practice at the University of Aberdeen's biomedical physics laboratory aims to recenter the history of MRI invention and development, shifting it from the supposed "center" (the metropolitan research centers where the principles of MRI were first discovered) to the supposed "periphery" (at the University of Aberdeen where MRI was transformed into a viable clinical technique). The marginalization (to make peripheral) of this piece of history is related not only to geography but also to the role played by manual labor, affectivity, and memory. In recent years, scholarly research on image-generating technologies, molecular biology, and astrophysics has begun to embrace a multisensorial turn in laboratory studies thanks to a focus on the body as an essential instrument of inquiry in the lab and on scientists' bodily and affective engagement in the construction of knowledge.[65]

The philosopher Annemarie Mol has paid attention to matters of reality—and the reality of matter—studying the *body multiple* as it emerges from the material relationships through which it is enacted in a specific place and time. To give an example, she argues that the ethnographer does not separate the disease from the relationships, technologies, and practices that brings it to light: "She [the ethnographer] may talk bodies—but she never forgets about microscopes."[66] The activity of knowing the "body multiple" is spread across the instruments, habits of work, buildings, and attitudes rather than pertaining exclusively to a knowing human subject.

In her ethnography of atherosclerosis, Mol combines concepts and methods from different theoretical traditions, drawing from actor-network theory, historical epistemology, medical anthropology, and phenomenology. She analytically explores the mundane and material layers of the reality of atherosclerosis. Mol pays attention to the multiple realities enacted by the practices she investigates. Her take on knowledge as a compositional activity is indebted to actor-network theory.

From the late 1970s, a few scholars within the French-British tradition of science studies elaborated actor-network theory (ANT) to chart the relationships of human agency and the intricate technical and material relationships that enabled or influenced their actions.[67] The social actor was said to be an actor-network of all these relationships. There was no scientist without their being a scientist-microscope or a scientist-microscope-extended-set-of-laboratory-relations. ANT targets the dichotomous logic behind thought organized in "macro versus micro," "actor versus structure," "social versus technical," or "subject versus object." It is the association (the actor-network) that becomes the dynamic center of agency.

In this ethnographic account of MRI development at the University of Aberdeen I show how scientists "feel" in their bodies the struggles of coping with certain materials, theoretical problems, and everyday tinkering in the workshop space. In his work on an affective topology of the senses, philosopher of new media Mark Hansen sees the creative potential of affectivity: indeed, he defines affectivity as "the capacity of the body to experience itself as "more than itself" and thus to deploy its sensorimotor power to create the unpredictable, the experimental, the new."[68] Affectivity has to do with the transmission of intensities between bodies and technologies or (particularly if we think in actor-networks) between bodies and bodies. It functions as a conduit for the transformative and creative potential of lived experience. This entails a shift from the attempt to catch reality as it is (traditional ontology and ANT approach) toward a tuning in with the multiple temporalities encrusted in the layers and lines of lived experience.[69] Using laboratory ethnography and archival research, the present ceases to be a self-evident category to reveal how all fragments of lived experience are encrusted with multiple pasts.

In laboratory ethnography, we scholars not only work with and interact with scientists doing things but with scientists among machines and the relationships of the laboratory, with scientists doing things and feeling things, and with things. Machines and their hardware or software components are not just elements of emotional exchange, but nodes within a more general assembly of relays within a wider affective entanglement. In her work on the relationship between affect and artificial intelligence, the feminist cultural historian Elizabeth Wilson highlighted the degree to which machines and their creators are bound up with "a fusion of intellect and muscle and beauty and nerves."[70] The manual labor involved in the creation of each component of a new technology such as MRI (designing and assembling the hardware, writing the code for turning data into images) is not simply a way of taking care of the technological object but much more a way of taking care of future patients, who are the end users of this technology.[71]

The analysis of archival material brings to the foreground the aesthetic and affective tropes embedded in images and data visualization. Affectivity is connected to materiality, with reference not just to bodily processes, but also to the material world as a site of affective exchange between human and non-human agents (including machines and their components). In this exchange between a human and a machine, the machine has intensities and qualities of difference, but these are only an affect when they come into a human, where they begin to be part of the body. Design sketches, photographs, lab notes, and newspaper clippings, which might seem to be marginal at first look, can turn out to be the driving forces and narratives behind the development of a certain technology or scientific theory. These incidental things are repositories of memory, aesthetic choices, and affective labor, allowing a first migration of biomedical imaging to the laboratory from the arts even before any form of artistic intervention.[72]

In this chapter I have suggested a theoretical framework for thinking about and creating art–science collaboration. The gesture of opening the black box of scientific practice in the early development of an imaging technology, before the data-visualization pipeline is closed, brings to the center bricolage, aesthetics, and the affective relationships present in scientific experience. I complete this chapter with the following brief section on a call for holding art and science together in one eyesight machine, in a stereoscopic vision.

A Stereoscopic Vision of Art and Science

In June 1838, the Victorian scientist Charles Wheatstone published a paper describing a curious phenomenon he had just discovered. If you drew two pictures of something—say, a tree—from two slightly different perspectives, and then viewed each one through a different eye, your brain would assemble them into a three-dimensional view. This was, he noted, precisely how our vision works; each eye sees a slightly different perspective. Wheatstone created the world's first stereoscope to demonstrate the effect. A decade later, the scientist David Brewster refined the design, crafting a handheld device one could raise to one's own eyes. Photography had recently been invented, which meant Brewster's stereoscope could display not just hand drawings, but also photographs captured from real life.

Stereoscopy began to transform science and art. Thanks to the stereoscope, astronomers were able to obtain a view of the moon's surface using two pictures taken months apart from each other. New lunar features were revealed to the human eye. Stereoscopic photography was a means to achieving realism in science and medicine. Joseph Towne, one of the most skilled makers of wax moulages in the nineteenth century, used the new technology of stereoscopic photography for constructing his three-dimensional anatomical models. Stereoscopy was an embodied form of vision, in contrast with the detached and distant model put forth by the camera obscura.[73]

In 1920, the cinematographic pioneer Louis Lumière developed photostereosynthesis (*photo-stéreo-synthèse*), a now lost imaging technology able to produce dimensionally deep and multilayered images through a series of stacked photographs. In this process, individual frames were shot at extremely small depths of field at incrementally increasing focal lengths, which had the effect of "depth-slicing" a dimensional space. Serial exposures were printed as transparent positives on glass and stacked together to produce a composite 3D photo with the scene "entombed" in a volumetric translucent image. It was the exploration of depth rather than of movement that seemed to be at the core of cinema's birth.[74] In his genealogy of computer tomography (CT) and its way of seeing, doctor and anthropologist Barry Saunders recalls the study of early photographic and protocinematic experiments such as photostereosynthesis: "Lumière's experiments forefront more than mechanism and geometry. Adding his work to the genealogy of early tomographic devices highlights again the importance of embodied (craft-practical) gestures along with machinic (engineered, black-boxed) movements—and of representations' effects on modes of viewing."[75]

Although the stereoscope was killed off by newer, more bewitching media, stereo images never entirely vanished, living on metaphorically and then resurfacing with the advent of virtual reality.

I would like to refer to two instances in which the metaphor of stereoscopic vision is mentioned in two different theoretical traditions. The idea is that a stereoscopic image is able to conjure different images in the eye and the mind of the onlooker. The first is historical materialism taken from philosopher and cultural critic Walter Benjamin and bears upon his reflections on photography as a medium through which our experience and knowledge of the world is mediated in unconscious ways. The second comes from the philosopher of science Wilfrid Sellars and his differentiation between the manifest and the scientific image (see chapter 5).

In several of his works, starting from his 1929 essay on surrealism to the unfinished work *Arcades Project*, which he pursued until the end of his life, Walter Benjamin was concerned with images and their use. Ongoing scholarly debate questions what exactly Benjamin meant by the term *image*, whether the visual component did play a role or whether the image was confined to the sphere of language.[76] The image opens a *space* for conducting critical theory and practice. This image-space can make the past present, make close what is far, make every point of view less definite and stable, or, as Jevtić quoting Benjamin says, "It is not the subject that holds the image, it is the image that holds the subject."[77] Therefore, the image is a way to overcome the split between subject and object.

What is clear is that Benjamin's conception of the image relied on cinematic and precinematic visual practices such as stereoscopy.[78] The expansion of optical possibilities through instruments converges with the advent of modernity and industrialization. If Galileo Galilei's use of ground lenses as a telescope had already shifted our worldview in relation to our position in the universe, the introduction of photography and other vision machines in the second half of the nineteenth century led to a loss of faith in our ability to believe our own eyes.

For Benjamin, the stereoscope provides the model for a concept of vision able to create an in-depth view of history. In a 1923 fragment in his *Arcades Project*, Benjamin makes a first reference to the stereoscope, stating that its goal was "to educate the image-making medium within us, raising it to a stereoscopic and dimensional seeing into the depths of historical shadows."[79] Benjamin envisaged a process of image making that would end up in a stereoscopic vision. His collections of notes, photographs, and artifacts found in the Paris Arcades was meant to provide one-half of the image required, the other half being gleaned by his readers from their own historical memories. The two halves might then crystallize into a single mental image—a stereoscopic vision of the world.[80] Stereoscopic optics was a way of telescoping the past through the present.

As much as the optical unconscious is not available to our sight, the stereoscopic image does not exist in the world, but only in the mind's enhanced eye, being made through the combination of a viewing device (the stereoscope), a doubled image (the stereo card), and human binocular vision. The stereoscopic image evokes, but does not reproduce, three-dimensional perception. Thus, it provides an illusion of depth and dimension, but not an illusion of reality: "His dialectical image, like the stereoscopic image, is not part of the phenomenal world, but an image that is activated by present readers gazing upon the past."[81] It is an entirely imaginary scene—a potentiality—that cannot be envisioned otherwise. The stereoscopic image can enact an awakening in the reader/onlooker: a fragment from the past, read and seen in light of the present, triggers a dialectical image exposing another reality not otherwise available.

The legacy of the transformative power of the stereoscopic image and vision can be found again in the work of Sellars, who distinguishes between the scientific and the manifest image (see chapter 5).[82] His account of stereoscopic vision does not consider that the stereoscope was a technological device, a kind of prosthetic to the human senses, which created not just an image but a way of inhabiting the environment. Namely, in Sellars the two images should not be understood as material pictures, but rather as two frameworks for describing subjectivity in relationship to the world. The first framework results from the new physics, according to which the world is made up of neurons, strings, atoms; the second framework results from the world we grew up and live in, made up of solid objects, words, goals, free will. The manifest image, the philosopher Daniel Dennett argues, comes from the *Umwelt,* a concept from early twentieth-century biology encompassing not only the environment but also the things that matter to the organism for its well-being. The world of the manifest image is populated with affordances and opportunities. The manifest image is not the ideology of common sense; it has evolved across history to comprise quite abstract things, such as colors and money.[83]

Sellars argues that the two images should not be taken literally, for they are two distinct conceptual frameworks to describe and explain the position of the man in the world.[84] Given that one will never reach a complete description or explanation of humans in the world, we need to keep both views in focus, in a stereoscopic image. Despite what Sellars calls "the primacy of the scientific image,"[85] he argues for a "stereoscopic vision"[86] in which the descriptive and explanatory resources of the scientific image are enriched by the manifest image, so that the world described by science becomes the world in which we do our living.[87] For Sellars, this remains a goal that can be achieved only in our imagination. I argue that the communities of scientists and artists, working together, can foster and maintain a stereoscopic vision in how we approach the conundrum of what it is like to be both a biological organism made up of molecules and cells, and an entity equipped with intentionality, desires, thoughts, and values.

I Opening the Black Box

2 Histories and Practices in MRI Early Development

Encountering MRI

Inside the MRI scanner the patient lies still, her vision impaired by the required physical posture. She can move only her eyes and, because of her fixed horizontal position, the only things she can see are the roof of the scanner and its walls.[1] The technical procedure does not allow subjects to access their own MRI images; these appear on a computer screen in a separate room where the radiologist and the physician monitor the examination. The first things the patient experiences inside the scanner are the sound of the machine and the voices of the radiologist and the physician. No images. No eye contact. Exchanges are mediated by voices through headphones and eventually drowned out by the alien-like whir of the machine. This intense acoustic experience saturates the space inside the scanner with reverberations and vibrations.

The sound resonates in the patient's ears, and it is owing to this resonance that the feeling of her own body is created and endures after the MRI scan is completed. The magnet's voice opens her body as a site for resonance. The body is caught up and carried away by the magnetic sound, ceasing to be the patient's personal body and becoming a web of acoustic reverberations, their resonance captured in MRI images. Thus, far from being transparent and representational, MRI images are generated by an acoustic force whose "trace" is preserved in their regular looping beat, bearing witness to the pressure exercised by the magnetic field on the still body.[2]

The first encounter with MRI happens through sound and not through images; these are only later reconstructed by physicists and then read by radiologists and clinicians. MRI is a device with a specific voice produced by forces resulting from rapidly switched magnetic gradients interacting with the main magnetic field, a phenomenon that in turn causes minute expansions and contractions of the coil itself. The gradient pulse produces the characteristic rocking sound of MRI, and the intense vibration and loud noise are referred to as gradient noise.[3] The MRI signal is produced by the interaction between the patient's tissues and the radio-frequency pulses that are generated by the transmitter coil surrounding the whole body or parts of it. In an MRI image, both signal and noise are present: the signal is the voxel or pixel brightness in the image; noise is the random differences in pixel values generated by the patient's body. Noise disturbs the reading of the image and has to be eliminated to allow radiologists and clinicians to make a diagnosis. The process of turning the signal into a meaningful image, free from noise, is far from straightforward. Yet the process of turning data into visual output is the main aspect of MRI to be offered to patients as "fact."

Visualizing Data in MRI: How the Journey Starts

How then are biomedical images generated from hardware, and data from signal/noise? What is it that scientists see, particularly in the case of an emerging technology, before the image-generating procedure and the visual output become standardized?

The term *visualization* varies across knowledge domains, and it can have descriptive, aesthetic, instructive, explanatory, interpretative, evaluative, and persuasive intents.[4] These can also function as bridges between communities of users from different backgrounds (for example, scientists and artists) and their ways of seeing.[5] In this sense, visualization favors a common understanding despite users' different views. Visualizations are not simply an aid to science. They are how science often creates its objects, conducts its inquiries, and advances its arguments.

MRI technology was developed at the University of Aberdeen in the 1970s/early 1980s, first with the construction of the world's first whole-body MRI scanner and then with the invention of the spin-warp method for transforming data into images. More recently, the technology has been reinvented, with the ongoing development of FFC-MRI, which enables the visualization of information not available to conventional MRI scanners. But an invention is a retrospective construction, as sociologist Amit Prasad argues in his transnational history of MRI: "[T]he 'invention' of MRI was not a singular event, or a set of events, frozen in time (the early 1970s), but, rather, the result of entangled activities of a number of actors that extended over decades."[6]

Narratives around MRI technology are multiple and make use of a variety of approaches, from the historical sociological to the semiotic.[7] However, none of these accounts has considered the narratives that accompany and shape a technology in its early developmental stage. These emerging narratives are fundamental for grasping the social construction of a technology as an ever-changing set of processes. In part I of this book (chapters 2–4) I explore two different periods in the history of MRI in Aberdeen: its development and its reinvention.

I argue three points. First, data visualization in biomedical science cannot be discussed without attention to its sociocultural and historical specificities. As Sabina Leonelli claims in her study on data-intensive science, scientific practice should be studied by looking at the "situation," which is defined as "the dynamic entanglement of conceptual, material, social, and institutional factors involved in developing knowledge and clearly positions research efforts in relation to the publics for whom such knowledge is expected to be of value."[8] The process of turning data into visual output is profoundly historical, locally constructed, and co-evolving with the specific circumstances in which it is situated.[9]

Second, visualization is a relational process connecting concepts, data, spaces, and people.[10] Scientific data visualization emerges from highly specific situations and processes that are in themselves fragmented and recursive, exhibiting a rhizomatic pattern.[11] Third, patients are a driving force behind challenges, decisions, and efforts undertaken by physicists and other researchers engaged in developing a new biomedical imaging technology. Scientists also think through images. In some cases they envisage possible future clinical applications of the technology under development. By doing so, data visualization becomes a way of world making.[12]

The case study I examine here is local, historical, and informed by the materiality of images, data visualization, and ways of seeing. A sensibility to both history and context is crucial not just to scholars of technology studies, historians, or social scientists interested in a specific technology, but also to artists willing to use biomedical imaging or to tap into neuroscience. Artists benefit from becoming familiar with the local histories embedded in a technology and its ways of seeing—artists need to attend to the local and material history of the data-visualization process that created the visual output, for instance, a brain scan. Furthermore, images are entangled with memory and affect. Digging up archival objects, images, and instruments is a way to evoke and explore the affective dimension of visualized data as it emerges from the relationships between technologies, images, ideas, and people. The archival material explored in this chapter comes from various sources. The first is the publication papers and oral history interview held in the Special Collection of the University of Aberdeen Sir Duncan Rice Library. It is the official repository of published articles, manuscripts, slides, and photographs relating to MRI and other technologies developed by the team of physicists and engineers at Aberdeen led by John R. Mallard, including the physicists James (Jim) Hutchison and William (Bill) Edelstein, the biologist Margaret Foster (Meg), the MRI researchers (physicists David Lurie, Tom Redpath, and Glyn Johnson), the MRI researchers with an expertise in electronics (Robert Selbie and David Bussell), as well as the radiologist Frank Smith and the technician/radiographer Gordon Crosher. This team developed and tested the MRI body scanning machine and brought its widespread use to the medical profession.

Spanning the development and clinical use of MRI, positron emission tomography (PET), and other significant biomedical imaging technologies from 1965 (the year when Professor Mallard was appointed to the purposefully created chair in medical physics at the university) to the early 1980s, the selection of materials represents key moments in the development of such technologies in Aberdeen.[13] Data-visualization challenges cut across the various technologies and techniques developed by the research team. The papers authored by Mallard engage with the history of MRI development in Aberdeen, combining scientific accuracy with storytelling techniques and the use of paratextual elements. The second archive is Jim Hutchison's laboratory and personal notebooks that are now property of the Special Collections of the University of Aberdeen. The collection comprises a wide range of photographic material and slides that were processed by both Hutchison and Raymond Hutcheon, the department photographer at the time of Mallard. Hutchison's personal notebooks (called the VB books) are records kept by Hutchison since his childhood. In these notebooks (more than a hundred) he wrote down notes about his thoughts, ideas for future projects, and experiments.

The last archival source, far from being a dead storehouse of memory relics, is the recordkeeping system of Eddie Stevenson, the engineer behind the construction of many scanners in the biomedical physics department. His personal archive material—predominantly letters, design sketches, invoices, scrapbooks, or transparent folders filled with old photographs and newspaper clippings—tells the less known, more marginalized Aberdonian history of MRI invention, both confirmed and contested over the years. Both Hutchison's and Stevenson's archives reframe the history of MRI development. First, these archives reveal how the history of MRI innovation was a collective enterprise rather than a linear trajectory of improvements and discoveries led by a single scientist. Second, Hutchison's and Stevenson's archives show that the peripherality of aesthetics and craftsmanship are actually at the core of the narrative that brings Aberdeen at the center of MRI transnational history. An invention never happens in the way in which it is later publicized. For this reason, notes, visual material, and anecdotes that might seem to be marginal at first look—the "cursed" part of scientific research—turn out to be the driving force behind the development of MRI.

Mark I as a Boundary Object

A strange cylinder-shaped object, resembling a space shuttle, stands in the middle of a small room inside the Suttie Arts Space in Aberdeen. This is *Mark I* with its skeleton of four coils and its complex sets of copper wires, rods, and bolts. In stark contrast to today's neat and polished commercial MRI scanners, *Mark I* is open in its design, laying bare the intricacies of its structure to the eyes of the onlooker.

Mark I was developed in the Department of Medical Physics and Bio-Engineering at the University of Aberdeen. Upon its completion in September 1978, it became the world's first whole-body MRI scanner used to diagnose disease in patients—a major milestone in scientific achievement and a huge step forward in the delivery of health care worldwide.

In the existing photographic reproductions available in the archive, *Mark I* is represented much like similar biomedical technologies, both in terms of framing and in the spatial arrangement of the subjects. For example, it is interesting to compare and contrast the photograph of *Mark I* to the one of *Indomitable*, the world's first, but not clinically reliable, full-body MRI scanner, invented by the physician Damadian in 1977.[14] The first thing to notice in both is the closeness of the scientists to their beasts. One or two scientists (often smiling) are depicted standing next to the machine while another is portrayed as the experimental subject inside the scanner.

In the photograph of *Indomitable*, the inventor Damadian stands close to the machine like a reassuring version of a modern Frankenstein, his foot firmly on top of the bench bar as if flaunting his ability to tame his creature, which is about to take on a life of its

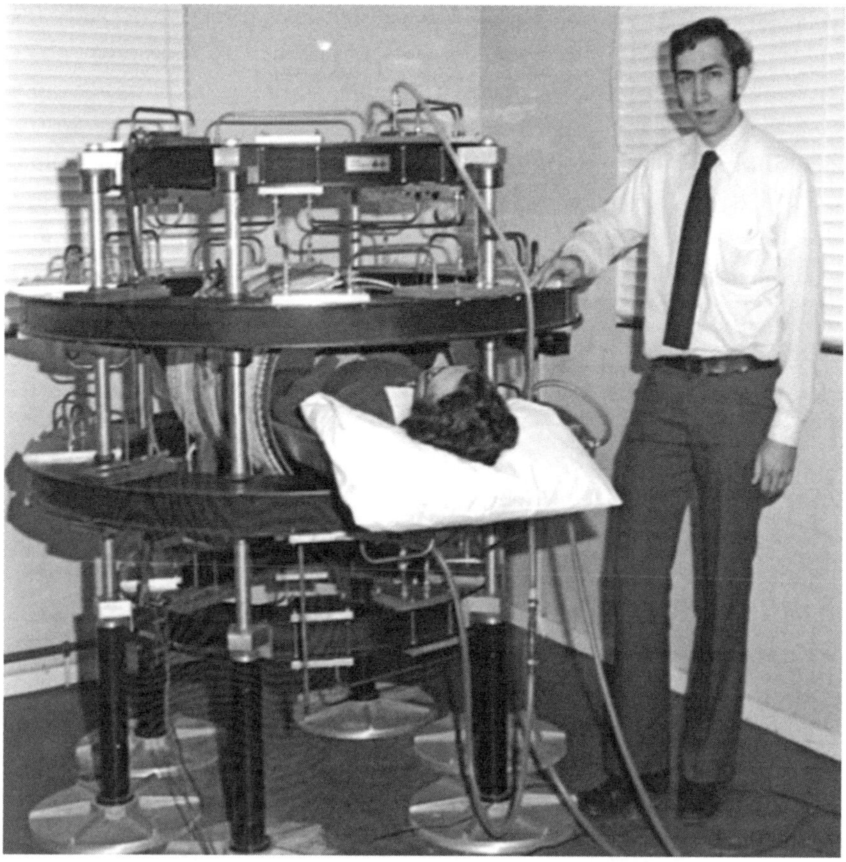

Figure 2.1
Jim Hutchison and Bill Edelstein with *Mark I* (1980).
Source: Courtesy of Margaret Foster Hutchison.

own. In the photograph of *Mark I* (figure 2.1), Bill Edelstein, the American postdoctoral physicist who was part of the team involved in its construction, also stands next to his scanner, his hand almost caressing it. The other postdoctoral researcher involved in the Aberdonian research team, Jim Hutchison, lies on a borrowed wooden patient tray inserted into the magnet, assuming the position of the experimental subject.

Hutchison, almost invisible in this picture, would later become the inventor of the spin-warp method, a new nuclear magnetic imaging technique fundamental in transforming data into images and destined to become the global standard for data–image conversion. In both photographs, the perspective is frontal and the proportions give a sense of the magnitude of the collective endeavor. In the case of *Mark I*, the enterprise was a leap in scale, leading Hutchison and the team to build a full-body MRI scanner, scaling up the imaging process from small tissues to a whole human without any stages in between.

With its six feet firmly on the ground of the Suttie Arts Space, *Mark I* is now quietly living its second life as a boundary object.[15] On the one hand, *Mark I* is a material landmark in the history of technological development in the field of biomedical imaging, a spotlight on the Aberdonian role in the transnational history of MRI innovation. On the other hand, it exists in the realm of fine arts, a sculpturelike object with aesthetic features of its own. The scanner inhabits simultaneously two temporalities (the past and the present) and two epistemologies (the scientific and the artistic). The instrument is located in an art gallery within a functioning hospital, where patients are treated and cured on a daily basis.[16] The closeness to the clinic, the drive toward the community of patients as the end users of biomedical technologies such as *Mark I*, was and still is the feature of MRI development in Aberdeen.

Stevenson played a huge role in the design and construction of several biomedical imaging technologies in Aberdeen across the decades, *Mark I* included. One of the objects in his archive is a postcard, handmade from an old-style black and white photograph depicting an agglomerate of small gray buildings in the foreground, and semidetached houses and trees in the background. Overall, a dull photograph. The card is signed by staff from the medical physics unit. On the front of the postcard, just below the image of the building, words in capital letters (with surplus suspension points and exclamation marks) warn: "IN CASE YOU FORGET WHERE TO COME BACK TO.....AFTER!!!!!" The ironic threat and irreverent tone of these words contradict the drabness of the picture. The reverse of the postcard explains that the ".....AFTER!!!!!" refers to Stevenson's honeymoon in August 1969. This is a personal photographic relic of the laboratory as a communal "home" to return to.[17]

Hardly visible in the institutional archive, the crucial role played by Stevenson within the laboratory comes to the fore in this photograph even more than in his numerous sketches for designing new imaging equipment. The laboratory has multiple configurations, being a physical space in which experiments and demonstrations are conducted, a normative place of investigation where scientific protocols are established and, as this postcard demonstrates, a contingent social group ("my lab") bound by specific research questions and endeavors.[18]

Today, *Mark I* silently welcomes the gallery visitor as an in-between object whose function has been elevated to more than just imaging patients. *Mark I* is an occasion for the lay public to encounter not only a piece of technological equipment used to visualize our body and brain, but a whole new world in which science and technological innovation is made visible as a historical and cultural endeavor. *Mark I* is present in two spaces: the Suttie Arts Space within Aberdeen Royal Infirmary, and the biomedical physics laboratory workshop. In the Suttie Arts Space, *Mark I* is present as a 3D model of the original, closely following the instructions and drawings laid out by Stevenson in his design sketches. In the workshop, *Mark I* is present in the form of material traces left on the floor (figure 2.2).

These traces are a remnant of the object in question. They are the means through which the scanner continues to be present in the daily laboratory life of researchers using the Aberdeen biomedical physics facilities. They bridge the laboratory's past and present. Therefore, thanks to its present dual location, *Mark I* lives its second life, acting

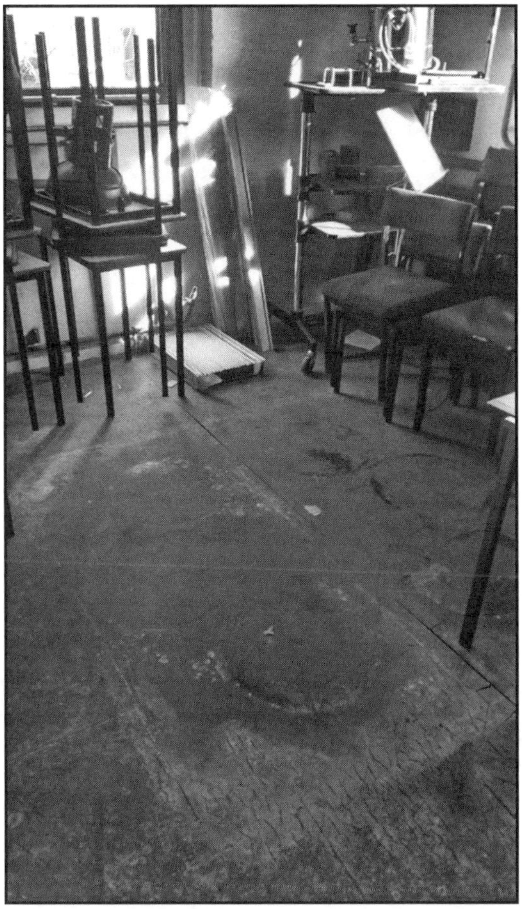

Figure 2.2
Mark I traces on the workshop floor. Photograph taken during laboratory ethnography, March 2017.

as a boundary object between different communities (researchers, clinicians, and public gallery visitors) and different times (past and present).

These minor material and visual elements are attempts to claim ownership for a history of technological innovation that would otherwise be recounted only by the official photographs hanging on the wall in the coffee area of the lab, each portraying the Aberdonian makers of biomedical imaging technologies together with their inventions. Photographs, sketches, paper clippings, images published in journal articles, and pieces of the machinery are ways of connecting researchers to the world, acting as life companions and provocations to think. As Turkle argues, thought and feeling are inseparable in these objects: "We think with the objects we love; we love the objects we think with."[19]

Material objects and traces, such as the *Mark I*'s floor imprints, are all glimpses of things that prop up the material and visual history of MRI trajectories in Aberdeen.

Glimpses appear and quickly disappear, leaving a trail—a trace—like an afterimage or an imaginative association.[20] To work through these material traces is to produce a series of scattered microhistories that are impalpable and tend to live only in the present. A glimpse is an experience. It is seeing less well, before the object becomes something to be observed, immobilized like a butterfly under glass or a corpse on the anatomist's table. Glimpses are affective memories, neural traces of something briefly seen, loved, and already lost, just before it vanishes. This history of the Aberdonian laboratory, therefore, is not an innocent one.[21] No vantage points of observation, no universal or overarching narrative, but an embodied vision built up with those intermittent, mercurial glimpses of truth.

The Drive toward the Patient in the Aberdonian Development of MRI

Archival material combined with interviews and ethnographic fieldwork single out the Aberdeen MRI laboratory as distinct from other national and transnational histories. It is the place in which MRI technology has been reconfigured across decades, always maintaining the focus on the clinical aspect of biomedical imaging—the drive toward the patient. Prasad recalls how in the 1970s, the University of Aberdeen, EMI (the British music company), the University of Nottingham, and London's Hammersmith Hospital were the main centers of MRI research in the UK.[22]

But it was the close connection between the research laboratory and the clinic—between physics, biology, engineering, and medicine—that made Aberdeen different from other places. This "techno-specificity" of Aberdeen is apparent in the words of Mallard:

> I had this strong commitment to patients. I always worked out to make sure that whatever I was doing was useful and, at that time, of course, all the physicists were going into nuclear physics, atomic energy research, things like that. But I wanted to be more down-to-earth, doing something immediately useful if possible. As physicists working on the development of imaging techniques, we could all get side-tracked into things that aren't of much use, but are interesting scientifically, but not necessarily with a very practical application.[23]

Although it is not possible to summarize into a single narrative the changes that medicine went through in the early twentieth century, it is clear that the term *biomedicine*, coined between the two world wars, was shorthand for identifying the work of scientists and doctors. The rise of biomedicine corresponds to the molecularization of biology and medicine and to the sharing of methods and techniques applied to study life processes and diseases.[24]

The passage quoted above makes clear that there was no institutional drive to bridge the gap between physics and medicine in the UK in the 1970s. Drawing upon his own personal recollections in a historical paper on the evolution of biomedical imaging, Mallard mentions the childhood memory of using his father's bacon-slicing machine. This experience ignited the imagination of the future scientist, who would later intuitively grasp the potential of digitally "slicing up" the human body for diagnostic purposes.[25]

This experience and intuition eventually led Mallard to undertake a career in biomedical physics rather than atomic physics as most researchers did in his day.

The creation of the chair in medical physics at the University of Aberdeen in 1965—the first in its field in Scotland—gave the research team the opportunity to establish a tighter connection between research, technological innovation, clinical practice, and patients. The process was anything but smooth, at least initially, and required the availability of technologies developed elsewhere. This was the case with the cyclotron, the UK's first radionuclide imaging device, which could be used for producing radioactive isotopes for nuclear medicine. Mallard built it at Hammersmith Hospital in London thanks to a grant from the Medical Research Council; he then struggled hard to relocate it to Aberdeen until he managed to get the army to move the machine.

Bringing medicine, biology, physics, and the clinic closer together was the driving force behind the success of the specific research program implemented in Aberdeen as Mallard recalls: "[A] biological program to understand the resonance signals went hand-in-hand with the physics and technological development of the imager."[26] The Department of Medical Physics and Bio-Engineering pioneered the clinical use of whole-body CT scanners and gamma cameras for nuclear medicine.

The patient, albeit not present as flesh and blood in the laboratory during the first phase of technological development of *Mark I*, was a reference point for researchers. References to the patients are not always explicit in the scientific papers published by the Aberdonian research team on the development of biomedical imaging technologies. This is not surprising, given that the clinical application of an emerging technology is not necessarily clear in the early stages of research before clinical trials can occur. The patient's body is often anticipated in the design sketches for the components of a new imaging technology or in the experimental trials in which physicists use their own bodies to test the apparatus. Furthermore, any references to the patient can take the form of pictures or words that are paratextual to the main technical argument advanced in a scientific article. For example, an article published by Mallard in 1965 in the *Journal of Nuclear Medicine* starts with a hardly known poem by the Irish poet J. R. Stephens (1880–1950):

> O little probe, O little probe,
> That moves slow to and from,
> Your eye sees what man cannot see,
> And it makes him wonder so.
> You find hot spots and cold spots
> That give to us a clue
> And makes the doctor wonder
> "What are we going to do?"[27]

Not particularly interesting from a literary perspective, this poem nevertheless references the principles behind techniques developed by Mallard's team in Aberdeen, such as those in molecular imaging—PET and single photon emission CT (SPECT).[28]

Tomography had been known since 1964 thanks to an analog system put together by Dave Kuhl in the US: the Aberdeen team, though, was the first to demonstrate and build a digital CT for nuclear medicine in 1967–1969: the system was nicknamed ASS for Aberdeen Section Scanner, an important step toward the application of this technique to X-rays.[29]

In the 1960s, Mallard knew that when radioactive iodine is swallowed, it is concentrated in the thyroid gland, and that by using a Geiger-Müller counter over the neck, one can measure the gamma rays and detect abnormalities in the function of the gland. A relatively crude image depicting the size and shape of the thyroid gland could be obtained. The gamma rays first had to be detected, then counted, and then plotted on graph paper as figure 2.3 shows.

It became a technique for localizing tumors because radioactive iodine did not concentrate in tumor tissue; thus, tumoral regions appeared as "cold" spots embedded in the "hot" gland.[30] This indeed is the principle behind PET imaging, in which areas of greater intensity ("hot spots") indicate where large amounts of the radiotracer have accumulated and where there is a high level of chemical or metabolic activity. PET

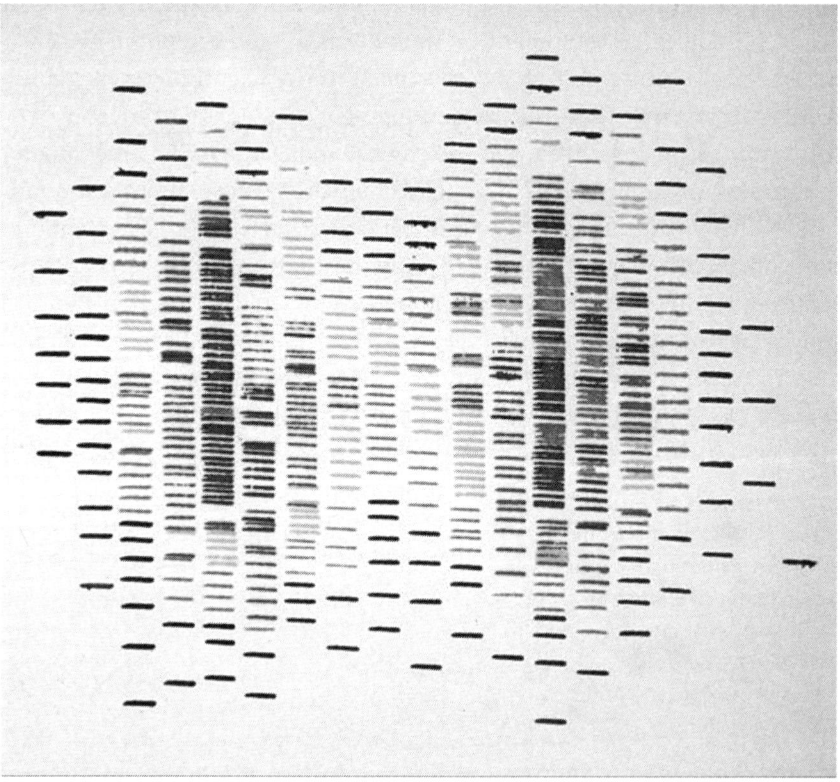

Figure 2.3

Isotope scanning and display, mid-1960s. PowerPoint slide taken from a presentation given by Professor Peter Sharp.

Source: Courtesy of University of Aberdeen. See plate 2.

scans, like other biomedical images, are exposed to the risk of false positives. In this sense, as the poem suggests, interpretation of the visual data is paramount since the doctor will then make decisions on how to proceed with the patient.

The closeness between the visualized data and the patient plays a major role in the development of biomedical imaging techniques. First, data visualization is not just about creating pictures that embellish the experimental results. The picture itself is a number, a way of measuring bodily parameters. Second, imaging is deeply connected to the patient's body and its condition of health and illness. Any results obtained after imaging are hard to read because the human body is extremely complex and the image itself is complex, because it shows both the pathology and the normality on the same surface at the same time.

The relationship between the biomedical apparatus (in our case, the MRI scanner) and the patient is closer than one might expect and influences the final visual output. For example, the comfort of the patient inside the claustrophobic scanner tube is crucial for ensuring that the patient does not make any voluntary or involuntary movements that might cause artifacts to appear in the final scan. Great attention is given to the design of the bed on which the patient slides into the scanner. The mirror placed on top of the scanner roof offers a gateway to the outside, reducing the feeling of claustrophobia. Headphones and a buzzer may be provided to allow the patient to listen to music or attract attention, to further minimize any discomfort caused by the experience of undergoing a biomedical scan.

It is not surprising therefore that the relationship between scanners and patients was in the minds of the physicists working on the development of an MRI scanner that could be clinically useful. In one of his articles published in a history-oriented medical biology journal, Mallard briefly discusses a line engraving depicting a procedure where all phantasies and follies are purged and good qualities are prescribed (figure 2.4).[31] At the end of his own historical account of MRI development at the University of Aberdeen, Mallard recalls also the centuries-old fascination for the phenomenon of magnetism, which was known already by the Chinese in the Middle Ages and then systematized centuries later when William Gilbert, physician to Queen Elizabeth I, published his text *De Magnete* (1600).

Although Mallard's paper does not cite the source of the image, the cultural and literary historian Sander Gilman discussed this picture in his book on the cultural history of madness and art in the Western world and identified the original picture as an early modern German sixteenth-century broadside by the etcher and engraver Matthias Greuter.[32] The broadside is a satirical depiction of "Dr. Wurmbrandt" (literally, worm distilled) and his cure for folly.

The picture, which is full of alchemic symbols, is a complex composition of two different scenes showing the patient first diagnosed (in the background) and then cured (in the foreground). The one that captures Mallard's eyes is the latter, in which a physician is sliding a patient, lying on a portable bed, into a furnacelike structure. The head of the patient is inside the furnace, the rest of the body outside. The top of the structure

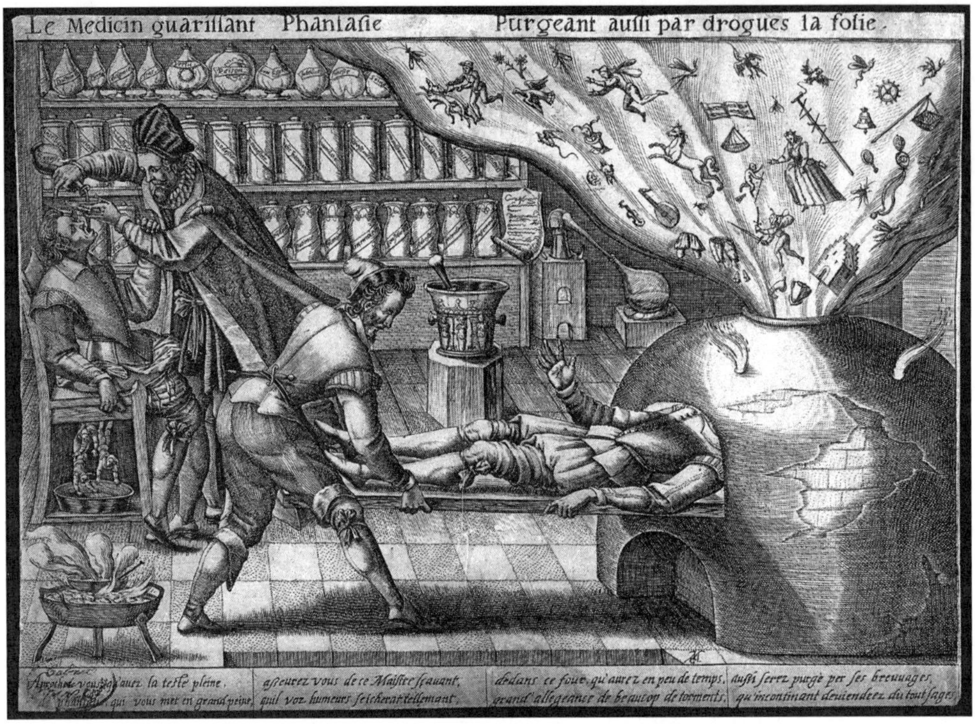

Figure 2.4
Line engraving by M. Greuter ca. 1600.
Source: Courtesy of the Wellcome Collection CC BY.

has an opening from which smoke billows out in a cloud. These are the "phantasies" (illnesses) being distilled or burned out from the patient's head.[33] The French version has the following text: "The physician exhibits fantasy, in addition to cleansing the drug of madness."[34]

In Mallard's own words, the scene and this furnacelike structure bear a striking resemblance to the MRI scanner: "At the beginning, it could not have been expected that the work of physicists in nuclear medicine—and later MRI—would lead to a step forward in the battle against mental disorders; a fulfilment of a medieval dream.... All those years ago, the conceptual relationship was predicted between the patient and modern imagers or scanners!"[35]

Without referring to any sources to support his idea, Mallard suggests that the drive toward the technological development of biomedical imaging scanners was present long before the technology was available. The picture allows the technology take on the mantle of historical necessity. Not only does Mallard avoid specifying what the "conceptual relationship" between scanners and patients actually means, but he also overlooks any close reading of the image, despite being accustomed to reading other types of images—those that belong to physics and medicine. A close reading would have helped to better interpret, and to challenge, this image as a straightforward pictorial representation of the doctor–patient relationship mediated by a scanner *ante litteram*, a machine for vision.

As an image the engraving exercises a rhetorical/persuasive function not related to any scientific argument and proofs, but rather to the place of that particular laboratory and ways of working toward clinical application rather than theory development, within the broader history of MRI development. This image functions almost as a *divertissement*; it is used quite arbitrarily for its vague metaphorical resemblance to the contemporary procedure of undergoing a scan. To say that the image of the scanner *ante litteram* partakes in the construction of the myth related to MRI development means that there clearly was the need for creating a myth around the historical necessity of turning the principles and properties of magnetization into a clinical device that can be used to diagnose patients. This engraving plays the function of narrating one of the key red threads underlying MRI development at the University of Aberdeen, that is, the centrality of the patient. The specific function stays even though, ironically, the iconology of the engraving is an explicit criticism to the promises offered and the procedures undertaken by a healing apparatus consisting of both humans and machinery.

There are several overlooked cues on how to appreciate the cultural-historical significance of this image. Besides Gilman, Jacqueline Vons (a philologist and historian of medicine) conducts a close reading and historical analysis of the French version of the broadside in light of Renaissance medical discourse and practice. The iconology of this picture is not straightforward. The image, far from being the original creation of an artist, is inspired by a cluster of similar copies and variants that were in widespread circulation in Europe during the sixteenth and seventeenth centuries. Both the background and the foreground of the image show rather terrifying and ambiguous procedures that seem to have little to do with medical practice and more with metaphorical cures and motifs around the idea of purging sins and folly.[36] The first procedure, in the background, takes place before a row of shelved bottles labeled "humilite," "obeissance," "honnestete," and other "good" qualities. A man, sitting on a chair, is forced to swallow a liquid (labeled *sagesse*, the French word for wisdom) from an alembic held by a practitioner and to defecate demons. Vons interprets the procedure as a purge unfolding in front of our eyes. Elements that belong to medicine and imagination are juxtaposed and mixed together to enhance the sense of a nightmarish world rather than one of objective reality.

The second, the "familiar" MRI-like scene, offers a representation of madness as being physically located in the head of the patient. This image represents the physical source of insanity by reference to one of Galen's theories in physiology, which posits that cranial sutures ("cracks" in the skull) are chimneys from which the humoral superfluities of the brain are evacuated.[37] If this function is impaired, the moods accumulate and cause disease. Another practitioner holds a patient (the same or another one) on a wooden stretcher while his head is placed in a furnace from which vices and phantasies are being expelled. By placing the patient's skull in the furnace, the doctor dries the moods and allows the vapors to escape.

Fire plays an important role in the procedure. Alchemists' fire was a viscous liquid that upon contact with air, would burst into flames and burned until it was consumed. It was nonmagical and could be created by an alchemist. In early modernity, Robert Boyle (1627–1691), the experimental philosopher of the seventeenth century and one of the fathers of the experimental method, did a series of experiments by *fire analysis*, in which he subjected samples to intense heat and subsequent distillation to reveal their elemental principles.[38]

The art historian Leclerc de la Verpillière argues that the only technique the print clearly refers to (always in a metaphorical way) is the process of distillation or sublimation, which was used in early modernity not only in alchemy but also in artisans' workshops.[39] Distillation is the process of separating the components or substances from a liquid mixture by using selective boiling and condensation. In the engraving, the physician is depicted as someone capable of pointing out to the patient the material substance of her illnesses. Sublimation is the phase transition of a substance from solid into gas without passing through its intermediate liquid phase. In early modernity the human body was often represented as an alchemical vessel that could take the form of a crucible, a still, or a retort. The techniques of distillation and sublimation hint, albeit in a simplified manner, at the process of alchemic transformation that was a prerogative of the human body as alchemical vessel.

The physiological process is accompanied by a more allegorical and moralizing memento, following Vons's interpretation: the released images (phantasies and illnesses, as Mallard correctly calls them) are dangerous for the social order as they evoke the arts, gallantry and love, and war games. To visualize something that lies in the depths of the skull means detaching the illness from the body in order to free the patient from the hidden source of their illness. This interpretation is supported also by looking at the original German version of the engraving, which is accompanied by a long text under the image. Sander Gilman translates this [as follows]:

> You sick men and women: If you wish to entrust yourself to a doctor, then entrust yourself to me. I am the best healer of the human race.... If my medicine is to refresh you then you must have faith in it.... But come! We will test it in my chemical laboratory. There I have set up my Brennhelm [a dome used for distilling]. Come. Present your head and do not be afraid. We will in a short while see the mist go up in full current with the thousand-fold contents of a fool's mind—contents which I noticed so well in you! Oho! They already come up. What distilling! What things fly out! What trash was stuck in your head! ... If I make you free of this illness then proclaim that I am a master.[40]

The machine becomes more than a simple aid in the hands of the healer. It becomes an agent, able to release what is entrapped deep in the psyche. Illnesses and phantasies, the psyche and the brain, are all conflated in the images puffed from the top of the furnace. The so-called predecessor of the MRI scanner has a moralizing function implicitly at work. The comparison between this medieval "scanner" and contemporary ones becomes plausible at a metaphorical level insofar as contemporary brain imaging techniques attempt to discipline the body via the images they produce. Recent appropriations of this image have taken it as an illustration of either broad concepts related to the mind and folly or of medical instruments and procedures.[41]

The argument against a certain technocentric vision of medicine put forth by the engraving becomes, through Mallard's remediation, an endorsement of the dream of constructing diagnostic imaging technologies for healing human beings. In the historically oriented papers, though, the use of literary and visual sources that, strictly speaking, do not belong to science practice (for example, the engraving or the poem) might hint at the unintentional desire to unveil the role played by broader cultural and aesthetic elements within scientific practice and innovation trajectories. Although Mallard might have lacked the words, references, and cultural background to articulate this intuition in a more sustained manner, the recurse to images, poems, and personal memories calls for paying attention to the role played by wider cultural motifs, aesthetics, affectivity, and craftsmanship in science.

Once dug up from archives or interviews, material objects such as the bacon-slicing machine, the picture from the Middle Ages, the poem, the postcard, and the imprints of *Mark I* on the laboratory floor function as paratextual elements in relationship to the history of MRI development in Aberdeen—living traces of the role played by the psychic apparatus of memory and affect in the development of MRI. They ask the viewer to consider the impact that one's own life experiences, origins, readings, habits, and encounters exercise upon a research project, line of thinking, article, or research group devoted to the development of a new technology. Almost parasitic, such objects corrupt the idea of the independent "body" (whether the body of an article or of an argument) by making it vulnerable to their action.

These material traces contribute to knowledge construction not just inside the laboratory but also in the wider public arena. By bringing to the foreground the historical and cultural tropes embedded in ways of visualizing human beings, these material traces enable a first migration of biomedical imaging from the laboratory to the arts even before any form of artistic intervention.

Opening Up the Black Box of Data Visualization in Biomedical Imaging

Latour, known for his work in science and technology studies, uses the metaphor of the black box to describe scientific practice—conducting science is constructing and closing a black box (or black boxing). Laboratory findings and events, for example, are often black boxed and presented as facts. "[Blackboxing is] the way scientific technical and social work is made invisible by its own success. When a machine runs efficiently, when a matter of fact is settled, one need focus only on its inputs and outputs and not on its internal complexity. Thus, paradoxically, the more science and technology succeed, the more opaque and obscure they become."[42]

Through interviews, archive research, and ethnographic fieldwork in the biomedical physics laboratory at the University of Aberdeen, it is possible to explore how scientists construct and frame discourses and material practices around data visualizations when a biomedical imaging technology is still under development, when its image output and data-visualization pipeline are not yet standardized: "To follow scientists in action one needs to go from final products to production sites, from cold stable objects to warmer and unstable ones. Instead of black boxing the technical aspects of science and *then* looking for social, economic and cultural influences and biases, one should be there *before* the box closes and becomes black."[43]

All the procedures to set up a protocol for the creation of images from data, the decisions to follow one research trajectory instead of another, the interface developed to enable a user-friendly analysis of the images, are black boxed in order to allow other professionals (radiologists, clinicians) to use the scanner. These are not in the position of understanding all the different technical components of the biomedical imaging apparatus but this does not matter to them insofar as the scanner works properly. Entering the laboratory where MRI and, nowadays, fast field-cycling MRI are under development means to investigate a biomedical imaging technology, its visual culture, and ways of seeing before the black box is closed. The final visual output of MRI imaging—the body or brain scan—does not immediately reveal the highly constructed nature of the apparatus or the procedure of visualizing data. On the contrary, the technology is made invisible and black boxed in a body scan.[44]

The moments before a biomedical imaging apparatus such as an MRI scanner functions properly are gateways to the sociotechnical and scientific labor behind the technology. Once the scanner works, only the input and the output can be accessed and made available to the public, but not the inner workings of the apparatus or the decisions or conventions implemented in the visualization pipeline. To open the data-visualization black box in biomedical imaging, one needs to uncover the moments in the history of MRI invention in which decisions on how to collect, display, and interpret data took place. However, visualized data published in articles are often referred to as "milestones" in the development of a new imaging technology or as "proof-of-evidence" of an experimental hypothesis. They are hardly considered in themselves.

By the end of the 1950s, the signals from a magnetic resonance imager could provide contrasting data between normal and diseased tissues. Mallard believed, "if we could build an imager that would image those signals we would be able to 'see' the tumour."[45] Early animal work with electron magnetic resonance developed first into a program for finding the nuclear magnetic resonance of water, and then into the project of building the first clinically useful whole-body MRI scanner. The assumption was that a new technology, able to detect a difference in the signals coming from ill and normal tissues, would enable visual access to the disease. Signal detection becomes an image, and tissue-contrast differences become the disease, both materialized by the image-generating technique. The implied conceptual leap is that it is possible to move from looking at the electron spin resonance signals coming from rats (the experimental subjects) to looking at the human body in its wholeness.

Multiple biomedical imaging technologies exist simultaneously without one replacing the other. The development of MRI in Aberdeen, for example, was concomitant to the development of PET and to the use of radioactive isotopes in nuclear medicine. Radioactive isotopes contributed to the advancement of the molecularization of life, a concept that is crucial to the understanding of the human body as a composition of cells, neurons, and molecules rather than organs only (chapter 4). Rheinberger defines the molecularization of life as a "new discoursive regime [that] did not simply replace an older one but became superposed on existing layers of biophysical and biochemical terminology to form a hybrid discourse of pervasive heuristic power."[46] The visualized object is based on the molecular tracer, an instrument of intervention rather than of mere observation and description. Interestingly, the tracer and the traced object cannot exist simultaneously. For the second to appear and become visible, the first has to vanish. As Rheinberger says, "radioactive labeling exhibits the paradox of the production of traces as such … : at the very moment that the trace is produced, the marker, by decaying irrevocably, abolishes itself."[47] By disappearing, the instrument brings a new epistemic thing into the realm of the visible.[48]

Scaling Up: From the Hand-Painted Image of a Dead Mouse to a Full-Body MRI Scan

When moving to Aberdeen in 1965 to take up the chair in medical physics, Mallard brought with him technologies and techniques that he developed at Hammersmith Hospital during the early days of nuclear medicine. For example, besides the cyclotron he brought the gamma camera (also known as the scintillation camera)—the first one ever built in Europe. Both techniques in nuclear medicine helped researchers to establish the difference (in the form of contrast) between malignant and normal tissues. The cyclotron production of radioactive isotopes for medical use brought together physicists, chemists, and physicians in an interdisciplinary field. The gamma camera was particularly useful for visualizing radioactive isotopes in vivo.[49]

In 1965, Mallard's team realized that the images formed by the gamma camera could be digitized—and therefore quantified—by dividing the area of the image into small squares (today's pixels) using two crossed multichannel analyzers for each side of the pixel along the *x*- and *y*-coordinates, respectively.

This represented a huge turning point in the development of nuclear medicine imaging in Aberdeen. In 1971 Lauterbur, who was already known for his nuclear magnetic resonance (NMR) studies in the field of chemistry, became persuaded that pictures could be made: "[If] we applied a field gradient of a known shape, we could back-extrapolate against the shape of the field gradient. We can make pictures with this thing!"[50] Just a few years later, inspired by Lauterbur's remarks, Hutchison and the team put together a permanent magnet and magnetic field gradient system to try it out. This led to the first ever NMR image of a whole mouse (figure 2.5).[51]

The colorful, pop-art-like hand-painted image of the mouse with a broken neck was produced in late March 1974 and presented in April at an annual academic physics conference held at the University of Nottingham.[52] The image acquisition time was

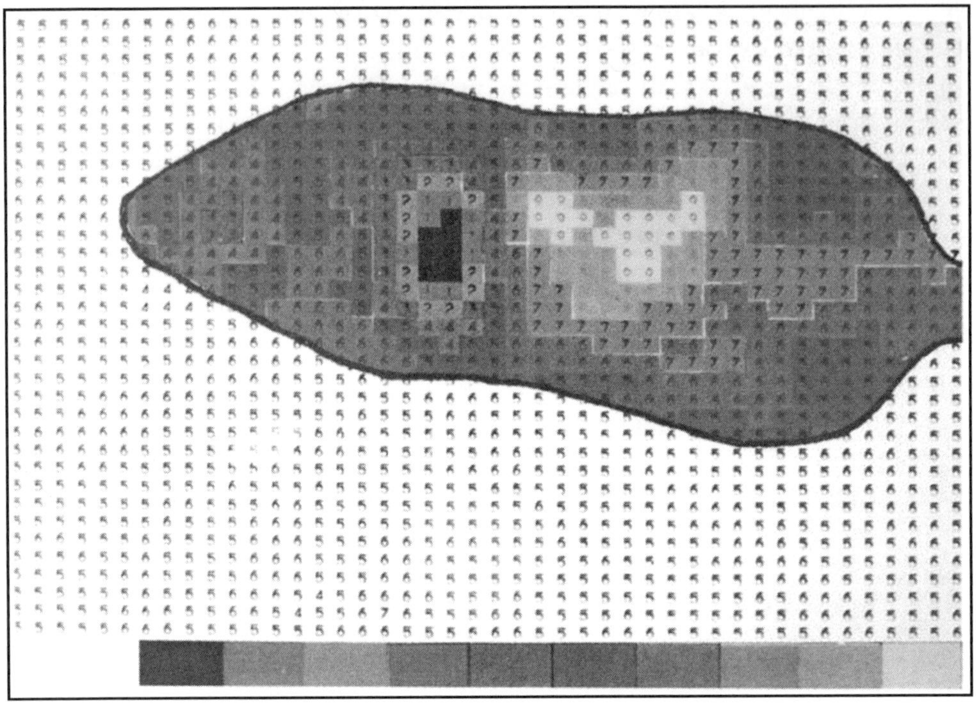

Figure 2.5
Map of mouse produced in 1974 and presented at a conference in Nottingham.
Source: Courtesy of Professor David J. Lurie, University of Aberdeen.

around one hour, during which the experimental subject had to remain completely still (and therefore had to be killed). This map, offering a dorsal view of the mouse, was acquired using twenty-five projections. The diagram accompanying the image shows the anatomical features of the mouse. The map is an example of convolution and back-projection techniques, which were deemed to be the most appropriate for NMR. The outline of the mouse, which had a broken neck as a consequence of being killed, is shown by NMR intensity signals related to the concentrations of protons in each pixel of the image. The colors represent average relaxation time (T_1)—the time it takes the tissue to return to a state of equilibrium after magnetization. The liver and brain are localized by the yellow and blue regions (longer T_1) throughout the thickness of the animal.

But the image also revealed something unforeseen—the long T_1 values around the neck fracture. Mallard commented, "To our astonishment, we saw also on the image the long T_1 values of the inflammation surrounding the fracture. The very first image had shown a sort of pathology!"[53] The long T_1 of the edema around the broken neck is imaged as the very black area. The light area, which represents the shortest T_1, coincides with the expected position of the liver. The two dark areas exhibiting a long relaxation time coincide with the expected positions of the brain and the lower neck. The white corresponds to noise regions. The two main difficulties encountered were, first, the problem of carrying out a full 3D reconstruction from 2D projections, particularly if one had to perform that on living samples; and second, the difficulty of guaranteeing a uniform magnetic field and gradients throughout the experiment.[54]

With its striking colors and series of numbers, the hand-painted image of the mouse was the world's first NMR quantitative T_1 image to show an abnormality. The image worked as a proof-of-concept visualization of biological data in terms of function rather than structure alone, and it was quickly believed that NMR would soon be in wide commercial clinical use.[55] The use of colors in the image of the mouse tunes in with the image generated by the mechanized automated scanner built by Mallard in 1957. Before biomedical imaging technologies such as MRI could be permanently placed within radiological units, the standard procedure followed by physicists was to print out both the numbers and the anatomical pictures. As Mallard remembers, "Our very first mouse image, we did actually publish it with all of the numbers and then we showed a colour version of it, converting those numbers into the different bands of colour that we decided to use. You could see an abnormality in the mouse from the colour change. You could see it in the numbers as well, but radiologists don't think that way.... Radiologists just weren't interested in the numbers. They never have been."[56]

The mouse map sits between mimesis and convention. It is realistic and artificial at the same time: pictorial yet based on measurements. The dichotomy between numbers and pictures is a thread running through the history of data visualization in biomedical physics. Brain scans, for example, are considered by physicists as "data" rather than images. Visual displays in science tend to render the object under study (whether a mouse, a cell, or a brain) in a space that is measurable and therefore quantifiable and mathematized.[57] This process of mathematization and transformation of the visualized object into numerical data is made explicit in the mouse picture that was produced at a time when powerful computers were not yet available. Nowadays, this process is inbuilt and therefore black boxed in computerized software.

The use of hand-painted strong colors (green, red, yellow) to represent the bodily interior reveals that physicists were not used to collaborating with radiologists on anatomical images.[58] Physicists did not have to look at images to produce a diagnosis. Images, however, were useful to radiologists and clinicians who ultimately could decide whether a new technology was going to be useful in clinical diagnosis. The power to attract funding so that a new technology, still in its infancy, could be transformed into a fully functioning prototype to be used for clinical trials, and ultimately commercialized, was in the hands of clinicians and radiologists.

Nuclear imaging involves encoding color or gray shade from gamma ray count rates or density. If count density modulates gray shade, it is very difficult to immediately recognize the absolute level. The coexistence of numbers and colors, anatomical details, and functional measurements was motivated by the need to appeal to diverse audiences. Physicists read the T_1 values, whereas clinicians and radiologists could look at the grayscale variations in the different anatomical regions of the mouse and "read" any abnormalities. But when bright colors were used, the stark contrast between them and the clear contours of

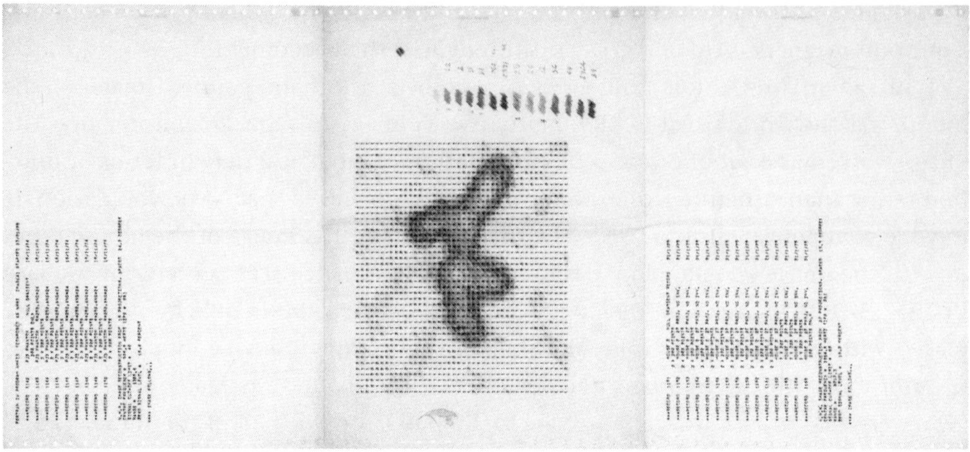

Figure 2.6
Map of mouse with color code produced in 1975.
Source: Courtesy of Professor David J. Lurie, University of Aberdeen. See plate 3.

the mouse meant even lay audiences, including potential funders, could grasp at a glance the internal structure of the body of the mouse (figure 2.6).

The color code used for displaying information in this image does not mirror in a straightforward manner the color conventions used at that time in visualization in the field of biomedical physics, or even in previous images produced by the Aberdeen team using a variety of techniques. Notably, the color scale does not normally include pink. This color was chosen to allow certain pixels to represent the experimental subject as an organic body rather than an ensemble of measurements and parameters. Usually associated with human skin, pink seems to be used here to convey the impression of an object (the mouse) in its wholeness.

The gradation has a degree of arbitrariness: it is organized by grouping yellow and orange for the liver, darker and lighter pinks for the body parts of the mouse not at the center of the physicists' and radiologists' attention (that is, the body parts that are not reproduced in the anatomical diagram), green and black for the area of the neck directly affected by the fracture, and blue and purple for both the brain of the mouse and the injured area.

The mouse is made visible and invisible simultaneously in the same diagrammatic map. The numerical data transposed into colorful pixels, paired with the sketchy anatomical diagram, convey a visual schematization that embodies yet eschews a realistic representation of the mouse. This visualization is a map that portrays hierarchical and power relationships between the types of matter composing it (including the body of the mouse, the colors, and the T_1 values). Although flattened onto a two-dimensional surface, the physiological vitality of the mouse is captured in this map in both its realism and abstraction. This image bears similarities with the representational aesthetics used in proto–Geographic Information Systems (GIS) land valuation studies that took place from the late 1950s through the 1960s.[59]

In his ethnomethodological study on the moral and epistemic relations between diagrams and photographs, science and technology studies scholar Michael Lynch examines photograph–diagram pairs in scientific texts, claiming that when the diagram is superimposed over the photograph, the authority of the document is undermined. He observes that the manually produced diagram exercises a disciplinary function upon the photograph it accompanies, taming the surplus of reality that the photograph embodies.[60] In the case of the diagrammatic map of the mouse, the diagram offers a crude schematization of the anatomy of the mouse with the purpose of guiding the reading of the image without overwhelming the viewer with colors and numbers. In this manually painted diagrammatic map, the realistic quality of the mouse exists only in the form of the outline of the diagram. The diagrammatic image of the mouse with a broken neck demonstrates how data are aesthetic-laden even before they leave the laboratory.

Both forms of display—the array of numbers and the anatomical picture of the mouse—reveal the location of abnormalities. It was radiologists' preferences that shaped the visual turn toward representing data as images, dropping not only the numbers but eventually also color in favor of adopting a gray scale. Radiologists, in fact, were used to reading and interpreting the body in black and white images since the advent of X-rays. Scientists continued to publish nuclear medicine data as both an array of numbers and an anatomical image until nuclear medicine technology was firmly placed in radiology units.[61] Since then, the data have been presented solely in image form. The decision to drop the numerical values from the image meant that the supposed immediate access to the body of the patient was masked, and additional knowledge about a patient's health would not be available.[62]

The passage from the image of the mouse to a whole-body scanner could not have occurred without other major achievements obtained by different research groups. Two were the prerequisites for building a human life-size scanner able to image patients: Damadian's work on samples of human tissues, and in the early 1970s, Lauterbur's recommendations on how to build an imager and his suggestion to put a field gradient across the patient so that the full spectrum of magnetization would become detectable.[63] There was a third contributing factor: by the time the mouse image had been created, the Aberdonian research team already had considerable experience in building scanners for nuclear medicine. They were also familiar with the difficulty of persuading clinicians of the usefulness of a new image-generating technique. Clinicians always want to make sure that whatever technology is developed, it will be clinically viable.

The picture of the mouse with the broken neck functioned as an interface, a Latourian "immutable mobile," between the two different communities of physicists and clinicians.[64] It was with this picture in his hands that Mallard gained support from clinicians and radiologists for scaling up research to build a full-body MRI scanner for clinical purposes.

One cannot understand the development of MRI without taking into consideration the other epistemic contributors besides physicists: the communities of radiologists and clinicians. The close connection between these research and clinical communities in Aberdeen provided Mallard with fertile ground on which he dared move from the mouse to a whole-body clinical MRI scanner:

> Now all the other teams were pure physicists working in pure physics departments so to them it was the physics problem that was important, to us it was the clinical problem that was important. We wanted to get it going on patients, they wanted to get it going as a physics experiment. So they all worked up from little fingers—I'm serious—little fingers to wrists, to arms to heads. Whereas we wanted to jump in at the deep end because we knew it was no good showing an image of a wrist to a consultant neurosurgeon and saying, "Look, this is going to help you find brain tumours."[65]

The visual persuasiveness of the mouse image was critical in convincing both clinicians and potential sponsors, first, of the diagnostic value of the MRI image of the mouse with the broken neck, and second, of the feasibility of scaling up the research project from imaging a mouse to building a full-body MRI scanner.

At a time when computers were not yet that powerful, the manual labor put into the image creation and display of the mouse image was part of its visual performance.[66] A color change was very obvious to the human eye. Image production, display, and interpretation were difficult in the early days of MRI as well as in nuclear medicine,

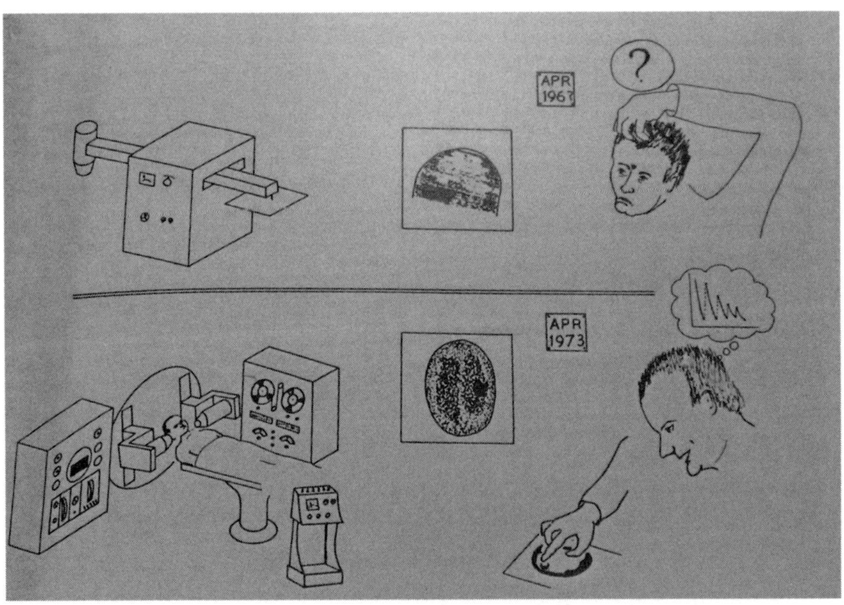

Figure 2.7
Artist (unknown), Impression of the improved diagnostic situation, 1974. Reprinted from John R. Mallard, "Radioisotope Imaging—The End of the Beginning," 26. MS3819/1/9171.
Source: Courtesy of the University of Aberdeen, Special Collections.

as shown in two radioisotope imaging diagrams, one produced in 1974 (the year the mouse image was created) and the other in 1979. The first depicts the improved diagnostic situation compared to that of the 1960s (figure 2.7).[67]

The improvement is not due to the use (or not) of color, but is the result of special views, data processing, and display optimization. Visualizing encompasses two processes: the first is viewing, which makes information visible to one's eyes; the second is seeing, which makes something visible to one's mind. Seeing involves the cognitive processes through which the onlooker transforms the received information into meaning, a mental representation of the information conveyed. This is what is expressed by the phrase "the eye and the brain of the observer," a recurring locution in many papers written by Mallard and his team.[68] The eye has to detect the change in color, and the brain has to process this so that a physicist or a radiologist can say if there is a tumor. Thus, the human eye is an important part of the imaging process.

The eye is good at detecting high spatial frequencies (fine detail and sharp edges of regions), but 1970s imaging technology captured only the low frequencies (broad contrast and shadowy regions). The problem for imaging was to avoid losing these high frequencies as much as possible. Human perception of differences in intensity is difficult to analyze due to its highly subjective nature. It was previously thought that the eye and brain determined whether a target is seen using a simple threshold model, in which the target and background intensity were compared and a difference above a certain threshold was registered. Mallard describes how the situation is actually far more complex and the observer's decision over whether a region is seen as a target must be described by overlapping probability density curves. The area under different sections of these curves corresponds to the probability of true and false positive and negative values. Perception experiments show that the observer's personality (specifically their aversion to risk) greatly affects the position of the threshold between these curves. This underlines the importance of repeating any test of an imaging system many times.

The second diagram is a representation of the radionuclide imaging process.[69] The diagram describes the radionuclide imaging process as a whole system, comprising a gamma-ray emitting radiopharmaceutical administered to the patient, a system that detects the distribution in space of gamma rays emitted from the patient, and an image of this presented to the eye and the brain of the observer by a display system. The detection system is essentially an information conversion and transfer device: each step in the process results in a loss of information, resulting in blurred and distorted images. The display renders the data transferred to it into a form that can be interpreted by the eye and brain of the observer as a recognizable pattern. If the display is poor, then information laboriously acquired by the detection system is wasted.[70] Given that the perfect imaging device does not exist, it is important to mitigate the flaws of each component of the system, whether physiological (the eye and the brain) or technological.

Both diagrams illustrate the vital role played by the eye and brain of the observer. The eye itself degrades the information and has its own response characteristics, while the brain has to reassemble this much-degraded information, recognize the pattern, relate it to known normal structures, and distinguish the abnormality. The eye and the brain are conceived of as two separate entities that collaborate to overcome the problem of subjectivity in relation to image reading and interpretation. Vision is not a passive process of secondary importance in respect to thinking. The only access to reality we have is through our senses. To perceive means to actively think.

The key role played by vision is in tune with the theory of vision proposed by the art theorist and perceptual psychologist of the same period, Rudolf Arnheim, in his texts *Art and Visual Perception: A Psychology of the Creative Eye* (1954) and *Visual Thinking* (1969).[71] Both works are heavily influenced by the principles of the Gestalt theory.[72] The eye never sees everything in front of it, but sees what is necessary. It sees only what it needs to understand where it is and what is around it. The eye makes continuous selections, focusing on constants in the environment or on its essential aspect; it makes deductions; it integrates between what appears and what is not seen; it anticipates and foresees what we will see if we turn back or move forward. The physiological act of seeing is accompanied by the brain's active interpretation of the object seen as an articulated system in its wholeness. Arnheim concludes that there is no substantial difference between thinking and seeing—the eye and the brain of the observer are both crucial for constructing knowledge. Vision is, therefore, the main form of knowledge of our culture: all of history could be rewritten through the history of vision.

In the 1960s and 1970s, research in nuclear imaging and radioisotopes focused on the problem of image production and interpretation by human perception before the advent of computerized image processing.[73] Humans are not very good at detecting contrast difference in small objects: there is a minimum detectable lesion size. The human eye also has difficulty detecting "cold spots" (as in the poem by Stephens, for instance, in the case of tumors in the liver). Furthermore, different types of imaging apparatuses tend to produce images of the same patients that suggest different diagnoses. Despite the improvements in technology and the advantage gained in using statistical rather than linear displays, research into image processing techniques (such as smoothing and filtering) have not had the desired clinical impact, and more work is needed to establish whether these methods actually improve diagnostic accuracy. This situation, which puzzled Mallard and his team since 1965, has improved thanks to the invention of the spin-warp method by Hutchison and Edelstein.

After the mouse image, the research team turned their attention to building *Mark I*. The coil was designed to carry the pulses of electric current to provide the magnetic field gradient along the *length* of the patient (from head to toe), *across* the patient (from left to right), and *through* the patient (from back to front). The subject was to be inserted horizontally between the two large middle windings into a cylinder that would have two of the gradient windings and the body radio-frequency coil. The vertical axis was designated the *y*-direction, *z* was directed along the axis of the patient, and *x* was horizontal across the patient. Water cooling plates and tubes were in place. The gradient coil form with the body radio-frequency coil were in the magnet. Although the design of the coil was important in the successful construction of *Mark I*, it was the spin-warp method that enabled the transformation of data from the scanner into images that could be read by the radiologist. *Mark I* could not count on a high-quality magnet, which is required by any MRI/NMR system, and the budget for developing the prototype obliged the research team in Aberdeen to build every single component of the scanner in-house. This meant spending a lot of time on mundane engineering tasks, such as avoiding spurious signals from AM radio stations,[74] but the technical deficiencies of the magnet prompted the team to find viable alternatives to the projection reconstruction method that was used in tomography.

Using Mallard's words: "The spin-warp technique was the real breakthrough for MRI."[75] The images obtained by 1979, before the invention of the spin-warp method, showed identifiable internal anatomy. The fault was in the line scan method used to localize the signals in the third dimension (through the patient from back to front). The spin-warp method gave for the first time an accurate distribution of the signals in the two dimensions of the transverse plane across the patient without suffering from the "noise" caused by inherent body movements. This method, which is still the gold standard for data–image conversion in MRI scanners across the globe, is applied to whole-body imaging, and fundamental mathematical relationships in the signal are readily transformed into an image. The hardware components of *Mark I*—the magnet, the gradient coils, the radio-frequency coils, the electronics, the patient support system, the data processing, and the system performance measurements—were not enough to produce artifact-free images of T_1 relaxation times from various tissues.[76]

As is evident in the images published to illustrate the workings of *Mark I*, artifacts due to the motion of organs such as the heart's beating could not be avoided. Therefore, after solving problems related to water cooling, signal quality, environmental interference, and more, Edelstein and Hutchison still had to struggle with the method of image reconstruction. The heart motion between subtractive signal acquisitions caused the vertical artifact visible in the image.[77] Edelstein recalls how he considered the opportunity of erasing the signal outside the body, which was known to be incorrect, like the signal from the body cavity. But mechanical objectivity could not be sacrificed in the name of obtaining better results. Artifacts in the image revealed the weaknesses of the scanner. Eventually, he decided not to manipulate the image: "I thought it better to leave it as is. First, that was more honest. Second, I thought of golf—if you lie now, then you have to lie every time you play in order to improve your score. If you tell the truth, then it may be easier to get better."[78]

The process of creating an image in the laboratory is a complicated affair involving many professionals. Edelstein describes the other techniques that he and Hutchison had to consider in the process of developing a new imaging method, from Lauterbur's projection reconstruction approach to Mansfield's echo-planar imaging. Edelstein had the intuition that an image could be created using the first gradient blip given the availability of different blip amplitudes for each signal acquisition. Between each blip, the frequency-encoding gradient waveform is turned on to a maximum value and then quickly turned off before the next blip. Signals are acquired between the blips.[79]

The integral under the blip produced the image information in the direction perpendicular to the projection direction. The new 2D imaging method, which was as efficient as Lauterbur's projection reconstruction approach, was developed by Richard Ernst and colleagues at ETH in Zurich.[80]

Interspersing the technical description of the milestones leading to *Mark I* and the image reconstruction method with personal memories related to his professional and family life, Edelstein recalls the "Eureka moment." Late at night on February 21, 1980, Hutchison and Edelstein took a couple of images of a bottle and then an image of Hutchison's chest. The new method was named spin-warp (as suggested) and aptly described the fact that the spin phases were twisted by the increasing blips.[81] The crucial issue was not only to obtain images with this new imaging technique but also to learn what was in the images and how to read them as Mallard highlights once more: "Could we image the liver? Could we image the kidney? We could, yes. What sort of images could we get of the brain and so on? Obviously, you've got to learn what your normal image is like before you can say, 'this is an abnormal image.' So we had to go through that stage; it took us several months."[82] Interestingly, Mallard recalls the crucial role played by the predictive drawings made earlier from laboratory measurements on animal tissue samples carried out by Margaret Foster.[83] Unfortunately, these predictive drawings are nowhere to be found.

After a period spent trying out the imaging technology on themselves to learn what was being imaged in each plane across the body, the first patient was imaged on August 26, 1980. As Mallard recalls, the image obtained revealed clinical information on a tumor metastasis in the spine.[84] From this moment, hundreds of patients were imaged. An old photograph shows the consultant in nuclear medicine Frank Smith acting as porter, carrying another patient, a contributor (with his body) to the research, from the Aberdeen Royal Infirmary to the MRI workshop (figure 2.8). The merging of the research laboratory and the hospital could not be more evident.

The patient in the photograph, an elderly man from Fraserburgh, is a visible but silent presence, surviving in the form of image data.

Building a whole-body scanner meant capturing the body in all its liveness—the heart beating, the blood pumping, vessels and lungs moving, and the patient inadvertently moving inside the scanner. This liveness, however, means artifacts are possible in the image. Without the spin-warp method, *Mark I* would have been a silent piece of technology, unable to produce a clinically useful visual output.[85] When the big companies started to produce scanners they initially referred to them as spin-warp imagers. Thanks to this method, images of good quality and clinical usefulness could be obtained from data, and problems related to movement artifacts could be solved in the post-processing of the image after data collection.

Mark I, the scanner used to image the full human body, was not the same as that used to image the mouse as figure 2.9 shows. This "benchtop" imaging apparatus was built by Hutchison using a permanent magnet at 0.06 Tesla.

It was thanks to a leap of imagination and through the results achieved in experiments conducted elsewhere, by other research groups, that clinicians were persuaded of

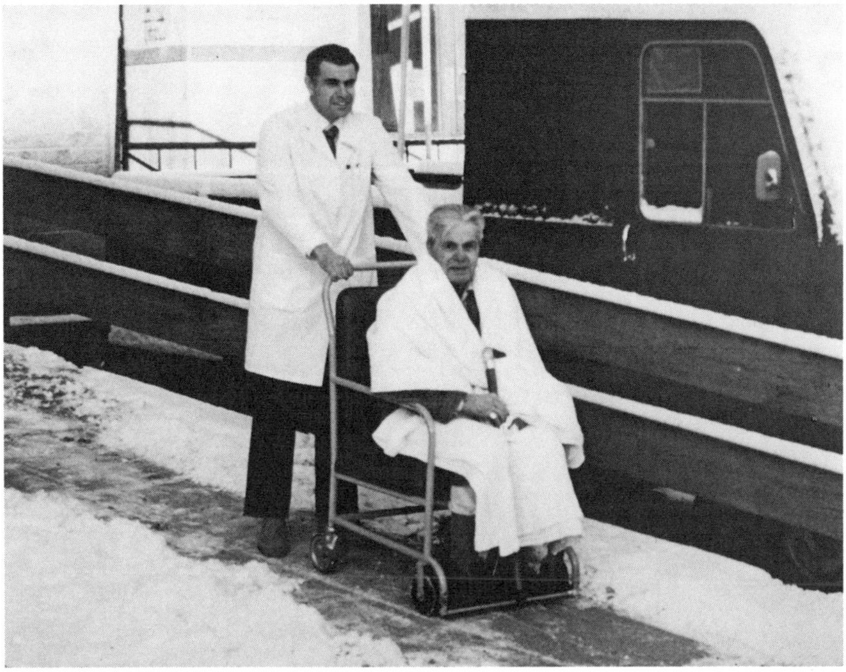

Figure 2.8
Frank Smith transporting patient, 1980.
Source: Courtesy of Professor David J. Lurie, University of Aberdeen.

the importance to scale up research and build *Mark I* in-house. Clinicians and researchers alike had to postulate that what was visualized in a mouse was going to be visualized in a human being too. Ultimately, only the value of T_1 in water protons in tissues is what connected the dead mouse with the living human body. Mallard, comparing the team's past work in nuclear medicine and MRI with current work on FFC-MRI led by David Lurie, argued that past research on MRI development was easier: "In a way our work was much simpler than what David Lurie is trying to do. I mean, the broken neck of the mouse that we imaged, that was it, it was a fact."[86] A fact is an assertion that some state of affairs or some statement is true, or some action has been done.

The mouse as "a fact," however, should be interpreted rather differently than the way Mallard interprets it. The mouse is an engendered reality—a fact that has been made, not something already given. A scientific fact is what we make real with our undertakings, not in the sense that scientific endeavor does not deal with reality but in the sense that it transforms reality.[87] The mouse was "sacrificed" (this is the terminology used by the team in describing the setting up of the experiment) because of the long exposure needed to build up an image. The mouse with a broken neck was *turned* into a fact and because of that became easy to control, transformed into a docile 2D diagrammatic picture that could be made available for scrutiny and analysis.[88] The picture of the dead mouse became the visual evidence for the feasibility and usefulness to scale up and move from imaging a mouse to imaging a full human body—a leap in scale and imagination.

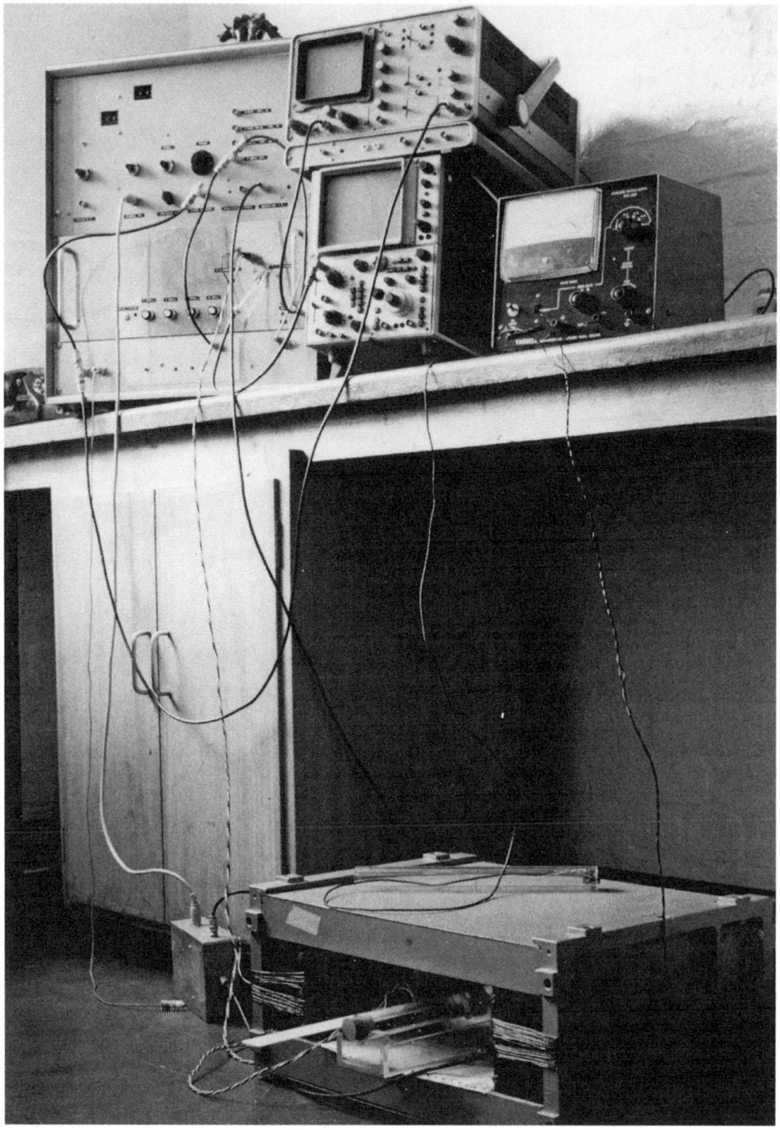

Figure 2.9
Mid-1970s NMR imaging equipment.
Source: Courtesy of Professor David J. Lurie, University of Aberdeen.

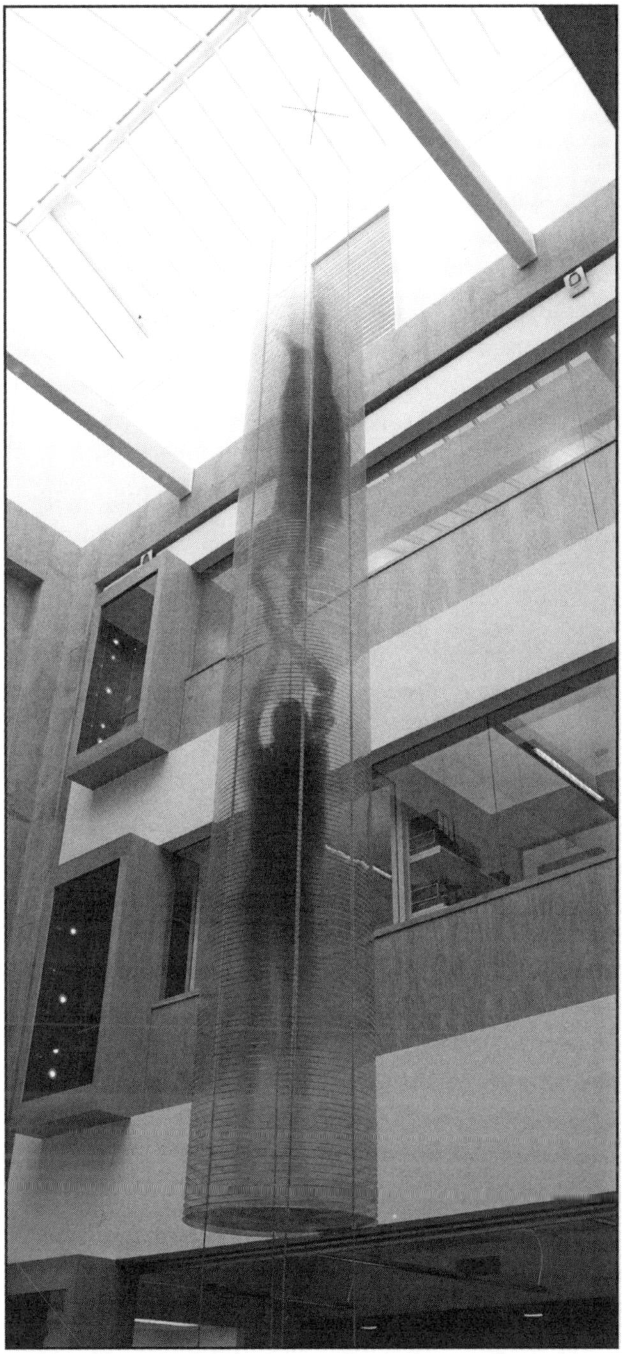

Figure 2.10
Marilène Oliver, *Doctor–Patient*. Silkscreen onto acrylic discs, 2009.
Source: Courtesy of the artist.

Hutchison's laboratory notebook contains the sketches and jotted down observations on how to scale up from the mouse image to a full-body MRI scanner.

The passage from the hand-painted image of the dead mouse with a broken neck to a full-body scan of a living human signified the passage from a 2D image with diagnostic potential to a full human body scanner that, thanks to the spin-warp method, was clinically useful. Mallard calls the history of biomedical imaging development in Aberdeen his personal "saga," as if it were a long story of heroic achievements. Here, I have recalled some of the steps and milestones that brought magnetism and medicine together for "the benefit of humankind."[89]

In the Ian Suttie Centre, a big sculpture stands in the middle inside the spiral revolving staircase: *Doctor–Patient* (2009) (figure 2.10). Made by the artist Marilène Oliver, artist and professor of printmaking and art and design, as a commission for the Centre, the art installation embodies the ideal and social impulse behind the development of a new biomedical imaging technology. Oliver has a long-standing interest in how medical imaging technologies enable us to materially contemplate our digitized selves. The installation is an MRI portrait of two digitized whole bodies, Mallard upside down, holding Suttie, the donor who financed the eponymous building. Both Mallard and Suttie had to undergo a scan in the MRI machine to obtain the head-to-toe slices.

This artwork perfectly embodies the material and visual histories of MRI invention in Aberdeen, a history in which the central position is occupied not by Mallard, but rather by the relationship between patient and doctor. From the art installation, no one can work out which figure is Mallard or Suttie, nor doctor or patient, for the bodily slices do not offer any form of personal identification. This relationship is portrayed as mutual, equal, sustained by two magnetic poles—the doctor and the patient—that cannot be conceived of one without the other.

3 Inside the Laboratory: From Signal to Coils, from Images to Bodies

> Well [smiling], an image of quality would have to be one that tells you everything, but it never does, does it? It only tells you part of the story, part of the story that can be detected. What we would really like to do is to be able to detect pre-malignancy, to be able to say "This patient is going to have trouble here," so we do something about it now before it gives trouble. But we can't do that yet, can we?
>
> —John R. Mallard, Interview, May 2017

That Obscure Object of Desire

It is a cold winter day in February 2017. I am sitting in the café area of the biomedical physics department at the University of Aberdeen, waiting to meet the physicists working on the development of a new imaging technology. The silent framed photographs hanging on the wall introduce me to the long-standing tradition and reputation of this department in the ongoing development of cutting-edge biomedical imaging technologies since the 1960s. I get up and take the stairs to reach the office where my meeting is about to start. I open the door, hesitant—I am not a physicist. Sitting around the table are seven male researchers of different ages. Each introduces himself, explaining in plain terms what he does. In turn, I introduce myself as a scholar of visual culture of science and medicine, holding a research grant awarded by the Carnegie Trust. I am interested in studying how data are visualized in the field of Scottish MRI biomedical innovation, both at the time of the construction of the world's first whole-body MRI scanner in the 1980s and with today's ongoing development of a new type of biomedical imaging technology, called fast field-cycling MRI.

A transparent cylinder wrapped in loops of conductive wire sits on the table. I know enough about MRI to recognize that this object, a coil, embodies MRI quite literally. A well-known simple description of an MRI scanner is "a coil within a coil within a coil within a coil." At its essence, an MRI scanner consists of multiple coils, each serving a different purpose, stacked or nested like a set of Russian dolls. Coils are crucial hardware components of MRI technology because they are used to create a magnetic field or to detect a changing magnetic field by the voltage induced in the wire. They are like small antennas. The perfect coil produces a uniform magnetic field without significant radiation. Different types of coils are designed and used in MRI systems for each body part. The object on the table is likely to be a volume coil for imaging the knee.

I do not ask about it, expecting someone to explain it to me at some point. Where to start when two actors do not know each other, do not speak the same language, have different educational backgrounds, and share no common history, no trading zone? The coil acted as an "immutable mobile," an object (or phenomenon) whose form and function remains stable across different contexts and places (see chapter 1).[1]

The coil became the mute, yet visible and palpable, communication through which the physicists first interacted with me, starting a silent conversation from material practice rather than from concepts. The object was never talked about in that first meeting, but as my ethnographic journey progressed, it became clear to me that different coils acted as my entry cards into the world of the biomedical physics laboratory, a material and representational practice of science in the making.

The coil, such as the one shown in figure 3.1, embodied the in-house knowledge and hands-on labor of the Aberdeen biomedical physics team. Since the times of the first prototypes of biomedical imaging techniques, scientists in Aberdeen have preferred to construct all the components of each image-generating prototype, controlling the production of each biomedical imaging technique themselves, without relying upon commercial manufacturers.

The seven physicists put on the table the visible material product of their ongoing research and history, without anticipating what I would encounter in the laboratory. They tacitly introduced themselves through the fruit of their hands-on labor. They presented themselves as makers of objects. In this laboratory physicists often *showed*

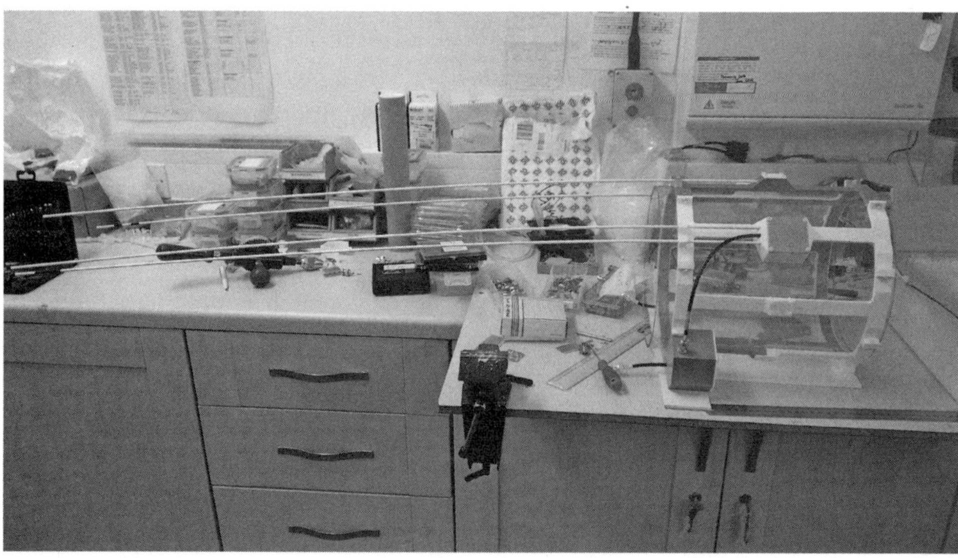

Figure 3.1
Coil printed with a 3D printer. Photograph taken during laboratory ethnography, April 2017.

me a different order of reality from what they *told* me through words. Any rhetoric on the latest achievements made by the research group is overshadowed by the materiality of science in the making: the time-consuming, iterative, painstaking everyday work to develop a new technology.[2]

Putting a coil on the table, rather than showing me a crisp, high-resolution MRI image, was a deliberate choice. Since I was there to understand more about data-visualization practices, I had assumed I would encounter graphs, diagrams, computer-generated images, models—all the visual objects that are ubiquitous in biomedical science; brain scans, with their detailed structural resolution or their brightly colored dots, are the first things encountered in popular science magazines and even in artworks that engage with this branch of physics and medicine. Yet these physicists started from a hardware component hardly recognizable by the lay public or even by patients. The coil is the interface between physicists and the body of the patient—the small physical antenna that during an MRI examination transmits a radio-frequency signal to the patient and/or receives the return signal, and transmits that data to a computer—which then generates images. No coils, no images.

MRI Development and Reinvention: Two Poles of One Experimental Trajectory

Technological innovation is commonly conceived of as a process that anticipates the future, driven by a vision of what might or should be. The emphasis is on progress. Contrary to the idea that imaging the future is the cipher of scientific practice, Rheinberger claims that science is "a process driven from behind," a concept he borrows from Thomas Kuhn.[3] Any scientific endeavor is performed with an overall goal, with specific objectives and anticipated outcomes in mind. However, the outcome, Rheinberger argues, is often something one could never approach directly, being the product of several steps forward and backward, of experimental breakthroughs and obstructions, rather than linear progress: "In order to remain productive, experimental systems must be designed and conducted in such a way that the creation of differences becomes the reproductive driving force of the whole machinery: thus they are to be addressed as veritable *difference machines*."[4]

The experimental system is an apparatus comprising techniques, inscription devices, shared tacit knowledge, and labor. It is a machine that produces variations, alterations, mismatches, repetitions. The truth, power, and vitality of the experimental system bears upon the nonalignment between the original intention of the experimenter and the product of research. An experimental system therefore thrives on uncertainty and surprise.

The history of MRI is not linear, as it stretches across places (research centers in the UK, the US, and Asia) and across times—from its invention and development in the 1970s and 1980s to today. At present, in the same laboratory where Mallard, Hutchison, and Edelstein made the first steps in biomedical imaging at the University of Aberdeen, researchers are working on the development of FFC-MRI, an emerging, noninvasive, low-cost biomedical imaging technique that enables the visualization of biochemical information at a scale not detectable by conventional MRI. These two periods in MRI—development, and then reinvention—are the distinct poles of the same experimental trajectory. The internal coherence of these two overlapping communities of invention working respectively on MRI and FFC-MRI in Aberdeen is a function of the in-house know-how of a research group that builds highly advanced biomedical imaging devices without relying too heavily on external manufacturers.[5]

In this chapter, I explore the features and limits of data visualization in FFC-MRI. I rely on the extensive fieldwork I undertook in the biomedical physics laboratory in Aberdeen and on semistructured interviews with researchers (physicists, clinicians, biomolecular chemists, neuroscientists, and a radiologist) involved in the development of FFC-MRI across different research centers.[6] I argue that the construction and then the black boxing of the data-visualization pipeline influence the relationship and exchange between data, technologies, the clinician, and the patient's body. Unveiling both the configuration and limits of data visualization in the field of biomedical research can be done by examining how a specific visualization pipeline and protocol are concretely constructed in the laboratory while a technology is still under development.

Fast Field-Cycling: Reinventing MRI

The attention to the patient's body is a driving force behind all biomedical imaging technologies developed by the Aberdonian research group and continues long after the construction of *Mark I* (the world's first whole-body MRI scanner, discussed in chapter 2). Its successor, *Mark II* (1982), was used to scan more thousands of patients across ten years, thus enabling the collection of a huge amount of patient data. This achievement was not enough to keep Mallard and his group within the market. Despite efforts to keep the research and design of MRI scanners in-house with Mallard's founding of a British manufacturing company, M&D Technology, this research group, which was at the forefront of MRI development until 1981, could not compete anymore. MRI research shifted to high-field-strength machines, and industrial production of MRI scanners moved outside the UK.[7] The awareness of not being able to compete with high-field MRI in the global market might explain why this research group decided to explore the properties of magnetism at low field as early as the 1980s. Rheinberger explains:

> Usually, a scientific object disappears from the scene because people lose interest in it, without another epistemic object replacing it in the strict meaning of the word. The loss of interest can—sometimes at least—be due to the fact that the object of concern reveals itself to be phantasmal. In the majority of the cases, however, it simply becomes marginalized and is being dropped because it ceases to keep the promise that it seemed to offer, without being shown either not to exist or to lead on a wrong track.[8]

A technological object (for example, MRI technology) can be abandoned and then replaced by another that is either more efficient, more convenient, or more precise for bringing a certain phenomenon into sight. Conversely, a scientific object like low-field magnetism disappears because it could not make good on the promise that magnetism brought: the possibility of creating high-resolution images of the inner workings of the body. This was the promise of MRI at high field.

Investment efforts therefore were channeled for research and technological development in high-field magnetism with the construction of increasingly powerful scanners. Historically, with each step increase in magnetic field strength, there has been a gain in sensitivity, contrast, and improved spatial resolution. Exquisite visualizations of structure, biomolecular activity, and function can now be obtained. The possibility of obtaining clear, high-contrast images of various organs, including the brain, contributed to the race toward ultra-high-field MRI. That aesthetic values play a role in data visualization was already clear at the time of Mallard's team. High-field-strength scanners create visualizations of the body that are crisp, detailed, and *beautiful*, to recall the word used by a theoretical physicist and a molecular chemist working in Olsztyn and Turin that I interviewed in the course of my fieldwork. The price to pay for such visualizations was a loss of the range of metabolic information that low-field magnetism provides. In order to access those beautiful scans, one had to choose to be blind to the other properties of magnetism.

An Unexplored Research Trajectory

In the 1980s, Aberdeen was active in free-radical imaging research. Free radicals are reactive molecules that can be found in the body as part of the normal metabolism and whose concentration can change in the presence of a disease. David Lurie (at that time under the guidance of Jim Hutchison and his wife, the biologist Meg Foster) and his team developed a method called proton–electron double resonance imaging (PEDRI). In 1987, Lurie and the team proved that PEDRI could be used to image the distribution of free radicals in bottles and in small animals, despite technical problems related to things heating up because the object was exposed to microwaves ("So there was a danger of cooking the thing you were imaging," Lurie explained bluntly).[9] The solution to that problem was achieved in collaboration with Hutchison, and consisted of a method called *field cycling*. Using field-cycle PEDRI, it became possible to image free radicals without overheating the subject—bottle or animal. It was this technology that would pave the way to FFC.[10]

FFC-MRI as a technical object could not appear until its scientific object (low-field magnetism) became visible again after decades of obscurity. Hence, FFC-MRI represents a thread of MRI that was left unexplored. Today, to find out more about FFC-MRI, researchers must refer to papers from as far back as the 1980s. In recent years, drawing upon their 1980s work on free radicals, physicists in Aberdeen have taken the decision to open up one of the black boxes of MRI by contradicting one of the fundamental laws of MRI: that the magnetic field has to be kept constant during image acquisition. This decision paved the way to that unexplored MRI research trajectory.

The Aberdeen group has developed two whole-body FFC-MRI scanners: the one with a range of 0.02–200 mT (figure 3.2) is now used in a variety of clinical trials from breast carcinoma to strokes and Alzheimer's disease.

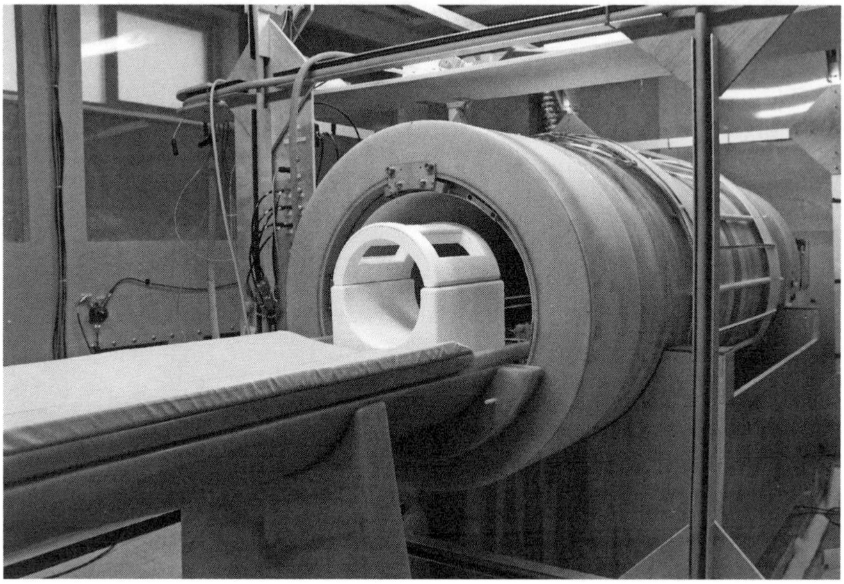

Figure 3.2
FFC-MRI prototype.
Source: Courtesy of University of Aberdeen.

FFC-MRI is a major shift in MRI technology. In conventional MRI, contrast is often derived from differences in the spin-lattice relaxation time constant, T_1, in different tissues. As shown in figure 3.3, diseased tissue often exhibits markedly different T_1 values compared to healthy tissue. In addition to differences in the values of T_1, it has been shown that the variation of T_1 with magnetic field—known as T_1 dispersion—varies between healthy and abnormal tissue.[11] By looking at T_1 dispersion it may be possible to detect disease sooner than would be otherwise possible.

Physicists tend to start from the signal and the coil to explain MRI. But water, which is the fundamental property in conventional MRI, is also the bridge connecting experimental and theoretical physicists, chemists, biologists, mathematicians, and clinicians working on FFC-MRI. All these researchers study the intensity of the water signal and how it depends on the relaxation of protons. In a biological system, water interacts with macromolecules showing a shorter relaxation time (T_1). When paramagnetic compounds are added, water interacts with them and the T_1 varies in relation to the applied magnetic field.[12] Since the earliest days of nuclear magnetic resonance (NMR) it has been clear that relaxation mechanisms would play an important role in all its applications. Seymour Koenig—physicist, anthropologist, and art historian; "a Renaissance man," as his obituary recites[13]—pioneered field-cycling relaxation as a technique to obtain information on both molecular structure and dynamics: "Relaxometry is a relatively new word for a long-established activity: measurement of the magnetic relaxation rates of solvent nuclei in aqueous systems to explore the nature of the solute entities."[14]

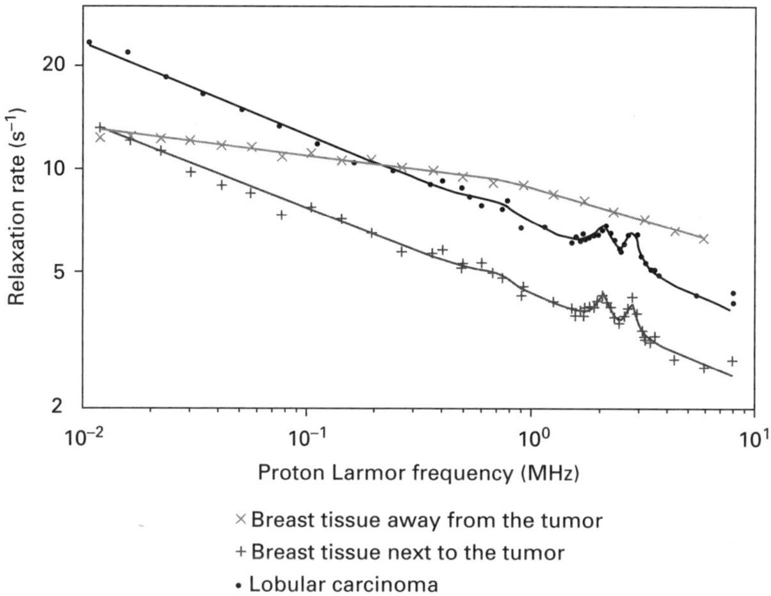

Figure 3.3

Dr. Lionel Broche, Comparison of dispersion curves from tissue samples of breast tissues, fibrous tissue, and breast cancer (from the same patient). The *x*-coordinate expresses the magnetic field strength; the *y*-coordinate, the T_1 value. The samples were obtained from surgery and fixed in formaldehyde (ethical approval given by the North of Scotland Research Ethics Committee). The curve profile changes dramatically between breast tissues and tumor.
Source: Courtesy of University of Aberdeen.

In fact, even the first detection of an NMR signal was delayed by several years because the chosen compounds had excessively long relaxation times. The most pronounced relaxation phenomena (in terms of field dependence) were to be expected at relatively low fields where low-frequency molecular motions can have a very large impact on T_1. The dependence of T_1 (B) on the field B was soon nicknamed the T_1 dispersion curve or, more recently, the nuclear magnetic relaxation dispersion (NMRD) profile. The first experimental curve of this type was published in 1950 by Ramsey and Pound.[15] In New York in the late 1970s, chemist Paul Lauterbur recognized the importance of paramagnetic ions in changing contrast in a biological tissue.

Reinvention

FFC-MRI is an emerging, noninvasive, low-cost biomedical imaging technique that breaks a fundamental law of MRI—that the applied magnetic field must be held constant during image acquisition. Unlike conventional MRI techniques, FFC-MRI uses a variable magnetic observation field, ranging from high values to very low values (weaker than the geomagnetic field). A single FFC-MRI scan obtains information comparable to one hundred MRI scan sessions; if one could line up one hundred high-field MRI scanners, only then would one get the information visualized in FFC. Rapid changes in magnetic field strength are at the crux of this technology (hence "*fast* field-cycling"), providing image quality that reveals a vast amount of new medical information.

FFC-MRI can be used to differentiate tissues that appear similar on conventional MRI devices thanks, first, to the greater endogenous contrast present at lower magnetic fields and, second, to patterns that emerge from the overall relaxation dispersion curves (T_1) of these tissues. FFC-MRI is the only method allowing the determination of the spin-lattice relaxation time constant ($1/T_1$) over a range of magnetic fields using one instrument only. There is no need to adjust the radio-frequency coil amplifier or to tune the probe at each frequency/magnetic field strength, as would be required if using a conventional MRI magnet system. Fixed-field magnet systems are not able to measure nuclear spin relaxation down to low magnetic field strengths due to sensitivity limits: the NMR signal-to-noise ratio decreases with the intensity of the magnetic field.

The main difference with MRI is that any conventional MRI system can only provide information about the sample's relaxation times at one (fixed) magnetic field. In FFC-MRI, field strength is switched rapidly during the collection of an image, then returned to a fixed magnetic field to read out the NMR signals. By obtaining FFC-MR images at a range of switched fields, it is possible to optimize the endogenous contrast contained in the variation of relaxation times with magnetic field strength—something that is completely hidden from conventional MRI, no matter the field strength.

Another contrast mechanism that is accessible to FFC-MRI but not standard MRI is an effect called the quadrupole dip, which provides quantitative information related specifically to protein concentration and dynamics. The ubiquity of proteins in the body and their role in disease makes the latter particularly attractive. FFC-MRI also offers radically new possibilities for exogenous contrast, via injected contrast agents precisely tailored to the new FFC-MRI instruments. These agents improve sensitivity and specificity by at least an order of magnitude compared to conventional contrast-enhanced MRI. This will enable the development of molecular imaging applications.[16]

MRI and FFC-NMR are both well-known and established methods. The combination of these techniques in FFC-MRI, however, is much newer and currently limited to a handful of research laboratories across the world. FFC-MRI aims to explore how relaxation rates change with magnetic field strength, an idea that has been successfully exploited in NMR for more than half a century and which is known to provide unique structural information on materials, noninvasively. In the 1970s, there was no commercial technology available that would allow acquisition of the relaxation value in relation to the magnetic field, but the research contributions by Seymour Koenig's group from IBM were known. As I mentioned earlier, Koenig contributed crucially to the development of a technology able to conduct these measurements in a variable magnetic field.[17] The information on relaxation times could be used to extract information on contrast agents or to create images at different field strengths, as the Aberdonian group does. These two approaches have always been in dialogue.

The applications of this emerging technology cover many areas, from materials to food science and geology. But FFC is particularly useful in biomedicine and especially in pharmaceutical and health care applications, where it has been used to study the conformational properties of aqueous solutions (formulations) and protein dynamics. Perhaps most important is its use in studies for the development of contrast agents for clinical MRI. With FFC-MRI, physicists are attempting to develop a new imaging technology for detecting biomolecular changes in strokes, several types of cancer, and early stage neurodegenerative conditions, potentially contributing to future clinical and research brain imaging standards.

The research project Improving Diagnosis by Fast Field-Cycling MRI (IDentIFY), funded through the EU Horizon 2020 program and coordinated by PEDRI developer David Lurie, involves partners from nine sites across Europe, led by the University of Aberdeen.[18] Although I focus on the work done by the research team in Aberdeen, which comprises mostly physicists, as well as a radiologist, a neuroscientist, and a clinician, I have also conducted interviews with other teams, particularly those in Turin (specializing in biotechnology and molecular imaging), Grenoble (health and medical sciences), and Olsztyn (theoretical physics and mathematical modeling), whose work directly influences the development of FFC-MRI in Aberdeen.

The objective of the IDentIFY project is to bring FFC-MRI to the stage where it can be used as a routine tool for clinical diagnosis. The main project packages cover four main areas: theory, technical aspects, contrast agents, and clinical applications. Particularly challenging is the theoretical framework needed to describe and understand the new biomarkers to which FFC-MRI gives access. Why does one see certain changes in the behavior of water in the molecules of diseased tissues? The challenge is to understand what it is that one observes, given that the theory of relaxation in tissue at ultralow field strengths, leading to models and biomarkers, is still underdeveloped. This challenge, led by the team of physicists in the Computer Science and Mathematics Department at the University of Warmia and Mazury in Olsztyn, Poland, is particularly difficult because FFC is a niche area requiring a high degree of specialization.

The second research area—technical aspects—led by Aberdeen chiefly aims to create and improve technology to enable FFC use at low and ultralow field strengths. The third—contrast agents for FFC—aims to increase sensitivity and ultimately allow molecular imaging. In the department of molecular biotechnologies at the University of Turin, organic and inorganic chemists conduct experiments in living mice using a relaxometer with a specially modified magnet to enable researchers to visualize a small living animal (like a mouse) rather than just solutions or tissue parts.[19] Finally, the clinical aspect, which is the focus of the French Institute of Health and Medical Research in Grenoble, is aimed at extending the range of clinical applications of FFC, with an emphasis on the brain, relying on the FFC-MRI tests conducted on tissue samples and in patients.

In science, visualizing something makes it real. Looking at FFC-MRI from the perspective of chemistry/biology rather than physics alone, one can say that FFC-MRI visualizes the dynamics of water molecules in a biological system. Water is found throughout the body—in cells, in the extracellular space, in the cerebrospinal fluid, and in joints and cavities. Yet the visualization is not of the cell itself but of thousands of different cells, profiles, vessels: water entering and leaving in different ways and at various speeds. Therefore, the time the water stays inside a cell can indicate health or disease or be a biomarker of, say, the aggressiveness of a tumor. What gets visualized then is an average of water movement.

Researchers therefore are not looking at the disease per se, but at water and its interactions with proteins. The challenge is to understand what this means in terms of present and/or future pathology. Technology looks only at a circumscribed aspect of the phenomenon under investigation, not at everything. Some technologies address the molecular level (for example, genes, proteins, and their interactions), but there are as yet no techniques for looking at the level of structure, scaffolding, or interaction at the *microscopic* scale. Biologists tend to think in terms of protein interactions and cellular level, but it is the world in between that can be explored by FFC-MRI.

The type of visual output obtained with an emerging technology is not merely a question of aesthetics nor is it just related to the epistemic function of the image, the knowledge that the image constructs and makes available. The visual output also has implications for the commercialization of an emerging technology. The colorful MRI image from 1974 of the mouse with a broken neck, displaying T_1 values, was crucial in convincing donors of the importance of scaling up research to construct a full-body scanner. Similarly, the visual output of FFC-MRI will influence the way in which this emerging technology is communicated to and accepted by the scientific and clinical communities. It is radiologists and clinicians first who need to be convinced of the feasibility of introducing this new imaging technology in routine clinical practice.

From Signal to Coil

A typical day in the FFC-MRI biomedical physics laboratory starts with physicists working around the hardware and software code components of the scanner to make sure that the signal is present and of good quality (see figure 3.4).

Signal-to-noise ratio is the most crucial parameter in any MRI-based scanner: "Fingers crossed it will work," "Good, I've got a signal," "The signal's miserable today, there might be a problem at the software level," "Are you magnetic? [referring to me, because every time I come to the laboratory the scanner does not seem to work properly]" say the physicists, with a degree of fatalism and irony. Physicists recalibrate the FFC-MRI parameters on a daily basis, because the scanner needs to be retuned every time. Even when the signal looks good to the human eye, the computer does not fall into the trap of thinking that the signal is useful. A good signal is one that shows a certain pattern: spatial information with a clear peak.

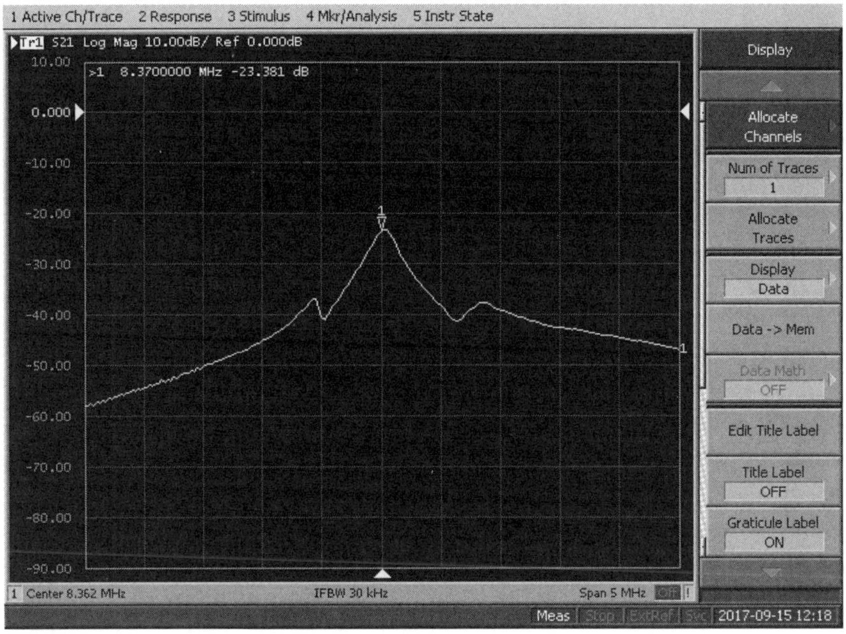

Figure 3.4
Signal quality. Photograph taken during laboratory ethnography, March 2017.

The rotating frame of reference—the position from which the magnetic field is observed—needs to be right, with no oscillation (when there is oscillation, it means that the magnet and the coil are not aligned) and with the same frequency as the magnet.

One young postdoctoral physicist in particular is always ready to satisfy my curiosity and keen on finding everyday metaphors to illuminate obscure concepts while I observe him at work in the laboratory. For instance, he explains to me: "If you're very off-resonance you don't get any signal, or your images shift in every direction. You need to know the frequency to get a good image. These"—he gestures to the shims, the devices used to ensure the homogeneity of the magnetic field—"should all start dancing."[20]

The coil receives the signal and then researchers need to encode spatial information into the sequence of the scan to be able to produce an image. The spin-warp method is the technique used to encode spatial information in two dimensions to then enable conversion of the signal into an image. The same researcher explains to me that filtered back-projection was the method used before spin-warp for encoding spatial information in one dimension. He praises the new method, highlighting advantages by means of adjectives that belong to the realm of aesthetic appreciation: "The beauty and elegance of this simple mathematical relation is the way in which the signal comes already prepared for transformation into an image. With the filtered back-projection, one has to throw away more information [filter], and artifacts are more likely. With spin-warp, maybe you don't acquire as much information, but at least you don't have to throw away what you acquire."[21]

The spatial frequencies in the MR image are contained in *k*-space; this abstract concept is usually represented as a matrix and is the first visual output combining all the signals that come out of the scanner. *k*-Space data are then mathematically transformed to generate the final image. A bad signal leaves its trace in the image: if just one pixel in the *k*-space matrix is bad, then all the pixels in the final image will be bad. Every signal measurement tells you something about the entire image.[22] Although the *k*-space cannot be used for clinical diagnosis, one can use it to diagnose whether there are any problems in the scanner at the level of hardware. Adjusting the signal is therefore a crucial part of the protocol that the physicists use to make the prototype FFC-MRI scanner stable enough to begin imaging patients.

All data are handled via a software interface used for signal and image processing. MATLAB, the matrix-based language used to express computational mathematics, makes data visualization possible—it is the middleman that makes everything work. As a programming language, however, MATLAB is not ideal in terms of its graphical interface. The chosen interface is a crucial component in the data-visualization pipeline because radiologists need an efficient workstation to convert data into standard formats and images, make annotations, and combine and compare all the variables.

For theoretical physicists, data are the fundamental units of research. The data and experimental setting must be organized into a pipeline that can be controlled so that a certain amount of knowledge is produced. Far from being static and raw, data—not hypotheses—are the true drivers of research. In the development of FFC-MRI, even data collected from the early work on free radicals in small samples of animal tissues contributed the basis for working at low-field magnetism. Data acquired during the setup and testing of the data-visualization protocol, the scanner prototype, or an experiment and data acquired during clinical trials constitute the in-between stage from traces to facts. Once the first experimental data are obtained, an equation is used to fit a straight or curved line as closely as possible to the data—this equation is the model. The model is put to the test with new experimental data; if the model deviates too far from these new data, a better model must be found.

Data are more important than facts in applied science. Rheinberger discussed the passage from traces to data in the age of molecular biology and spoke of a primacy of data over both traces and facts: "Data are there. They have become the primary entities that populate our infra-worlds of knowledge. The facts have to be made more than ever."[23] If facts are made, then they are more precarious than one is prone to believe. Data and their patterns—maps, curves, visualizations, and the like—have primacy over facts insofar as data can be stored, consulted, retrieved, and mobilized. Data are not the by-products of scientific research; rather, together with the instruments used to produce, visualize, store, and display data, they contribute to shape the phenomenon under investigation, to direct the observation in experimental practice, and to guide the interpretation of the data.[24]

Knowledge does not necessarily take the form of concepts or theories. It can be embodied in instruments, protocols, or images. This foundational knowledge is part of the attempt to reduce complexity to control the variables and parameters required to set up an image-creation protocol. In data visualization, the focus is always on a fragment of reality (whether a tissue, area of a certain organ, or behavior of a molecule) or on different fragments that are first isolated and then rearranged so that a novel configuration might offer the answer to a problem.

Manufacture and Bricolage

The development of a new biomedical imaging technique and its visualization pipeline is a skilled practice informed by action—by the hands bringing an image into existence—rather than just by abstract representation or by the transmission of information and rules. In Aberdeen, physicists in the biomedical physics and bioengineering department control every single phase of the construction of biomedical imaging systems. This peculiarity, which took root in the late 1960s at the time of Mallard and his research team, is still a feature of Aberdeen, which remains one of very few research groups working on MRI across the world that is able to develop a scanner from scratch. In the laboratory workshop, the first thing one encounters is not the prototype of the new FFC-MRI scanner, but its minor yet crucial components: the coils. The first step toward an image that can be diagnostically valuable is to make sure that the signal-to-noise ratio is good. The coils are an integral part of this. The geometry of overlapping in coils is essential. Two loops cannot talk to one another: the coils are independent, each picking up signal from the local environment, but each coil must not pick up too much noise. This is a prerequisite for obtaining a pure signal.

A research fellow in the group showed me an old photograph of himself working on the design and development of coils in 1988. Sitting in his office full of posters and photographs of a past golden age in which he was at the pinnacle of his research productivity, this physicist describes himself as a craftsman: "I'm the artisan. I'm the cobbler holding shoes. I've made a wide range of things. I've built [radio-frequency] coils, I've built grading coils, coils for [continuous wave] MRI systems. That big cubic coil array round the point-two tesla [pointing at a photograph on the wall], I built that."[25]

Bricolage is a crucial component of any scientific innovation. The messy environment of the workshop, with tools, wires, cables everywhere, and researchers bent over the table, busy in the construction of coils for different body parts, convey the idea that invention does not necessarily occur in the *minds* of the scientists but much more in their hands, "in the experimental system they create, at the bench," as Rheinberger said.[26]

The skill and know-how required to construct the technology for detecting, collecting, and displaying data, and the related protocols for handling them, is a form of embodied knowledge. What Leonelli says in relation to biology is valid for physics too:

> Embodied knowledge is expressed ... through the procedures and protocols that allow scientists to intervene in the entities and processes of interest; the ability to implement those procedures and modify them according to the specific context of research; the skills involved in handling instruments, models, and organic samples; the perception, often based on the scientists' experience in interacting within a specific space (such as a laboratory), of how to move and position oneself with respect to the models and materials under study; and the development of methods to facilitate the replication of experimental results.[27]

No experiment would be materially possible without embodied knowledge.

The "do-it-yourself" attitude is both a virtue and a necessity for the Aberdonian research group. There are only five scientific groups in the world working on FFC-MRI development. Big manufacturing companies are not keen on very risky projects like FFC-MRI, preferring to invest a lot in higher-field magnetism because that is what clinicians are pushing for. This makes even more urgent the creation of a worldwide community of researchers working on FFC-MRI. The skills that are necessary to build MRI scanners are very difficult to find. With a glint in his eyes, this researcher expresses his hope to push the field-cycling community toward open-source hardware called OSI.[2] The open-source model and community-driven platform would enable scientists across the world, especially in developing countries, to build their own scanners without relying on manufacturers.[28]

All the physicists I interviewed in the course of my fieldwork pointed out that FFC-MRI is a *new* technology, rather than a straightforward development of MRI. FFC enables the visualization of the dynamics of water molecules in diseased tissues, thus being part of the framework of investigation on the chemical and functional properties and dynamics made possible by imaging technologies such as fMRI and PET. For this reason, the name FFC-MRI might be provisional, with the "MRI" part dropped in the near future to better highlight the uniqueness of this technique and to sell it more convincingly to potential investors. The embryonic FFC-MRI scientific community has a crucial role in persuading clinicians to implement their new biomedical imaging technology, whose visual output, clinical application potential, and even the uncertainty of its name define it as an emerging technology.

Joyce correctly pointed out that decisions about machine design in the early days of MRI were shaped by decisions about how to best visualize data;[29] the same is true today. The coils are the hardware components closest to the body of the patient. They are the bridge between the signal, the patient's body, and the researcher. The coil must be as close as possible to the anatomical part that is to be imaged.

Like the coil, the bed—or couch—is another crucial hardware component of the scanner and forces researchers to bear in mind the patient's body while they are developing the scanner prototype. For the construction of *Mark I*, Eddie Stevenson had to design and build a patient-friendly couch. The couch for the FFC-MRI prototype is even more important because there are no commercially available couches for low-field MRI: "First of all, just the visual aspect of the scanner. It's very striking to see people come into the room and say, 'Wow, I wouldn't like to go in there,' [laughing] because it looks tiny, homemade, and uninviting. And I know that MRI companies put a lot of effort into the design and appearance of the system and so on. So, I'm sure there will be a lot of things to do, just for the visual aspect of the machine itself."[30]

The ideology of the "normal" average body influences the design of key scanner components. Soon after starting to image volunteers, the physicists realize that the couch they 3D printed is too narrow for imaging people with large bodies. The couch needs to be redesigned to avoid it becoming an object that discriminates volunteers based on their body size.[31] Gender also plays a role. I experienced this after being asked to try the bed of the scanner before physicists and clinicians started conducting trials on breast cancer. For the first time, I was given a voice in the laboratory: I was being asked to articulate my needs and bodily experience *as a woman*, not just as a potential patient.

In the laboratory, physicists tend to focus on the single components of the machinic assemblage rather than on the machine as a whole. For instance, attention is devoted to the single coils or the amplifiers that are crucial components of every biomedical imaging technology or on the individual parameters that need to be controlled and calibrated to obtain meaningful visual output. There is a stage in which the ensemble of the scanner prototype and its various hardware and software components, including the visualization pipeline, reaches a configuration stable enough to allow researchers to interact with the machine rather than with its single components. At this moment, the scanner starts being interpellated as a thing in the laboratory endowed with an internal animating principle, rather than as an inert passive object.[32]

This turning point from the passivity of the technical components to the scanner as something with agency is present in both the invention and the reinvention of MRI and is closely related to the attention given to the patient during the scanner's development. For example, *Mark I* started to be treated as an ensemble even before the scanner was constructed—more precisely, when the possibility was envisaged of scaling up from the mouse scanner to a whole human MRI scanner. The scanner already existed *in potentia*, in the minds of researchers. The second turning point occurred with the invention of the spin-warp method, which enabled the production of clinically readable images, thus shortening the time required for a scan when imaging patients. With FFC-MRI there are again two main turning points, as I witnessed firsthand in the laboratory: first, the moment at which the first image counts as a proof of concept; and second, the moment when patients start to be imaged. These two moments are closely related.

Proof of Concept

Creating an image that can work as a proof of concept is not as straightforward as one might think. The labor required to collect, clean, store, and analyze data and then turn the data into visual output is enormous. Researchers test and discard various techniques and options to speed up the image acquisition process, improve the clarity of the signal, or build better hardware and software components crucial to the process of turning data into a diagnostically valuable image. A proof-of-concept image is possible only once the protocol is clearly set out to make the scanner stable enough that a readable image can be obtained and the patient can be scanned.

The philosopher of information Luciano Floridi argues that the primary objective of any communication system is to transfer messages from a source to a destination as accurately and quickly as possible.[33] However, like any communication system, visualization pipelines are subject to errors and noise. For instance, until physicists were able to solve magnet shimming and insufficient signal quality, they would obtain images with "zebra artifacts" (alternating dark and bright bands) or of very poor quality. Although the zebra artifact can be removed in post-processing, the quality of the image still suffers.

One day, after months of daily struggles in the Aberdeen laboratory around the scanner prototype, one of the physicists was able to show me what they called a proof-of-concept image.

"I expect I will be asked 'what for?'" he said, referring to the reluctance of the medical community to accept that further development is needed. "Why should we care about FFC-MRI, given that we have high-resolution MRI? I will then show this image at an international conference on MRI to prove that this scanner works."[34] The image, a T_1 map of bottles containing different concentrations of a salt solution, proves that the prototype they built is able to measure the T_1 parameter. It is generated from five separate images previously created and labeled "bottles1," "bottles2," and so on. These are the actual images from the scanner that show how the signal varies. Figure 3.5 gives a visual representation of the variation of T_1 between the different bottles. The bottles are arranged in order of concentration, with the most concentrated at the bottom and the least concentrated at the top. Except for the top three bottles, which contain pure water, each bottle contains an aqueous solution of manganese chloride (a salt). The value of T_1 depends on the amount of salt in the water, with higher salt concentrations having the lowest T_1 values.

In tune with the use of color in Mallard's era, here too color speeds the transmission of information to the onlooker and reduces the cognitive effort required to understand the image. The gradation of yellow in figure 3.5 is a clue to the change in signal between each bottle, as a number is assigned to each brightness level (for example, 0 for pure black, 2 for pure white). Color also plays a communicative and rhetorical role. Much like when Mallard showed off the colorful image of the mouse to radiologists and potential funders to convince them to scale up to imaging a whole human body, the first proof-of-concept FFC-MRI image must convince colleagues working on high-field MRI of the possibility of obtaining useful images working at low field strengths.

The physicist, not the radiologist, validates the image as a proof of concept. Dummy objects used to calibrate scanners, like the bottles used in this experiment, are known as "phantoms." The term has been adopted in the medical world to mean any test object that mimics the human body in some way. Very much like coils, phantoms are also three-dimensional models, and like images, models belong to a network of production, interpretation, and communication: they can be abstract or concrete, physical, or symbolic.[35]

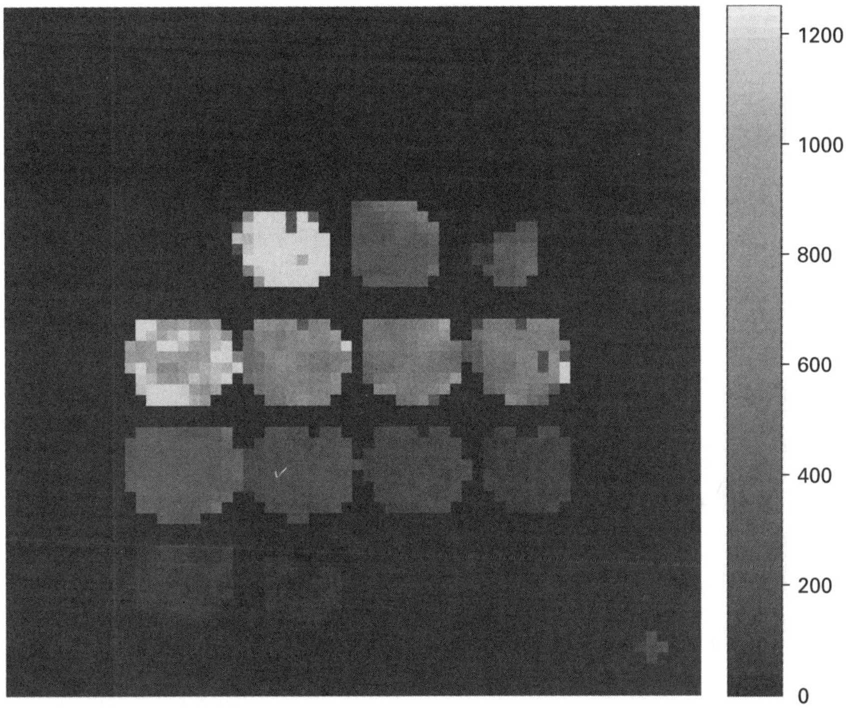

Figure 3.5
Dr. James Ross, T_1 Map, 2017. PowerPoint presentation slide.
Source: Courtesy of University of Aberdeen.

Phantoms of course do not replicate the human body, but they can represent simple versions of certain organs and their functions. They can either concentrate on a specific area of interest in the human body or they can have clear anthropomorphic attributes. For example, the bottles in question are inanimate objects that, thanks to the water they contain, are able to animate the scanner and allow its calibration. Phantoms are crucial for testing and calibrating scanners and making sure that patients do not get harmed. At its core, the phantom is the patient in disguise. It is an anticipation of the patient's body, although, as the young postdoctoral student whispers before I leave the laboratory, "patients are much more difficult to image than bottles of water."[36]

Soon after the proof-of-concept image validating the technique of FFC-MRI, the principle investigator (PI) of the IDentIFY project comes in and announces that on November 21, 2017, the university aired a press release announcing that the first patient had been imaged with the FFC-MRI prototype.[37]

Night Science

In their everyday laboratory activities, for instance while developing an imaging protocol, scientists conform to what the French molecular biologist and Nobel laureate François Jacob described as *night science*: "Night science wanders blind. It hesitates, stumbles, recoils, sweats, wakes with a start. Doubting everything, it is forever trying to find itself, question itself, pull itself back together. Night science is a sort of workshop of the possible where what will become the building material of science is worked out."[38]

Data and night science are both drivers of research. Instances of night science are recursive moments of interruption from the main research trajectory to explore other viable pathways. In published outputs that are not driven by a historical sensitivity, night science is omitted. Ethnographic laboratory fieldwork, laboratory traces such as scribbles jotted down by scientists, as well as artists' practices can suddenly illuminate night science and bring it to the foreground. The development of FFC is continually traversed by instances of night science. The decision to contradict one of the rules of MRI in order to explore dimensions of magnetism left aside by research at high field is a clear example of how night science within the mainstream research program of high-field MRI can become a distinct research trajectory. Night science is not just about experiments going awry but also about unexplored research trajectories, assumptions suddenly interrogated, and known techniques applied in new ways to produce unexpected results.

Night science becomes visible at the laboratory bench. For example, a variety of techniques are constantly being tested out to improve the speed of image acquisition in FFC, an important part of the protocol. One such technique is magnetic resonance fingerprinting (MRF), a very recent technique first developed in a laboratory in Cleveland, Ohio, and presented in an article published in the journal *Nature* in 2013. This technique is designed to allow the rapid acquisition of quantitative multiparametric maps (longitudinal relaxation T_1, transversal relaxation T2, proton density weighted sequence PD) with a high level of robustness and reproducibility while reducing complexity in imaging. Despite being a powerful diagnostic and prognostic tool, MRI is slow compared to other biomedical techniques, and it is qualitative, not quantitative. The contrast between tissues is the primary information used to characterize an underlying pathology. If the contrast value cannot be quantified, then its evaluation and interpretation lack objectivity; in addition, the resulting data cannot be standardized or normalized, meaning that they may be too variable to be useful in some clinical scenarios.[39]

Through multiparametric maps acquired simultaneously, MRF is designed to enable tissue characterization with quantitative parameters to help detect and analyze early tissue changes, a crucial goal of FFC-MRI. In his analysis of the context in which nuclear magnetic resonance first appeared, the physicist and historian of science Klaus Hentschel argues that "The NMR signal is thus like a fingerprint of the substance under examination."[40] Each tissue should have a unique set of NMR parameters (T_1, T2, PD, and so forth), like a fingerprint.

For the sake of clarity, in conventional MRI two separate processes take place during relaxation: longitudinal relaxation (T_1) and transversal relaxation (T2). Each MRI image consists of a T_1 component and a T2 component. It is possible to switch off most of one of either components, creating a T_1 weighted or T2 weighted image respectively. The proton density (PD) weighted image enables the visualization of the number of protons per volume. In order to achieve this, both the T_1 and T2 components must be switched off.

If one knew all these parameters, one could calculate exactly how that tissue would appear in an image for any given scan. MRF uses (mostly) standard MRI techniques combined with conventional pattern-recognition algorithms. The backbone of the MRF method is its dictionary and how well that is designed. The dictionary is created by simulating many thousands (or more) of possible experiments using specific equations (called Bloch equations) and storing them in a lookup table (the so-called dictionary).[41] Thus, there are three main steps in MRF: constructing the reference dictionary, acquiring some images, and using the dictionary.

In an informative article on MRF,[42] the fingerprinting aspect of the technique is said to be analogous to the fingerprinting identification process used in forensics to profile and identify persons of interest. The dictionary is a database in which tissue parameter combinations are collected. In forensics, the database is where all known fingerprints are stored and associated with other parameters such as the person's name, eye color, and date of birth. In MRF, the dictionary is generated using algorithms to predict the signal evolution. MRF varies the acquisition parameters such that each tissue generates a unique signal evolution. After the acquisition, a pattern-recognition algorithm explores the dictionary to find the best entry representing the acquired signal evolution of each voxel. The fingerprint contained in a voxel is compared with all the entries in the dictionary. If there is a positive match, the tissue represented in the voxel is identified and all the known parameters relative to that fingerprint can then be retrieved from the dictionary and assigned to the voxel.

Interestingly, the initial motivation behind the development of this technique had nothing to do with improving acquisition speed but rather with improving patients' well-being inside the scanner.[43] Conventional MRI produces a loud banging noise that can cause the patient to experience anxiety and annoyance, making the examination all the more difficult and stressful to endure while having to lie still. The noise of the scanner can also interfere with functional studies of brain activation. Some researchers realized they could exploit the new MRF technique to convert digital music files directly to the encoding gradients.[44] This meant that instead of the usual alien-like noise, the scanner could be made to play music. In the first such experiment conducted, the scanner was a 3T whole-body scanner, with music produced by switching magnetic fields while quantifying multiple important tissue properties. The audio waveform was processed to minimize the peaks of the waveform and constrain it to a band of amplitudes.

The idea was, therefore, not to mitigate or eliminate the noise of the scanner, but to make it pleasant, improving the patient's well-being inside the scanner. MRF-music, as the technique became known, enabled quantitative images to be generated with a pleasant-sounding acquisition. Thus, the centrality of the patient can lead to developments in technology and unexpected outcomes.

Fingerprinting does not describe how to acquire data from hardware to signal like the spin-warp method does. It is just a signal processing trick. And the images obtained do not need to look good—only a barely recognizable image is needed. But when enough images have been collected, the necessary parameters can be computed.

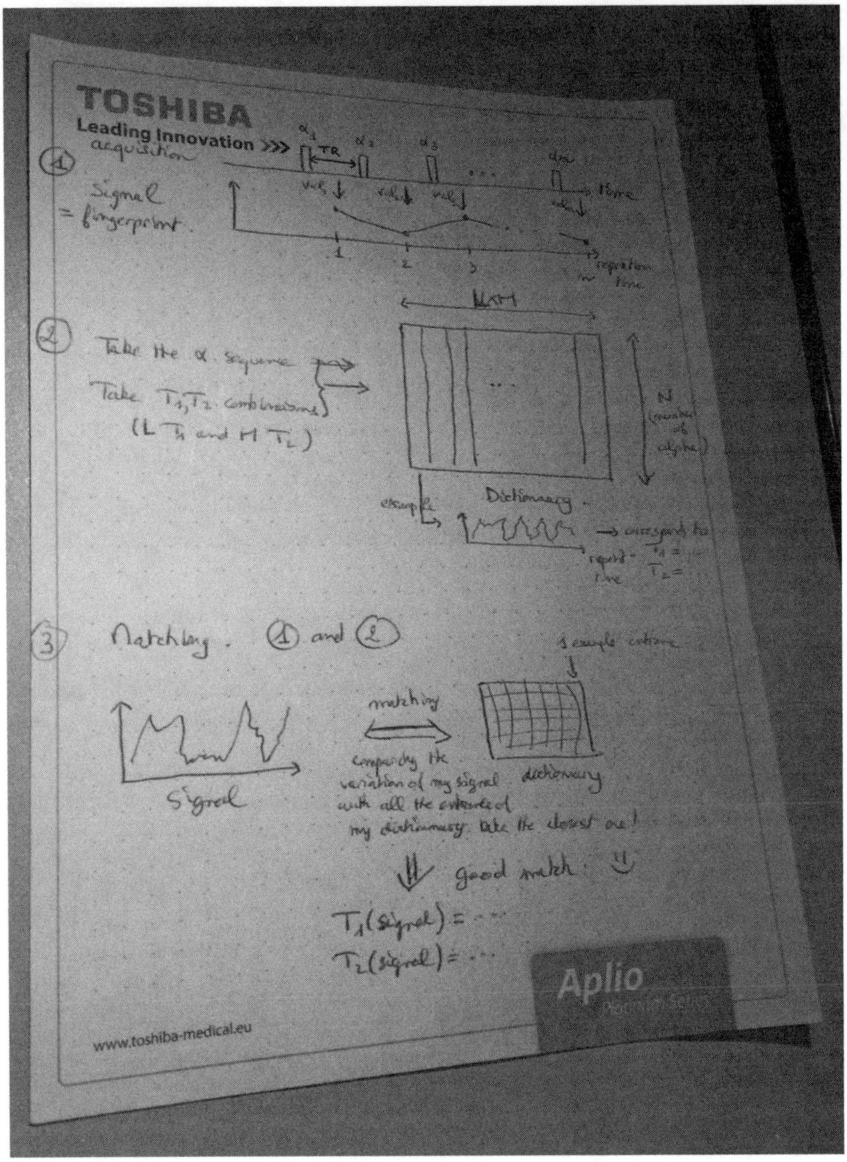

Figure 3.6
Handmade sketch of fingerprinting technique. Photograph taken during laboratory ethnography, April 2018.

During imaging, the signal from each tissue in the imaging volume should vary according to the Bloch equations. The signal from the experiment is matched to one from the dictionary, telling researchers exactly what the NMR parameters are. A pattern of data is put into the dictionary to see if it can be recognized. MRF allows you to measure more parameters at once than conventional MRI. You can regenerate the dictionary if it does not contain the pattern, but you only need to go back to the data collected by the scanner, without having to image the object again.

With MRF, one does not need the full data set, just as someone's identity can be identified from a partial fingerprint; and creating the dictionary does not take much time. However, what you get out is based more on what you put into the dictionary than on the data acquired. If the content of the dictionary is too far away from the data, this becomes a problem.

The effectiveness of the fingerprinting technique is communicated by the images it generates. However, a sketch made by a researcher on a piece of paper shows the principle of fingerprinting as a *process* rather than a result (figure 3.6).

This type of informal writing is an instance of night science. Akin to what Rheinberger calls "scribbles," this writing is a way in which an experiment occurring in a certain space and time is reenacted (and abstracted) onto paper to increase its communicability and (sometimes) the exploration of data.[45] Scribbling should not be confined to written notes because it can coincide with operations of calibration made onto laboratory equipment with the temporary images and visualizations that do not make it into the standardized final protocol.

From Images to Patients' Bodies

Once the proof-of-concept image is obtained, the physicists start testing the scanner with experimental subjects—either volunteering themselves or imaging patients in trials set up in collaboration with clinicians and radiologists. Two in vivo images obtained of a subject's head in April 2017 prove that the scanner can image human-sized samples without suffering from image distortion or poor signal-to-noise ratio. As soon as they managed to obtain a satisfactory image, they started talking much more about the patient, imagining the patients inside the scanner. Before, their discussions focused much more on the technology, the components of the scanner, and the software. But now the human component has returned. "Imaging the first patient with a neurological condition is going to be quite daunting," one physicist confided to me.

The patient, with all her intimidating corporeality, health condition, needs—in a word, her *aliveness*—appears in the discourses and practices of physicists tinkering with the FFC-MRI prototype. The vitality of the human body threatens any control effectively exercised upon neurons, cells, and molecules, whose vitality can be isolated, studied, manipulated, and even grown. The patient body cannot be managed with the same ease. For instance, some patients who agreed to act as experimental subjects in the FFC-MRI project were not able to undergo a scan because the couch of the prototype was too small for them. In some cases, patients can suffer from claustrophobia; therefore, reducing the data acquisition time becomes paramount in the visualization protocol and pipeline. The FFC-MRI prototype exposes the inner working of the machine body, its interior architecture.

The biological variability of nature in vivo is a threatening challenge not only to physicists but also to neuroscientists and clinicians involved in the FFC-MRI project. The transition from the proof-of-concept image to clinical application of the technique is challenging because the new imaging technology is tested on stable samples. Whenever a perturbation is observed in experiments using such samples, one knows that it comes from the hardware or software rather than from the sample. Once the imaging apparatus has been calibrated sufficiently and tested so that it is reliable, the sample introduced into the experimental setting is biological. The problem is that no two biological samples are ever quite the same; for example, in patients with a glioma, researchers need to be aware of diffuse glioma types and malignancy grades and that the differences in the signal come from the complexity of the sample.

FFC-MRI is to be tested upon the alive, vital bodies of patients and their health conditions. Although FFC-MRI technology seems promising for studying the progression of neurodegenerative conditions, the testing will start by imaging a small cohort of patients admitted to hospital having suffered strokes. In such patients, one of the most important issues is understanding the situation as early as possible after admission. The main problem is what happens immediately after the stroke. When the clot is dissolved, oxygen-rich blood returns to the tissue and initiates a series of pathological free-radical reactions, which damage the tissue. The protein content, geometry, and overall structure of the tissue all change, affecting the behavior of the water and rendering it detectable by FFC-MRI. In this respect, FFC-MRI might turn out to be a useful first-line care technology.

The decision to image stroke patients instead of those with neurological disorders is motivated by the necessity to quickly produce clinically viable results that demonstrate to radiologists and clinicians that FFC-MRI works. Figure 3.7 shows images of a patient with a suspected cerebral vasculitis (essentially inflammation of the blood vessel wall) who initially presented with suspected stroke. Two images (a and b) are conventional MRI images obtained at 3T. The other images are FFC-MRI T_1weighted images obtained with evolution fields of 1 mT, 6 mT, 37 mT, and 200 mT. T_1 at low field shows similar contrast as what was obtained on the high-field images.

The interesting thing therefore is that the physical mechanism behind the contrast we observe is different. The FFC-MRI images show regions where the slow timescale molecular motion of water has been altered. Taken in combination with the other techniques one starts to get a more complete picture of what is happening.

In stroke, one does not know whether the stroke started five minutes ago or half an hour ago, or whether the area of tissue surrounding the stroke—the so-called penumbra—is dead, dying, or salvageable. Often, it is not possible to use an MRI scanner for safety reasons, and in many cases, the scan obtained with other imaging techniques such as CT might not reveal any abnormalities. But a physicist I interviewed in December 2017 explained that even if FFC-MRI does not tell us more than MRI can, if it produces a useful image it will demonstrate that it is a safer, faster, low-cost MRI. As radiologists and

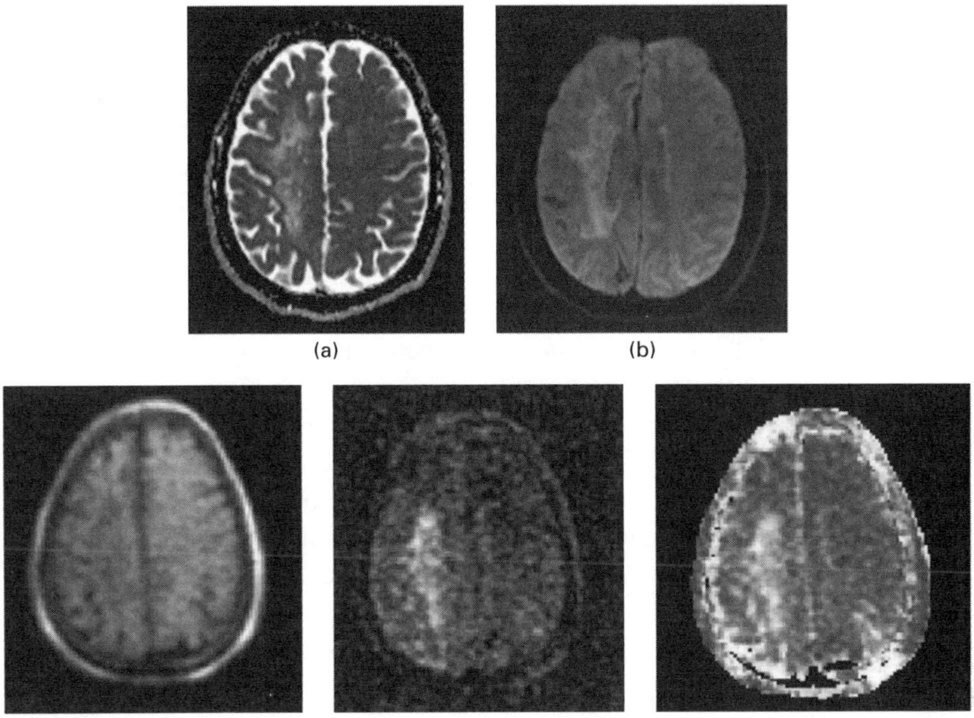

Figure 3.7
Dr. James Ross, (a) and (b) MRI images obtained at 3 Tesla; (c) and (d) FFC images obtained with different evolution fields; (e) composite FFC-MRI image, 2019.
Source: Courtesy of University of Aberdeen. See plate 4.

neurosurgeons begin to whisper to each other in hospital corridors, a buzz builds around FFC-MRI that this technique could be very useful for patients.

While the Aberdeen group tests the prototype on human beings, the Turin-based research group focuses on studying the complex interplay between the magnetic field, the biodistribution of the agents, and the dynamics of the water molecules, with the objective of designing a powerful contrast agent for use with FFC-MRI scanners. The patient is absent except when press releases are published on the research center's achievements. On those occasions, researchers receive phone calls and emails from patients with cancer hoping that the research breakthrough will immediately turn into a new cure or drug for their specific disease. In Turin, only small animals are used for FFC-MRI research. In Aberdeen, the advantage is that the studies and trials can be conducted with human volunteers. Scaling up from the animal to the human is still one of the main issues, as it was at the time of Mallard. The Aberdeen researchers conduct experimental work in vitro on a range of very small biological tissue samples first, before scaling up to the patient in vivo.

The Turin laboratory conducts biodistribution measurements of the contrast at high field strength, using a 7-Tesla scanner, and then they visualize small animals with a relaxometer.[46] With the 7-Tesla scanner, the image comes first, then the quantification. The region of interest (ROI) is drawn by hand because the researchers know where they want to look and they know what to expect. Although the ROI is hand-drawn, it can be edited on the image as many times as necessary once it has been acquired. After drawing the ROI, they apply equations to obtain the curves that give them the dynamic range of T_1 values. The same information is obtained with the relaxometer, although this starts from the profiles—from the quantification rather than from the image. The use of both the 7-Tesla scanner and the low-field relaxometer enables the chemists to evaluate the contrast.

The profiles visualized in Turin inform the Aberdonian research group's studies on human volunteers. Turning these profiles into images makes them readable by the radiologist and therefore clinically useful. In comparative analyses between tissues, the researchers already know which is the healthy tissue and which is the diseased one. What is still to be understood is what gives rise to the different shapes of dispersion curves and why a certain shape corresponds to a specific disease. The meaning of the shapes at the cellular, molecular, and tissue levels remains difficult to establish. "So," I ask a biologist, "what exactly is the meaning of the shape of the curves?"

"Well, we know that the dispersion curve is probably the different motions of molecules and that these motions can't be studied by standard MRI.... But we don't know exactly what the shapes of the curves are telling us."[47]

There are no straightforward models in biomedicine. The existing ones for FFC-MRI have been developed using control samples and phantoms, with uniform and stable characteristics, whereas in actual tissues there is little homogeneity. The patient's body and its biological variability are perceived by physicists in Aberdeen as a challenge to the visualization pipeline and to the workings of the prototype. In Turin, biological variability refers to animals, not to humans, but similar challenges are faced. For instance, the unpredictability of how the tumor develops in the leg of the mouse is an uncontrollable variable that sometimes affects the timeline of the experimentation pipeline itself. The biological variability that puzzles both physicists and chemists once again reminds scientists of the presence of the subject's body, be it a mouse or a human being.

Understanding Quality in Biomedical Data Visualization

The curve of the graph visualization produced with FFC can be analyzed using Galison's framework of the image and logic tradition present in the field of twentieth-century microphysics (see chapter 1). The curve of the graph, which is an average, rather than a direct visualization, belongs to the second tradition. Being able to move between these two traditions and to produce good quality image data (not just measurements or just images) is paramount to enabling physicists to reach out to different communities—radiologists, clinicians, patients, and the lay public.

Producing an image of quality is one of the main goals for any professional working with biomedical imaging technologies. Data are visualized, displayed, and interpreted by different experts for a variety of purposes: to assess whether the hardware and software components of an experimental machine are working properly (glitches are often revealed in the image), to prove a theory (the image as proof of concept), or to make a diagnosis. What precisely is meant by an "image of quality" is a vexed question that depends on the user of the image, for example, whether they are a physicist or a clinician. Typically, the end users (clinicians) are given the final data-visualization output but are not shown the labor behind it. They do not see the decisions made, the written code behind the interface software, or the conventions at work in a visualization pipeline.

In biomedical imaging, the quality of the signal is the first means by which information can be transferred effectively, properly, and quickly. Overall, the understanding of quality in visualized data differs between conventional MRI and FFC-MRI. Compared to high-field-strength scanners, *low-field scanners* have *lower* signal-to-noise ratio, *lower* contrast, and *lower* resolution, which make it difficult to match the image quality of *high-field MRI*. An image of quality is an image that does not show any artifacts, unwanted aspects like lines across the image, or unexpected noise. It is the signal-to-noise ratio for physicists, as one tells me: "An image that is pure doesn't exhibit any artifacts.... It is also an image that displays the desired information. It is not necessarily an image that is of incredibly high resolution. Rather, it is functional information that can be extracted from the T_1 dispersion curve."[48]

For both MRI and FFC-MRI, one cannot talk about the quality of the final image without considering the quality of the signal.

To obtain a pure image, the signal has to be pure with no spatial encoding, that is, with no information mixed up with the signal. When you listen to the radio in the car, you tune in at 97 FM (the carrier frequency), which is 8.5 mHz in MRI; what the radio does is remove the radio frequency so that you only get the music. You are not interested in the radio waves, in the radio frequency, but in the music. It is exactly the same in MRI: the carrier frequency is proportional to the magnetic field, and on top of that carrier frequency is the spatial information that makes up the image. Although most of the time no one is concerned with the carrier frequency, physicists are when it comes to FFC-MRI, because the carrier frequency tells them precisely what the magnetic field is. The carrier frequency changes slightly at the exact moment the magnetic field changes, making it possible to distinguish what part of the image is noise and what is useful signal.

The issue around quality ties in to the readability of the images by its end users: radiologists and clinicians. Physicists are aware that what they understand with quality in relation to an image does not necessarily coincide with radiologists' and clinicians' views.

Me: Who's going to interpret the images you produce?

Physicist 1: We're about to embark on clinical trials. The images will be interpreted by a radiologist, so they will very much be assessing the *images*. We know what we like to see, but perhaps we don't know quite so much what doctors like to see. Hopefully we can adjust to meet whatever their expectations are.

Physicist 2: To me it's really subjective [what an image of quality means]. It's in terms of signal-to-noise ratio for a physicist—an image of good quality is an image where signal-to-noise ratio is quite high. ...

Me: How about if you ask a clinician?

Physicist 2: I guess that one of the things they'd say is that resolution has to be high as well ..., so you also need to have a resolution that's fine enough to be able to detect the pathology. And you depend on the pathology, so that's the problem.[49]

The patient does not appear in most of the physicists' discourses around the quality of image data, although it is the body and the brain of the patient that provide the experimental system with the data required to produce a visual output. Unsurprisingly, given their closeness to patients, radiologists highlight the importance of the image in relation to patients. The visual output must meet the (sometimes implicit) expectations of radiologists and clinicians. For radiologists and clinicians, an image of quality is able to show them what they need to know; in short, it is a reliable image showing what is happening in a patient.

The type of spatially resolved visualization in figure 3.7 (e) is to be preferred to a graphlike visualization for it tells the onlooker the extent of the disease, that is, where it is located and what structure it is close to. A graphlike visualization (such as the one shown in figure 3.3 for breast tissues) cannot be used to create a trading zone with radiologists and clinicians who need to visualize information spatially.

Color plays a crucial role in transferring information within the community of physicists, but not necessarily in the community of radiologists. Mallard wondered whether using a gray scale with an adjustable contrast enhancement, rather than color, was an effective means of increasing diagnostic sensitivity without distorting the information. He argued that although no one had yet proved that color provided extra information, in his experience it did. In the development of FFC-MRI, color comes into play only at certain stages of the data-visualization pipeline, for example, in the proof of concept of FFC-MRI, similarly to a colorful image of the mouse.

How do data become information? According to the philosopher of information Luciano Floridi, to become information, data need to be well-formed, meaningful, and truthful.[50] Being able to convey information in an appropriate way through images and other forms of visual media is paramount to achieving understanding. When the onlooker can see an entire data set in a single glance, the perceptual experience of seeing enacts a cognitive process (the eye and the brain of the observer, which Mallard talked about in his papers) that might lead to the generation of new hypotheses, such as about the correctness of the data set.

The theorem of data-processing inequality states that the information contained in the final visualization (for example, a brain scan) cannot contain more information than the original data set.[51] Floridi argues however that in a visualization pipeline knowledge can be reused to break the condition of data-processing inequality. In the case of brain scans, for example, an external subsystem (like a reference atlas or other parameters) could contain extra information about the data, thus throwing further light on the brain scans. What remains open to debate and further investigation is the perceptual and cognitive response of individual viewers who are part of the visualization pipeline. This brings in the problem of quality of visualization (or of information).[52]

Floridi's definition of information and the physicists' understanding of quality in data visualization highlight how, like any communication system, the visualization pipeline is subject to errors and noise. The concept of information as well-formed, truthful, and meaningful data seems to be quite static and at odds with the concept of information as, literally, *an act of giving shape*, rather than just as the result of something (data) put into a form that is not necessarily or exclusively visual.[53] Scientific visualization is also to be understood as an activity carried out by people, instruments, and the traces they leave, as a process "without a definite referent and without origins."[54]

Floridi's definition of information, which does not include any historical context, seems to work better when that which is visualized is a stable and well-defined object. It seems to work less well when the data visualization cannot be circumscribed into a straightforward interpretation. As much as images are life forms, however, visualization too is a vital process capable of producing new relationships among things, data, spaces, and people rather than simply illustrating what it is not in sight.[55] Floridi's approach to information as well-formed, meaningful, and truthful data is that it does not seem to consider that knowledge is situated and partial; therefore, a given visualization can never present the whole picture.

Radiologists, molecular chemists, and biologists, who are all also involved in the development of FFC-MRI, have a rather different concept of an image of quality than physicists do. Radiologists understand quality as usefulness. An image of quality is an image that is reliable (not open to misunderstanding and ambiguities), an image showing what the radiologist needs to know in order to then take clinical decisions. This type of image is performative for the radiologist. It makes her practice safe by showing (telling) her what is going on with a patient. Molecular biologists think in terms of molecules and numbers. An image of quality is an image that enables discrimination between healthy and diseased tissues.

In contrast, for molecular biologists the visual component of data visualization is less important than the numeric one:

> Considering my background as someone who thinks more in terms of molecules, I would not define an image of quality as a high-resolution image, but as one that is predictive of the metabolic state of the organ or pathology I am observing. I think a quality image is an image that is able to discriminate well between a healthy tissue and a diseased tissue.... The image, too, is data—a number we actually measure much more than see.... It is true that the image is useful, of course, because one can say it is here rather than there, it is the left side rather than the right, it is in a kidney rather than in another organ. But the signal intensity is important too, so the number inside the image is very important—as is the case in our FFC, obviously.[56]

There are two crucial points in this passage. First, the old dichotomy between image and number, which has run throughout the history of MRI, comes to the foreground again. The image is less reliable than the number. The image runs the risk of reducing FFC-MRI to a technique for localizing the disease and visualizing the structure of organs in tune with what conventional MRI does. The image component is required by radiologists, not by physicists. Second, FFC-MRI is entangled with predictivity. It is about visualizing the metabolic state of the organ or of the pathology under observation at a very early stage when it is not yet symptomatic. In FFC-MRI, an image of quality shows what it needs to show, especially when the equipment is far from the best. The quality is to be understood with reference to the clinical read-out potential that one can extract from the image.

Sometimes, however, the final image is not easy to interpret and communicate. This is the case of the curve of the graph in FFC-MRI. The theoretical physicists are still struggling to establish the meaning of the shape of this curve and its relationship to clinical applications. The curve of the profiles is an unknown epistemic thing.

Epistemic things are the "material, functional units of knowledge production…, techno-epistemic processes that bring conceptual and phenomenal entities into being," situated at the interface between the material and conceptual aspects of science.[57] As an epistemic thing, the curve of the graph is vague enough to push research ahead, being latent within and emerging out of the technical conditions embedded with the experimental system. What makes this project relevant and truly innovative in comparison to other scientific projects is that, in the words of a molecular chemists who leads one of the work packages, "the knowledge expansion is not just horizontal—with this project, researchers encounter the unexpected, bumps into the unforeseen, into phenomena that they cannot explain. The result is unknown."[58] The right amount of vagueness therefore rather than theoretical precision is key to a powerful experimental system. Uncertainty, being at the core of the interpretation given to the shape of the graph obtained with FFC-MRI, is the focus of the next chapter.

Ultimately, data visualization, even when the interpretation is not yet straightforward, is based on and is about patients' bodies, real or imagined; in the early development of an imaging technology the patient's body is "anticipated" through the body of scientists testing the apparatus or through phantoms. The production, interpretation, display, and communication of visualized biomedical data impact the health care pipeline, decision making, and interventions on patients' bodies. At the molar and the molecular scales, the body of the patient is simultaneously the constant reference point in the laboratory and a daunting present absence. It is through the graph of the T_1 relaxation time—through this type of data visualization, with all its vagueness, uncertainty, and yet authority—that the relationship with the patient is mediated.

4 Visualizing Uncertainty in MRI Reinvention

> [Although] we have some idea of what is involved in the act of walking (if only in general terms), we have no idea at all what happens during the fraction of a second when a person takes a step. Photography, with its devices of slow motion and enlargement, reveals the secret. It is through photography that we first discover the existence of this optical unconscious, just as we discover the instinctual unconscious through psychoanalysis.... For it is another nature which speaks to the camera rather than to the eye: "other" above all in the sense that a space informed by human consciousness gives way to a space informed by the unconscious... the inconspicuous spot where in the immediacy of that long-forgotten moment the future nests so eloquently that we, looking back, may rediscover it.
>
> —Walter Benjamin, "Little History of Photography"

A few months after my ethnographic journey inside the biomedical physics laboratory in Aberdeen took off, I started to become acquainted with the researchers' work and with their *ways of seeing*. Carefully moving my body between the scanner prototype, wires, amplifiers, and computer console where the two postdoctoral researchers jotted down notes for the experiment or wrote bits of code, I eventually learn to recognize the objects I am regularly shown—different types of coils, probe, and hardware and software components of the scanner. I am getting familiar with the relaxometer used to scan small tissues samples rather than human beings. The relaxometer does not produce images but graphs representing the evolution of the magnetic process, the amplitude of the signal.

I am learning to "see" the signal produced by the main scanner. I recognize whether the signal appearing on the screen is bad or good, meaning a signal with a certain pattern showing spatial information with a clear peak. I am becoming acquainted with phantom objects. I frequently watch one physicist undergoing several scan sessions to test the prototype. I learn to spot the zebra artifacts in the image—gray lines traversing the scan.

Yet, in spite of all I am learning, I am puzzled when the physicists show me the first proof-of-concept image or the profiles obtained with FFC-MRI. I cannot quite share the enthusiasm of researchers, their "eureka" moment. I find myself in the somewhat hilarious situation that Bruno Latour captures so well in a picture in one of his books.

It is a picture of the lay person entering the laboratory and scratching her head after being shown the graphic rendering of certain data (in Latour's image, a sinusoidal curve). An authoritative researcher says loudly at the perplexed laboratory visitor: "This is what you are looking at, *do you see?*"[1] The lay person looks again and again, scratching her head, wondering what it is that she is actually looking at. The image does not seem to match the words of the expert. An act of faith—blind trust—in the authoritative researcher should take place. The phenomenon talked about by the researcher is embodied in that visualization. The fact that the phenomenon under study, the "thing" talked about by the researcher, is made visible in the graphic does not necessarily mean that it is understandable by someone outside the laboratory or even by other scientists.

Like the hand-painted image of the mouse created by Hutchison and his team, the visual output of FFC-MRI is not only the epistemic thing created within the given experimental system, but also the interface through which physicists communicate with other stakeholders, whether researchers from other disciplines, potential funders, clinicians, or patients. Undoubtedly, when I look at the graphs produced with FFC-MRI during my fieldwork, I am learning to look at a new thing. However, what I am looking at is not quite what I read in the articles on FFC-MRI or see inside the scanner (a phantom object or an experimental subject). Am I getting closer to the reality of things I am looking at? What does it mean for a professional (physicist, biologist, clinician, neurosurgeon, radiologist) to see a biomarker of a pathological condition?

After a deluge of biomedical images of the inner structure and workings of the body, the FFC-MRI graphs leave both experts and nonexperts baffled. What exactly are we looking at? These "strange profiles," to use the expression of one of the biochemists involved in the project, are numbers rather than images. These visualizations are graphs in which the curve signaling a change at the molecular level shows a specific shape. They do not resemble structural or functional images obtained with conventional MRI or fMRI. These high-contrast images render the inner regions of the body visible, affecting not only our view of corporeality but also our own understanding of health and disease. The body composed of organs, muscles, blood, and tissues is at a molar scale. These graphs signal a change in the way in which the body is theorized. The body ceases to be a transparent organism, becoming instead an ensemble of molecules, whose behavior might be predicted by looking at data hidden in these curves.

In this chapter, I show how FFC-MRI is placed within the broader discourse, imagery, and practice of biomedicine and its ways of visualizing life in its unfolding at a molecular level. FFC-MRI is presented as a novel technology to visualize biochemical changes at this level that are believed to be related to certain diseases even in their early stages. The image of a biomarker allows the evaluation of the potentiality of an event (being ill) to govern not the reality but the probability of a given condition developing. At the beginning of the twenty-first century, genes, cells, bodies, technologies, and research areas become imbued with potential. I argue that potentiality is the implicit framing underpinning the development of FFC-MRI and the challenges related to its data-visualization pipeline and output. I put FFC-MRI, its way of seeing and intervening in the patient's body, within the framework of personalized and predictive medicine. The drive toward the patient, which characterized MRI invention and data visualization at the time of Mallard, is moved forward and at the same time reconfigured by FFC-MRI under the new framework of potentiality.

What do the "strange profiles" render visible? What do they hide? Is there anything unrepresentable in the field of today's biomedical imaging and neuroscientific research saturated by data, information, and visualization?[2] Whether it is stochastic uncertainty, model uncertainty, or uncertainty about the future, finding ways to convey uncertainty is one of the most important challenges in data visualization today. As I discuss in chapter 6, these are some of the challenges that the artist in residence at the Aberdeen biomedical physics laboratory has to tackle in her response to FFC-MRI, an emerging technology whose visual output is not yet standardized.

A Leap in Scale: From the Transparent, Molar Body to the Potential, Molecular One

Transparency and the Optical Unconscious

Technological innovations in medical imaging affect the representation of the body's interiors and the authority of the subject who performs the looking. Media theorist José van Dijck demonstrated how old and new technologies for investigating the structure and functions of the body, far from offering mechanical and objective recordings of the bodily interiors, enable and perpetuate illusion and voyeurism and transparency.[3]

Whereas in the early days of biomedical imaging, body and brain scans obtained with CT and MRI were not able to display clear contours of the imaged organs and bodily parts, the sociologist Regula Burri, who has done extensive research on biomedical imaging, argues that "today's images are high in resolution and contrast, thus making the sophisticated technology 'transparent' and able to disappear behind the image."[4] Hence, the paradox is that the imaging technologies that have contributed to the affirmation of the transparent body have become transparent themselves, creating in the lay public the belief of direct and total accessibility to the body and the brain.

But total transparency is an unattainable goal, regardless of the technology used to access and visualize the inner workings of the body. At the turn of the twentieth century, X-rays, cinema, and psychoanalysis, which were all discovered or invented in 1895, disclosed the interior of the body without the need of dissection (X-rays), depicted the movement of life (early cinematographic experiments), and analyzed the depth of the psyche (psychoanalysis). They fostered a new type of visuality that thwarts the trope of the transparent body, as Akira Mizuta Lippit highlights in his study of the hidden interiors of cultural life: "These three technologies introduced new signifiers of interiority, which changed the terms by which interiority was conceived, imagined, and viewed. They transformed the structure of visual perception, shifting the terms of vision from phenomenal to phantasmatic registers, from a perceived visuality to an imagined one. From visual to avisual."[5]

X-rays, cinema, and psychoanalysis haunt the myth of transparency and full accessibility to the body and the psyche by means of a mechanical-aided vision. It is another nature, another reality that emerges through the use of photography, cinema, and X-rays.

Referring to photography, the cultural critic Walter Benjamin argues that although we know what walking is and what it looks like,

> ...we have no idea at all what happens during the fraction of a second when a person steps out. Photography, with its devices of slow motion and enlargement, reveals the secret. It is through photography that we first discover the existence of this optical unconscious, just as we first discover the instinctual unconscious through psychoanalysis. Details of structure, cellular tissue, with which technology and medicine are normally concerned—all this is in its origins more native to the camera than the atmospheric landscape or the soulful portrait.[6]

When Walter Benjamin looked at photographs to theorize the optical unconscious, he trusted photographs to do the work of revealing the unseen aspects of sight itself. Our experience of ourselves and of the phenomenal world(s) is increasingly mediated by photography and ubiquitous image-generating technologies. Benjamin explored the ways in which this mediation occurs at the level of the unconscious. Although his definition of the optical unconscious remained relatively undertheorized and at a germinal stage, it was sparked by technological experimentation occurring in his time, such as the studies on animal and human motion conducted by the photographer and amateur scientist Eadweard Muybridge and by the physiologist Étienne-Jules Marey.[7]

Photography and filming techniques give us access to what is not directly perceivable by our sensorium, either because it is too rapid or because it is too small. For example, in the days of early cinematographic experiments on movement, filmmakers and scientists collaborated, using microcinematography, chronophotography, and time-lapse techniques to slow down or speed up processes, to magnify structures. Often the visualized phenomena were fleeting traces of something that was not there anymore. As psychoanalysis introduced us to unconscious impulses, so the camera introduced us to the unconscious optics. The camera recorded aspects of reality that did not fit the natural optics. When we magnify images, when we present a fragment of reality in slow motion or close up, we are not just displaying known elements from the world, but we make visible new structures of matter, a new order of reality.

The concept of the optical unconscious should be extended to encompass other image-generating technologies, not just analog photography. Digital and analog, algorithmic, and optical vision coexist in FFC-MRI. Technologies such as MRI and FFC-MRI produce visualizations that are not based on "the position of the observer in a 'real,' optically perceived world," to use a concept that the art critic Jonathan Crary explores in his study on the historical formation of the observer in the nineteenth century.[8] The technological shift in the medical gaze is called a "cyborg visuality" by the sociologist of science Amid Prasad who points out that the type of vision involved is mathematical and algorithmic rather than human.[9]

In contrast, like in conventional MRI, in FFC-MRI too there are instances of embodied vision. Researchers work on their PC keyboards, digitizing the code with their fingers, visually checking the code on the computer screen, sometimes jotting down notes, scribbling numbers and graphical representations on paper, and then analyzing the shape of the signal appearing on screen. It is a type of digital and embodied visuality that leaves the computer screen to stretch out in the world.[10] Image data are constantly interpreted and manipulated by humans.

The optical unconscious creates the object rather than merely revealing it. In line with the early cinema studies on motion, FFC-MRI too is a form of reconfiguring our perception, not of movement but of phenomena that are not directly available to our senses. FFC-MRI gives us images—*spaces*, one could say—that our direct sensory experience and perceptual ability fail to grasp. With FFC-MRI a new order of reality, previously unnoticed, is made available: that of the dynamics of water molecules. The vitality of matter at molecular and atomic scale becomes accessible. The entanglement between technology and human vision mediates the way in which we relate to the body. In particular, the technological unconscious emerging with FFC-MRI, albeit not yet codified, revolves around the concept of potentiality—the passage from the transparent and molar body to the potential and molecular body.

The Potential Body

Potentiality is a recurring theme in biomedicine today. Genes, cells, bodies, as well as technologies, are increasingly imbued with the dimension of the "potential." Since the advent of the Human Genome Project in the late 1980s, knowledge, expectations, and technologies in the fields of biomedicine and biology have been reorganized around the concept of potentiality rather than just transparency. The shift is from the visualization of the body as transparent to visualizing biomarkers indicating the possibility of a pathology. The body of the patient becomes the potential site of a future condition that might (or might not) develop. In February 1979, during the period of MRI development in Aberdeen, after the creation of the dead mouse image but before the construction of *Mark I* and the invention of the spin-warp method, Meg Foster in Mallard's team created a map depicting the yet-to-be *Potential T_1 Man* map (figure 4.1). This map represents a thread traversing the two moments in the Aberdonian history of MRI development and reinvention.

Potentiality in this map has a specific meaning. It refers to the spin-lattice relaxation time value in different bodily tissues.[11] In technical terms, conventional MRI measurements were carried out using an instrument that measured the relaxation times of small samples of tissue taken from animals. These maps are designed to give an idea of the spread of normal T_1 values. Visually, the concept of the Potential T_1 Man was rendered as a two-dimensional outline of the male human body with the various organs and tissues distinguished by colors signifying changes in the T_1 value.

This image belongs to a broader transnational cultural history of representations of the human body (brain included) from the early modern anatomical atlases through to X-rays and biomedical imaging technologies. At a visual level, it embodies the transparent body, but at the same time it envisages the future potential clinical value of MRI as

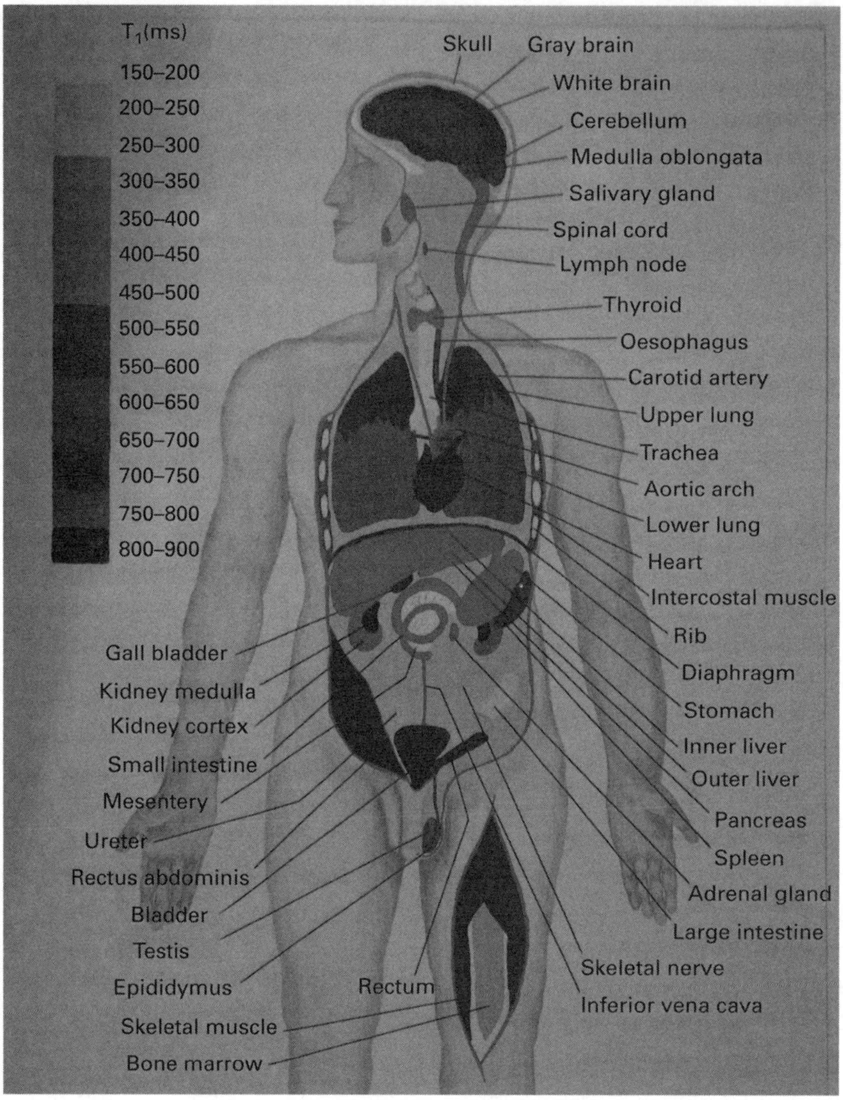

Figure 4.1
The Potential T_1 Man map. Reprinted from, Mallard, "Nuclear Imaging," fig. 30. Record 3819/1/125/1. *Source*: Courtesy of the University of Aberdeen, Special Collections. See plate 5.

a technique to visualize pathological conditions associated with changes in water balance in various regions of the body. At a more abstract level, the Potential T_1 Man map visually conveys the coordinated efforts of physics, medicine, and biology to shape and deliver health care by molecular imaging technologies. Color effectively conveys one of the striking features of the map, which is the high variation in T_1 values across different tissues all in their natural state, a discovery made possible by a novel medical imaging system. The driving force behind the new human is not yet potentiality (in the sense of predictive medicine), but it is also no longer exclusively transparency.

Simultaneously concrete and abstract, well-defined and fluid, the Potential T_1 Man map acts as a boundary object: "Boundary objects are objects which are both plastic enough to adapt to local needs and the constraints of the several parties employing them, yet robust enough to maintain a common identity across sites."[12] This map facilitates communication between the different sociotechnical worlds/communities it inhabits (physicists and biologists, physicists and clinicians, animal and human tissues, bodily parts and the whole body).

The diagram of the Potential T_1 Man is neither a faithful nor simplified version of man imagined by biomedical technologies. Rather, it creates a new way of visualizing the T_1 value in the anatomy of the human body, rearranging colors, numerical values, and anatomical details of a rabbit onto a two-dimensional map of a human being. The diagram is not a schematic representation of an entity that exists out there but rather a performative visualization that both creates and organizes relationships among data coming from animals, a new technology, and the human body. The diagram makes visible dynamic relationships. It does not only inhabit different present worlds facilitating communication among existing communities (as a boundary object would do), but it also helps to envisage a future machinery (a full-body scanner) that would reconfigure the relationships between physicists, radiologists, and patients.

This map was yet to be realized at the time of Mallard. The in vitro measurements of tissue samples were taken from one rabbit and then drawn onto the man map in an attempt to portray the variations in T_1 value.[13] These data *may* be applicable to human beings thanks to an NMR imaging machine capable of displaying T_1 information. It must be remembered that in February 1979, *Mark I* was still under construction. The Potential T_1 Man map did not, in fact, show potentiality but rather was used to illustrate what physicists and clinicians thought the *Mark I* scanner would be able to do in the next future. This image embodies the gesture of "scaling up" from the animal to the human. The colorful image is a two-dimensional transposition of a series of measurements taken from the world of animals and from human tissues to a future application potential. In the late 1970s, therefore, the concept of the Potential T_1 Man functions just as a goal to strive for rather than an already accomplished result. Although the ideal and ideology of the transparent body never fully disappear in contemporary biomedical discourses and practices, it is the category of potentiality that becomes prominent.

The sociologist of science and medicine Nikolas Rose explores the consequences for an understanding of the body and life at the molecular level. The passage from the transparent body to the potential one mirrors the passage from the molar body (composed of organs, tissues, and limbs) to the molecular body (composed of neurons, cells, and molecules invisible to the naked eye). This passage signifies a shift in the way life is conceived as Rose explains: "Starting, perhaps, in the 1930s, there was a shift from a molar image of life—of organs, flows of organs, of muscles, of blood and of tissue, represented by the paintings and drawings in anatomical atlases of the eighteenth and nineteenth centuries—to a gaze that envisions the body at the scale of the interactions between molecules."[14] The clinical regard of the doctor, the postmortem examination, and the visualization in the anatomical atlas were all interventions made on the molar body. In contemporary biomedicine, the molar body is increasingly superseded by the molecular body giving rise to a new gaze and a new conception of life that is an amalgamation of biology, technology, and sophisticated visualization techniques.[15] Molecular thought signifies a shift from the anatomical body, understood as a unified totality, to self-contained atomized components organized in new assemblages disconnected from the whole.[16]

FFC-MRI witnesses this shift from the transparent to the potential body and from the molar to the molecular one. FFC-MRI belongs to the category of the technologies of life that Rose describes as a configuration of instruments, persons, practices, and knowledge that are governed by certain assumptions about human beings and that work together toward a goal. For Rose, these technologies "embody futurity.... They try to bring potential vital futures into the present and seek to make them amenable to calculation, and then amenable to transformation in the present in the name of an enhanced future. And they are future-oriented in another sense.... They shape and they thrive on a promissory culture of hopes and expectations... of individuals, of their families, of governments, of scientists and researchers, of health care organizations and insurers."[17]

It is important therefore to understand the biopolitical implications of visualizing that which does not yet exist but *might* become in the future. The change in scale, from the molar to the molecular level, as Rose argues, corresponds to a change in "our capacities to engineer our vitality, our development, our metabolism, our organs, and our brains."[18] In biomedical practices, potentiality indexes a gap between what is and what might, or even should, be. Such a gap creates a space for understanding and intervening on human life at the molecular level.

Data Visualization and Uncertainty: What Are We Looking At with FFC-MRI?

With this new technology, scientists now aim to make visible the early stages of a disease that is not yet symptomatic. But what exactly are we looking at? To answer this question, one first needs to frame it correctly, using the work of historians of science and technology on objectivity and its meaning across history. In their book *Objectivity*, Lorraine Daston and Peter Galison embark on a multidisciplinary history of scientific objectivity by examining a wide range of images from atlases in medicine and the natural sciences.[19] The main argument is twofold. First, objectivity has always been historically contingent, it has meant different things across history. Second, making sense of objectivity requires an understanding of visual representations in scientific practice and of their entanglement with changing epistemic values and concepts of truth.

The three epistemic virtues related to the concept notions of objectivity are truth-to-nature, mechanical objectivity, and trained judgment. The first, truth-to-nature, represents the type rather than the individual specimen. Daston and Galison state, "It is an image of the characteristic, the essential, the universal, the typical."[20] This type of objectivity aims to extract a universal truth from what can be observed by the naked eye. Human vision has both to select what to observe and to conduct an aesthetic transformation of the represented object. Mechanical objectivity, which appeared with the invention of photography, is concerned with the mechanical, automated representation of an object. Attention is given to the reproduction of particulars rather than universals, as it was for truth-to-nature. In this second realm of objectivity, the reproduction of a tree, for example, is organized as much as possible without the biases of human intervention and attempts to capture the tree as it is—the individual specimen rather than the type.

The third epistemic virtue, which emerged in the early twentieth century, is trained judgment, a type of objectivity "moralized," as Daston and Galison define it. Trained judgment blends mechanical objectivity (from highly specialized instruments) with the human involvement in decision making related to data selection, visualization, and interpretation. One example is an X-ray image that requires both expertise and training in order to be made, read, and interpreted. The expert is able to use their skills and training to interpret the raw data obtained with instruments in such a way to identify in the observed phenomenon meaningful patterns, family resemblances, and aspects of the phenomenon that can be detected but not understood by the instrument on its own.

The three configurations of objectivity can coexist. There is no sense of a progressive replacement of truth-to-nature with mechanical objectivity and then trained judgment. The visual output produced with FFC-MRI is an example of trained judgment. Human and expert intervention are required for setting up the protocol to create the graph. Specific skills and training are required along the whole data-visualization pipeline, not just to create the visual output but much more to interpret it and put it to use among different communities of experts (not just physicists or biomolecular chemists but also radiologists and clinicians). The visualization pipeline analyzed in chapter 3 consists of the human and machinic components, represented by the hardware (the scanner and the various coils), the body of the patient, the signal, the software code, the console employing the matrix-based MATLAB language, and the graph of the T_1 parameter.[21]

The graph produced by FFC-MRI looks very different from the crisp, high-contrast scans obtained with structural MRI. The viewpoint of science historians is again useful for understanding the difference between the two types of visual output. Building upon Galison's distinction between the two traditions present in physics (the image-based and the logical) that I discussed in chapter 1, the historian of science and technology Borck distinguishes in the neurosciences an anatomical–microscopic tradition, based on the structural image, and a graphic tradition based on tracing or writing.[22] Two examples of instruments that belong to the first and second tradition are, respectively, structural MRI and electroencephalography.

In terms of the representational space it generates, FFC-MRI seems to be closer to the writing tradition because data are presented in the form of a graphic map conveying physiological processes and changes. The graph is not the direct product of an inscription device as is the case for a graph from an electroencephalogram; however, FFC-MRI does belong to the writing tradition insofar as "the recorded signs have to be analyzed, decoded or read rather than simply looked at."[23] FFC-MRI does not quite match either tradition because it is part of a third visualization regime that can be named, following Borck—the biomolecular one—which integrates both traditions. A multiplicity of instruments is better qualified to investigate phenomena that are not easily graspable as in the case, for example, of neurodegenerative diseases.[24]

Different instruments produce different visual outputs. The shift from high-field to low-field magnetism was accompanied by the shift from high-contrast images of the brain and body to profiles that visualize the dynamics and changes in the water content of tissues, whether intracellular or extracellular. The type of instrument used to investigate an organ (for example, the brain), a process, or a pathology affects the space of representation and the way we see what we see. Often the problem is the correlation between the output produced by the instrument and the object to be measured/detected/visualized. With functional MRI, for example, the problem is the lack of an indexical, direct, and straightforward correlation between social behavior and brain activation.[25]

The visual output produced by FFC-MRI is a graph expressing dispersion curves as shown in figure 3.3. One curve, the T_1 dispersion curve, has a particular shape and a typical behavior depending on the sample. So the molecular dynamics of the sample affects the behavior of the curve (see figure 4.2).

The aesthetics of the curve—aesthetics as the science of what is sensed and imagined—is an instance of *profiling* a condition of pathology in the organism. The absence

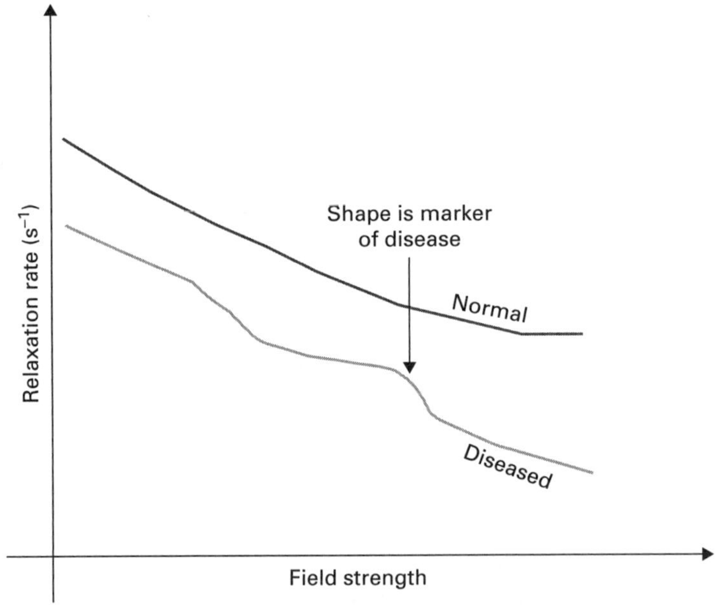

Figure 4.2
Reproduced from Professor David J. Lurie, PowerPoint presentation slide, fiftieth Anniversary Medical Physics, November 2, 2018, University of Aberdeen.
Source: Courtesy of Professor David J. Lurie.

or difficulty of establishing a direct correlation between the visual output (the profiles) and the phenomenon under investigation (a condition of pathology) returns with FFC-MRI.

A key member of the IDentIFY family is a physicist from the French Institute of Health and Medical Research in Grenoble. Her in-depth and multidisciplinary expertise in medical physics, neuroscience, glioma, and MRI made her aware of the challenges of interpreting the dispersion curve.

Physicist: I use the T_1 value every time, but understanding the origin of this T_1 value is really hard. This is *big science*, so to say, because the origin of the T_1 value comes from the interaction between spins, nuclei, and matter.

Me: Do you mean this is a question that can only be answered if one recurs to quantum mechanics?

Physicist: Yes. The problem is that we need to know what kind of interaction we are detecting and measuring: there are physical interactions, dipolar interactions, quadripolar interactions. For example, we need to know what the contribution of proteins is, the contribution of water, what is intracellular, what is extracellular, what the contribution is of the water exchange between different compartments. It's not easy.[26]

One of the major issues is what *kind* of information one wants to extract from the dispersion curve (for example, the amplitude of the quadrupole dips or the shape of the dispersion curve).[27] Leonelli explains that an object (in this case, the dispersion curve) can become a datum "when it is viewed as potential or actual evidence for one or more prospective knowledge claims, and given the unpredictable variety of claims which data might be used to corroborate, their evidential value can vary."[28] A change in the shape of the dispersion curve is not necessarily directly related to something happening in the tissue; in biology, several different pathways may lead to the same kind of change in the dispersion curve. So the dispersion curve alone is not a very insightful source of information. Its interpretation requires a knowledge of what kind of pathology causes a specific change in the curve, which can only come from clinical studies. Data visualization plays a crucial role in determining what is regarded as "raw data" and what becomes accepted as a "fact" or discharged from laboratory practice.[29]

The problem is that the *form* of the profiles (the shape of the curve) can affect the response and the decisions taken upon the *body* of the patient. The information inferred from the dispersion curve will be transmitted to radiologists and clinicians—the end users of the technology.

In Poland, the theoretical physicist who leads the work on the theoretical framework and modeling was ready to answer my question on the relevance of the relaxation curve.

Me: Can you please explain the relevance of the relaxation curve for visualizing cancer?

Theoretical physicist: We do not conclude whether some particles have cancer or not from the relaxation curves but from image[s]. You must *see* the cancer; you do not draw a conclusion on the basis of the shape of the curve. However, knowing the shape of the curves helps you to decide at which magnetic field strength you should take the image. But in the end you have an image, and when you look at it (like in a traditional MR scan), you can see objects that have different relaxation times. And this is the output of the examination.[30]

The series of numbers obtained with relaxometry needs to be put into an image in order to identify the required information about the pathology. The shape of the T_1 relaxation time curve functions as the interface between research in physics, its biomedical application, and the eventual adoption of the technology in the health care system. Like the picture of the dead mouse, the FFC-MRI graph is the means through which physicists share this emerging technology with researchers from other disciplines (biology, chemistry, engineering) within the same experimental systems or outside them (radiologists, clinicians, funders, patients).

Looking at the shape of the graph produced with FFC-MRI is not a neutral act. Both the act of looking and the visualization itself play a role in "materializing the biological process under investigation as a system, and in making that system something that can be considered real, or something that we can engage with as real," as Burri, Carusi, and Aspradaki said in their study on the ontological and epistemic roles of visualizations in contemporary medical practice.[31] The "real" to which the authors refer is not a preexisting phenomenon but what the different actors (researchers, clinicians, patients) perceive, experience, and interact with as real: "something that is negotiated over, struggled over, formed and transformed."[32]

The theoretical framework can contribute to refining the experimental observation, improving the experimental protocol, and interpreting the collected data. Theoretical physicists, in particular, are attempting to figure out the reasons why the curve of the graph in diseased tissues has a different shape than it does in normal ones. This comes down to studying the molecular dynamics, intermolecular distances, and applying quantum mechanics, as the theoretical physicist explained to me:

Me: Do you have a mathematical model at quantum level that explains what you do?

Theoretical physicist: With the mathematical explanation we can say more things about the correlation between the visualization and the visualized phenomenon. It depends on how one looks at that. One could say that it is not important at all because you can rely only on the statistics and just believe in the statistics.

Me: What do you mean?

Theoretical physicist: For the purpose of somehow building the equipment, it may be sufficient to collect the statistics. Frankly speaking, I suppose that at the end of the project it will be like that. [She pauses.] Anyway, people want to know things.

Me: I do, too! For instance, why is the relaxation time for pathological tissues slower than for healthy ones?

Theoretical physicist: Because there is a different water dynamic.

Me: Fine, but explain to me, please—show me the way how the water dynamics leads to slower relaxation…

Theoretical physicist: Well, then you will reach the next level of questions and end up using quantum mechanics. But other people do not need to go into this type of mathematics. What for? It's only me who represents the theory part and frankly speaking all that counts in the end is whether you have a nice image of a well visible pathological change or not.[33]

Beautiful data reveal the truth. Aesthetics and the image-based tradition in physics are needed to relate the graph to the pathology. It seems that observing and measuring the slope of the curve is just one step;[34] the other is trying to understand what it means—using "the eye and the brain of the observer," as Mallard once recommended when researchers working on biomedical imaging were striving to interpret the visualized data.

The skepticism expressed by the theoretical physicist is hardly surprising given that we are witnessing the rise of "a data-centric approach to science, within which efforts to mobilize, integrate, and visualize data are valued as contributions to discovery in their own right and not as a mere by-product of efforts to create and test scientific theories."[35] Even in the other research groups not everyone seems to agree that the theoretical framework is a crucial part of the project and that quantum mechanics should be used, given that it is fundamental in MRI. The opinion of one of the physicists more driven to experimental practice and instrument making than theory is that quantum mechanics is just one regime in physics and perhaps not the most useful one from a clinical perspective:

Physicist: To be honest, the theoretical framework is not that necessary for the success of the clinical application of FFC-MRI.

Me: What do you mean, exactly?

Physicist: Well, you have certainly heard of the different "regimes" in physics. The classical one, used for the macromolecular world, and the quantum mechanics approach, used to describe atomic-level physics. Theoretical physicists are interested in the fundamental reasons why in FFC-MRI certain differences take place.

Me: How about clinicians? Are they not interested in this question?

Physicist: They might be, but at the end of the day clinicians do not necessarily *need* to know the reasons why certain phenomena occur in order to make a diagnosis and decide on a treatment. It is also a time issue: we need to produce results.[36]

The physicist's position here is that an experimenter's confidence in the reality of what he is manipulating can be independent of commitments to a serious explanatory theory. What is interesting in this exchange are two things. First, there seems to be a difference in the *rhythm* of the experimentation, theory, and clinical practice.[37] Researchers involved in experiments and clinical work agree that the epistemic thing they see is "real." Therefore, they work on producing results regardless of the theoretical framework employed to ground the empirical work. In short, the form of reasoning of experimental practice has a different pace and relies on a different form of argumentation than that of theory. Second, MRI can (and theoretical physicists would say it *should*) be approached using quantum mechanics, given that MRI relies on the quantum properties of atomic nuclei.

Quantum mechanics plays a role especially when MRI is described quantitatively. For example, it governs the nuclear interactions that are responsible for relaxation. Although relaxation is consistent with classical mechanics, the observed rates of relaxation are not. Only if these are calculated using quantum mechanics do they match the experimental results. Normally, however, relaxation rates are measured rather than calculated from first principles. Hence, examples like this do not warrant the use of quantum mechanics for nonphysicists.[38]

Quantum theory became established in the 1920s as the most fundamental approach to understanding nature at very small scales, specifically, matter and energy. In essence, quantum theory provides a mathematical description of a world very different from that which we experience on the macroscopic or even microscopic scale. This theory does not provide exact deterministic predictions, only probable outcomes.[39] The use of statistics and probability to describe physical events in the early decades of the twentieth century contributed to the erosion of classical mechanical physics and more generally of the science of determinism.[40]

The introduction of probability affects not only the discipline of physics but even more so existing conceptions of nature, subjectivity, and society, posing the question of what is real under this new regime. Medicine, biology, and physics are connected by a regime of probability, which is the cipher of the introduction of quantum mechanics and statistics in the field of physics. The world of medicine and health care will adopt many quantum principles. The ability to detect molecular changes early, before debilitating symptoms of diseases appear, is appealing to both clinicians and pharmaceutical companies in view of treatment options and outcomes.

The Eclipse of the Real

The main challenge with the ongoing development of FFC-MRI has to do with the theoretical framework required to understand the shape of the curve of the FFC-MRI graph. In more general terms, the data-visualization conundrum at the core of FFC-MRI points to the limits of data visualization in biomedical imaging and the necessity of having a "nice" image capable of revealing the early stages of a pathology or the effects of an intervention on an organism. In her analysis of MRI and its use in health care, sociologist Kelly Joyce points out that over-reliance on visualization technologies to discover biomarkers for diseases potentially undermines the use of other nonimaging diagnostic tests and creates a "blind spot."[41] Biomarkers are linked to visibility. FFC-MRI still relies on imaging, albeit not on high-contrast images like those produced with MRI.

When we take a closer look, the problem shifts from "What are we looking at when we observe these profiles?" to the question of how FFC-MRI is going to impact the world of medicine and health care. The patient has always been the driver of MRI invention and reinvention. To address the problem of the limits of data visualization in FFC-MRI, in this section I put to work selected passages in which the philosopher and critical theorist Giorgio Agamben engages with the implications of the new regime in physics characterized by the introduction of statistics and probability in the study of phenomena. Needless to say, Agamben's remarks cannot be applied to FFC-MRI in a straightforward way. However, they do offer a critical framework to tackle the problem of what is the *modus operandi* behind some emerging biomedical technologies such as FFC-MRI. To some extent, the theoretical framework that is needed to sharpen experimentation and get to the core of FFC-MRI has to do with the challenge of understanding the broader background against which FFC-MRI operates.

A few words on Agamben, who is mostly known for his scholarly work on politics rather than on aesthetics or science: Agamben engages his readers with some of the most pressing contemporary concerns, from the concept of sovereignty and the rights of citizens to the concept of life itself.[42] The method he uses is "paradigmatic" as it uses the paradigm, which is a real case serving as an exemplum, to understand our present and its concealed grids of power and control.[43] At the center of Agamben's interest is the attempt to reframe the present situation (*status*) of the refugee. In support of "the Agamben of poetics, culture and signification,"[44] the question of the status of a certain subject/object is a chief preoccupation in Agamben's interventions in the fields of aesthetics and art, just as in his reflections on politics. When it comes to aesthetics, Agamben tackles the question of status in a literal sense: how do images, concepts, and objects come to acquire the power and authority they have? How can another object/subject/event disrupt this authority?

Science and technology do not occupy a visible place in Agamben's *oeuvre*, but they emerge in his reflections on the relationship between technological processes, the body, and the apparatus:

> I shall call an apparatus literally anything that has in some way the capacity to capture, orient, determine, intercept, model, control, or secure the gestures, behaviors, opinions, or discourses of living beings. Not only, therefore, prisons, madhouses, the panopticon, schools, confession, factories, disciplines, judicial measures, and so forth (whose connection with power is in a certain sense evident), but also the pen, writing, literature, philosophy, agriculture, cigarettes, navigation, computers, cellular telephones and—why not—language itself.[45]

Agamben's reflections on science and technologies are scattered across his writings in the form of brief remarks, images, and metaphors (the embryo, the speed of light). However, in the booklet *Che cos'è Reale? La Scomparsa di Majorana* ("What Is Real? The Disappearance of Majorana"), published in 2016, Agamben dwells on questions concerning the status of reality and the introduction of statistics in the panorama of contemporary physics, and the impact of this revolution upon the social world.[46] In this work, Agamben conducts a sustained interrogation around the status of reality, a critical category that contemporary physics seems to have neglected and even eradicated from its own horizon with the introduction of probability, statistics, and the development of quantum mechanics.

The starting point for Agamben is related to the disappearance of Ettore Majorana, one of the greatest theoretical physicists of the twentieth century and collaborator of Enrico Fermi, the creator of the first nuclear reactor. The case of Majorana's disappearance becomes paradigmatic for reflections on reality (meaning the range of phenomena that exist in space and time independently from being observed) and on our way of acting in it. Majorana had been working on neutrino masses, and after meeting with Werner Karl Heisenberg (the father of quantum mechanics) he published his work in 1933, which later became the basis of current atomic physics.[47] The nuclear forces he theorized bear his name today. In 1938, Majorana mysteriously disappeared while going by ship from Naples to Palermo, leaving no trace but a few letters and a couple of unpublished essays.

Agamben does not treat the case of Majorana as a detective chasing evidence would, but he builds upon the ideas exposed by the physicist and upon the letters he sent to different people before disappearing. In these three letters, Majorana mixed up contradictory elements in such a way that reconstructing what happened in reality is impossible. Like a quantum particle, Majorana reappeared and disappeared in different places simultaneously. Not only that, he produces a certain event (the disappearance) as improbable. Agamben points out to us that the only datum in our possession is the disappearance itself, but it is an improbable datum, in the literal sense of the term; that is, something that cannot be proven on the plane of facts. In other words, Majorana has disappeared to the extent that no one has ever found him. That the disappearance was intentional remains a probable fact: a hypothesis, but not a certainty.

Probability is not reality but what could become real. The passage from probability to reality is linked to the choices made and the variables encountered. Before deepening his analysis on Majorana, Agamben discusses studies conducted by diverse authors such as the writer and philosopher Simone Weil, the mathematician Cardano, and the philosopher Pascal. Of the latter, Agamben recalls the calculation of risk since it offers a clear example of how a line of reasoning based on probability can influence real life. Risk is calculated, for example, to measure the value of an unfinished game, in order to divide the compensation in the best way or, one could say, as close as possible to how one would have divided it had the game been played. One always gives a direction to one's own action in reality after analyzing different possible pathways to follow. Probability is never realized as such, but it allows reality to be intervened in and governed.

Agamben seeks to question the fundamentals of quantum theory, which are based on the assignment of the status of reality to probability. According to quantum theory, it is impossible to establish the exact state of an atomic system; at most—explains Agamben, quoting Majorana—one can "determine the probability that a measurement performed on a system prepared in a given way will give a certain result," and then significantly adds: "The result of any measure seems therefore to concern rather the state in which the system is carried in the course of the experiment itself, than the unknowable one in which it was before it was disturbed."[48] Reality suddenly becomes "unknowable"; man is merely a spectator of a world in evanescence. When the determinism of classical mechanics is abandoned in favor of the indeterminacy principle, what remains of reality?

Majorana, Agamben argues, intuited that probability and statistics were about to introduce a new regime designed to govern not only the laws of physics but also those of society. This point is put forth in one of the last two articles written by Majorana and published posthumously in 1942, titled "Il Valore delle Leggi Statistiche nella Fisica e nelle Scienze Sociali" (On the value of statistical laws in physics and in social sciences).[49] In this article the author establishes an analogy between physics and the social sciences, constructing an interdisciplinary communication experiment targeting not only scholars from these two fields but the lay public too.[50] Majorana maintains that quantum mechanics is an irreducible statistical theory, since it cannot describe the time evolution of a single particle or atom in a controlled environment at a deterministic level. This lack of determinism at the level of an elementary physical system motivated him to suggest a formal analogy between statistical laws observed in physics and in the social sciences.

Discussing the not immediately evident implications of Heisenberg's indeterminacy principle, Majorana writes that the result of a measurement concerns "the state in which the system is brought during the experiment, and not the one in which it is before its detection."[51] The alarming consequence of this operation is not, according to Majorana, the indeterminacy of the atomic system, but the manipulation that it undergoes during the measurement. Ultimately, the experimenter is legitimized to design a chain of phenomena commanded by the modifications he wants to make.[52]

Quantum thought imposes a statistical description to events involving the entities that populate the quantum world (subatomic particles and their spin, direction, and observation). As far as social and economic disciplines are concerned, statistical laws are elements of investigation in economic and social modeling and are characterized by the same epistemological status of irreducible probabilistic laws as quantum mechanics. At the time of Majorana, in the late 1920s and early 1930s, this intuition made for rather revolutionary reading because the dominant paradigm to describe the interactions between economics and physics was that of the mechanics of celestial bodies—a deterministic type of paradigm. Majorana suggested that the inherently statistical nature of the processes that describe quantum phenomena supported the idea that statistical laws could be incorporated into the process of scientific modeling of social phenomena. Majorana thus pointed out the true meaning of the indeterminacy principle, which is, Agamben argues, "not to limit knowledge, but to legitimize the experimenter's intervention as inevitable." The weakening of the real corresponds to the empowerment of man over it.

Far from being a science devoted to the experimental knowledge of reality, statistics is a science interested in enabling human beings (the experimental scientist, the doctor, the physicist, the social scientist, the politician, and so forth) to take decisions under uncertain circumstances. This is the biopolitical background against which stands a biomedical imaging technology like FFC-MRI, following Nikolas Rose's remarks on biopolitics: "Biopolitics, since at least the eighteenth century, has been future-oriented.... In the face of such futures, authorities have now the obligation, not merely to 'govern the present' but to 'govern the future.' Such futurity is central to contemporary problematization of the brain."[53]

FFC-MRI, in a similar fashion to other risk technologies in the world of health care, has a specific relationship with the present and future dimension when it comes to how they manage uncertainty and enable the calculation of risks/probabilities to make predictions. FFC-MRI is set out to assist researchers in the quest for biomarkers enabling the early diagnosis of certain conditions (for example, neurodegenerative diseases) before they become symptomatic. This emerging technology and its way of seeing, then, are perfectly inserted within the paradigm of personalized and predictive medicine by seeking to control (govern) the spectrum of uncertainties that patients might or might not have to face. Precision medicine is an emerging approach for treatment and prevention that considers individual variability in genes, environment, and lifestyle for each person. Precision medicine makes true predictive analytics possible. One is a requirement for the other.

Practices of seeing and their visual cultures have always been crucial to medicine. Evidence-based medicine relies on the recording of visible symptoms and on an understanding of "seeing," which coincides with diagnosis.[54] In the case of predictive medicine, "seeing" is accompanied by statistics in the categories of "potential" and "probability."[55] Potential is the undefined and unrealized set of all possible variables and states of a given problem or argument. Probability is the mathematical distillation of all those potential outcomes into a singular result, the most probable observed outcome to a given set of variables in each argument. With predictive medicine, a branch of medicine that aims to identify patients at risk of developing a disease, the relationship between data, images, and patients is organized around categories of probability, potentiality, and risk.

Biomarkers and the Uncertainty of Interpretation

What are the implications of uncertainty in the interpretation of the graph for diagnosing and treating the molar body of the patient? The problem of data visualization, interpretation, and display examined in the early days of MRI is still present in FFC-MRI, although it assumes another configuration. The history and practice of medicine show how the restoration of a condition of normality and healthiness was always at the core of medical intervention, and clinicians have always strived to predict the potential development of a disease from the patient's present circumstances and therapy. However, the anticipation of what might happen next was based only on symptoms and signs that needed to be read. Representations of the body in premodern medicine,

Foucault argued, were mute: the truth of disease could be deciphered only through a parsing of signs.[56]

With the advent of anatomical dissections, the body could speak for itself, revealing its secrets and being open to comparison with other bodies. The boundary between normality and pathological deviations from the norm could be constructed thanks to the practice of dissection and the availability of anatomical atlases. The standardized body was further established in the nineteenth century with the birth of clinical medicine and anatomical pathology and the possibility of exploring the interior of the body noninvasively, using instruments such as the stethoscope. Correlations could then be established between the symptoms on the surface of the body (visible) and their organic location (invisible to the naked eye).[57]

In recent decades, we have seen the passage from the anatomical to the molecular body and the availability of a wide range of technologies for visualizing and manipulating structures and processes at the level of cells, genes, and molecules. All this has allowed medicine to enter a new paradigm that entails the understanding and management of the normal, healthy, and alive body. Furthermore, the patient's physiological, genetic, and environmental data help clinicians to tailor prevention and treatment strategies to the needs and characteristics of the individual patient.[58]

Personalized medicine is a framework for medical care that involves the use of medical imaging technologies and the modeling and simulation of a disease on the basis of its underlying mechanisms. Personalized medicine is connected to predictive medicine. Revealing a personalized "disease signature" in a patient early on, before symptoms become observable and/or detectable, can open the way to predictive medicine, a medical intervention tailored to the patient, before a disorder becomes manifest or when it is still in its early stages.

Predictive methods, such as genetic testing and neuroimaging, are used with the aim of determining the probability of a certain disease developing in a person by identifying specific measurable signs (biomarkers) associated with the disease. However, they also entail instituting measures to either prevent the disease altogether or to significantly decrease its impact upon the patient. Usually, by the time a diagnosis of, say, a neurodegenerative disorder is made—by the time the abnormalities are visible on structural, metabolic, or blood flow scans—the patient's pathology is too advanced to respond to treatment. Therefore, the hope for the future is to use techniques such as biomedical imaging (including FFC-MRI) to identify pathologies at a much earlier stage than currently possible, when they are amenable to treatment, thus protecting people from progressive diseases that destroy their quality of life.

Neurodegenerative diseases and brain cancer are the two main focuses for FFC-MRI. With neurodegenerative diseases, the hope is to be able to identify early, low-level brain pathology and treat it before it develops in severity. With tumors, the hope is to open up a window on new therapies targeting subcellular dynamics. Current therapies for brain tumors seem to be condemned to fail in spite of the increasing number of biomolecular and imaging technologies available. The preferred method of cure is still open surgery, but tumors can reappear after removal due to molecular and cellular adaptations such as peritumor invasion, nontumor microenvironments represented by noncancerous cells present in the tumor, or tumor heterogeneity.

The major bottleneck however is the inaccessibility of the brain. The drive to find pathologies that evade biopsies or surgical removal but that might be accessible through FFC-MRI is contributing to the sharpening of observational techniques that can guide biopsies. Being able to decipher pathological drivers to predict behavior, find the relevant target, and then follow up with appropriate therapy will be a major shift in medicine.

The goal of biomarker research is to keep exploring and deciphering the brain through a multiplicity of technologies and techniques in view of renewing the classical model of biomedical research. Biomarkers shape the vision of "personalized, predictive and preventive (or PPP) medicine."[59] According to François Berger, chair of neuro-oncology and unit director of INSERM, Grenoble (partner of the IDentIFY project), the toolbox to renovate the classical model of biomedical research and health care should include techniques such as deep brain stimulation (DBS) and brain fingerprinting.[60] DBS is an increasingly relevant paradigm for nonlesion, high-precision, "physical" neuromodulation therapy for conditions such as Alzheimer's and Parkinson's diseases and dystonia. Brain fingerprinting is a computer-based technology designed to determine hidden information in an individual's brain by measuring electrical brain wave responses to words, phrases, or pictures presented on a computer screen.[61] The effort is to implement a synergy between macro/micromolecular, MRI/optic imaging detection, and the use of large repositories of brain imaging data. The integration between multimodal imaging (MRI, robotic imaging, magnetoencephalography, optical imaging, nuclear medicine, electrophysiology) and biomolecular investigation (molecular analysis, cell biology) at the level of individual complexity can provide rich information on the brain's condition and foster the development of individual precision medicine.

Yet physicists cannot quite explain the nuances of the biochemical molecular changes detected by FFC-MRI. Although they still hope that this emerging technology will contribute to early fingerprinting of certain diseases, the term *fingerprint* is not always considered the most appropriate to use, even within the same community of physicists. The type of language used by two physicists working side by side on the clinical relevance of FFC-MRI is imbued with the categories of visibility/invisibility and surface/depth:

Physicist 1: I'm not entirely sure of the biological aspects, of what's going on or not, but what we believe is that before degeneration, before the disease really takes hold, there must be some chemical change that takes place that we hope to be able to pick up on.

Me: What are you hoping to detect?

Physicist 1: We may be able to see some early fingerprints, some sort of profound change in the chemistry of a particular tissue before it becomes dysfunctional. And what we hope is that as it evolves, FFC-MRI may be able to pick up on biomarkers that may otherwise be invisible.

Physicist 2: Yes, but be careful. Remember that relaxation time, although it is a physical process, is not straightforward in terms of *interpretation*.[62]

The interpretation is not straightforward because in terms of pathology, the T_1 parameter does not tell clinicians something directly in terms of what happens in the tissue. Clinicians are interested in what kind of processes are happening in tissues, for example, if there is a fibrosis, if the cells are dying, and so on. Some or all of these biological phenomena will impact the dispersion curve, but the dispersion curve does not *directly* reflect what happens in the tissue. This means that *the dispersion curve is not a fingerprint of what happens in the tissue*.

Behind closed doors, one of the researchers in molecular imaging of the IDentIFY project took some time to share with me his own understanding of the predictive value of FFC-MRI, beyond the rhetoric that they all need to use in front of potential funders:

Me: How can we know which is the best treatment or the best drug for this specific patient?

Researcher: I put together various genetic and morphofunctional information, I stratify information within a group, and I say "This type of drug would work better on this patient; on this other one, a classic type of treatment is better," and so on.

Me: So, the predictive value lies in those terms—it refers to how one extracts, *from the images*, biomarkers that alone or together with others can be predictive of the development of a pathology, or to the patient's response to a specific therapeutic treatment. Am I correct?

Researcher: Well, in this context, one might push the concept of predictive medicine even further. There will be a new frontier. The new frontier will be to say how imaging can report on the so-called premetastatic niches.

Me: I'm not sure I understand.

Researcher: Let me try to explain. A person normally does not die of the primary tumor because if we spot the primary tumor in time—hence the value of early detection—with a surgical procedure one can take away everything, margins included. The problem is that the tumor generates cells that metastasize, find their path, go into the vessels, and create tumors in other organs. What is known with certainty is that one type of cancer always metastasizes in the same organs, for example, lung cancer metastasizes in the bones, in the liver, and in the brain.

Me: So, if one could say "Look! It will be in that area of the liver that cancer cells will metastasize …"

Researcher: Yes! And, if I have a drug, a treatment able to block the proliferation of cancer cells, well then I have considerable benefits, not only before the tumor becomes symptomatic but before a cell arrives. The tissue must have been prepared. There must have been something, so to say, that has opened up the path, something that has created spaces, [which] has permitted the cells to take root—that is, to join and then multiply in that area. We hope that FFC-MRI can give us biomarkers for this. At the minute, it is the stratification of the patient with respect to the treatment.[63]

Although FFC-MRI is already producing clinically relevant results in relation to brain strokes and several types of carcinomas like breast cancer, biomarkers for brain tumors like glioma and neurodegenerative conditions such as Alzheimer's disease are still lacking. The drive toward research on biomarkers for Alzheimer's disease is hardly surprising given that it is one of the plagues affecting the elderly population, with a massive cost on the National Health Service. To convince investors and clinicians of the usefulness of an emerging technology like FFC-MRI and to enable its future commercialization, researchers need to prove that the technology is able to give answers to questions that existing technologies cannot. In this respect, one of the most promising areas is the early diagnosis of neurodegenerative conditions.

Water present in the human body—central to both MRI and FFC—acts as an informant of chronic diseases, because it emits specific electromagnetic signals that can be read and deciphered. However, using the FFC-MRI prototype for patients with neurodegenerative diseases like Alzheimer's is challenging because there are no good models of what happens in the human brain. Cognitive impairment arises from the physical degeneration of the brain—if one has fewer neurons, it shows up in tissues. What happens in animal brains however does not reflect that. The brains of animal models of Alzheimer's disease do not shrink as much as human brains with the disease.

The questions that remain unanswered are, Does atrophy relate to water dynamics? And is protein aggregation a cause, consequence, or side effect of Alzheimer's disease? Protein aggregation is a common feature of many neurodegenerative diseases, Parkinson's and Alzheimer's included. To fulfill their different functions, proteins have to acquire the correct three-dimensional structure. If the folding of proteins fail, aggregation might occur. Dysfunction and accumulation of two proteins, which are, respectively, the beta-amyloid peptide and the tau protein, is believed to be related to the onset of Alzheimer's disease. However, the process that leads these two proteins to aggregate is still not clear.[64] In short, what drives the disease remains largely hypothetical.

In May 2018, clinical trials commenced with the aim of using FFC-MRI to find biomarkers for brain tumors like glioma and neurodegenerative conditions such as Alzheimer's disease. In undertaking research on Alzheimer's disease using FFC-MRI, the priority is to collect a huge amount of data on the dispersion curve values in patients with the disease, contributing fresh data to an already existing database and leaving a more nuanced analysis of the data to a later stage. A pilot study was conducted in Aberdeen by clinicians, biomedical physicists, and radiologists specializing in multimodal brain imaging and involves a cohort of thirty patients who have been diagnosed with Alzheimer's disease.

The study uses data coming from Generation Scotland, a resource of human biological samples and data provided for medical research by the people across Scotland born in 1936.[65] These people (over 30,000) have given their informed consent to participate in a series of academic and commercial research studies by providing blood, other samples, clinical measurements, and information about their health and lifestyle.[66] Thanks to these volunteers, a wide variety of conditions including heart disease, diabetes, chronic pain, and mental health have been studied to date. The goal is to use a variety of imaging technologies (structural and functional MRI, and FFC-MRI) and to store the images produced alongside other kinds of data in a comprehensive database containing socioeconomic, genetic, and neurological parameters. The advantage is that the cohort is particularly stable because the 1936-born participants have been routinely monitored across their life span.

The study on patients with Alzheimer's disease reveals one of the major bottlenecks of FFC-MRI: data processing. First, unlike a stroke, Alzheimer's disease is not a single event but a diffuse condition; this makes it very difficult to assess. Second, not being able to see anything in the patient imaged with FFC-MRI does not necessarily mean there is nothing to be seen. Algorithms are needed to extract quantifiable data; only after that would researchers be in the position of saying whether there is something to be seen. Human vision is not enough to evaluate which region of the image is interesting.

After processing, storage is another variable to consider. Once fed into a database, data are turned into authoritative images that serve to formulate a diagnosis or a prognosis. Brain atlases (which are of crucial importance in the study of neurodegenerative diseases) are organized around databases, possibilities contained in images, and metadata related to the brain. According to Anne Beaulieu, a scholar of science, technology, and culture with a long track record of work on the logic of the interface in relation to brain imaging and neurosciences, the atlas is at once the shaper and the embodiment of scientific authority.[67] The use of probabilistic atlases invites the onlooker to read the image of the brain as a result obtained after calculations across a database and in terms of possible outcome—for instance, the variation indicative of Alzheimer's disease.[68] The logic of the database conceives of images not as objects but as interfaces that build relations and allow data exploration.

The database will enable researchers to conduct multivariate statistical processing of physical and sociocultural–economic biomarkers, that is, "biosocial medicine of the human subject," as the anthropologist Joseph Dumit and sociologist Regula Burri call this "emerging bioscope."[69] The absence or excess of data is equally problematic. By making visible certain things through acts of visualization, data compression, mathematical transformation, and schematization, other things recede into the background and become invisible. It might be that patients themselves become invisible and mute—Alzheimer's disease is a condition in which patients often cannot speak for themselves. Furthermore, in spite of the rhetoric promising discoveries of clear predictive indicators, susceptibility biomarkers, and treatment targets for neurodegenerative disorders, such goals are not easily achievable, and efforts focused too strongly on them may also dry up funding from elsewhere. The effort to intervene in people who do not present any symptoms yet might reduce research and health care resources otherwise used to improve the conditions of those who are ill.[70]

In her book devoted to the exploration of the challenges embedded in research and conceptualization of Alzheimer's disease, Margaret Lock states that the causes of neurodegenerative diseases remain elusive despite several decades of investments in research and discusses the "imperialism of probability" with which we live today. This new imperialism of probability has superseded the science of determinism, which was dominant in the sixteenth and seventeenth centuries and has become eroded by the introduction of probability mathematics. In Lock's reading, the imperialism of probability has been fostered not only by the introduction of probability mathematics (and later with quantum physics) but also by the "massive expansion of literacy, computation, bookkeeping, the invention of the census, and the idea that people can be systematically divided into various groups or populations, ultimately for the purpose of governing society."[71]

Computation and the other categories mentioned by Lock are all related to the problem of the data deluge—the idea of constructing databases in which a massive amount of data can be stored to then be retrieved for analysis at a later stage. The risk however is to face a deluge of data that remain mute and unworkable because of the lack of the proper theoretical framework. The problem is the one I stated at the opening of the chapter: What is the "thing" that FFC-MRI visualizes? What does the biomarker actually reveal? In her study on the role played by responsible research and innovation applied to the development of emerging diagnostic technologies for Alzheimer's disease, Marianne Boenink argues that "a molecular biomarker requires, first of all, technologies to observe and measure bodily functioning at the molecular level. Such molecular observations only become 'markers,' however, when they are clearly associated with relevant clinical events. Establishing such associations requires huge databases that connect molecular findings with medical files, and tools from bioinformatics to analyse the correlations between them."[72]

It becomes very hard to draw a line between knowing and not knowing, to give a reading of a clinical condition, a reading that is inherently fragile because it has been exposed to the deluge of data and counternarratives that other biomarkers might provide. As the sociologist Ulrich Beck argues, the introduction of the categories of risk, potentiality, and probability to anticipate a condition of pathology signifies "the controversial reality of the possible."[73] These words, which resonate with the concern over the status of reality, were the cipher of Majorana's research in the reading offered by Agamben.

Problems arise not just at the level of modality (real/possible) but also at the level of scale. In contemporary biomedical laboratory practice there is a co-presence of molecular and molar exactitude. This co-presence of the two scales for imaging, talking about, and understanding the body, however, does not show up at the public level, for the answers are at the molar level; that is, they concern patients in their entirety: their bodies, brains, and circumstances of life.[74] Data, in contrast, are often related to the molecular body, even when they are arranged in patterns and correlations that move beyond the level of molecular organization. The issue of scale shows up when researchers try to understand the meaning of data patterns—their evidence. To do so, they need to be able to ascertain the reliability of data; their reliance upon previous knowledge of the phenomenon under investigation; and the relationship between the data, the sample or the body of the patient, and the experimental setting.

Chapter Final Remarks

Back at the beginning. At the end of my interview with John R. Mallard, I pause to look at the medals and awards on display in the living room of his house in Aberdeen. His wife is almost asleep in the armchair next to him. Speaking softly, she says to me, "If John does not have an aim, he is lost. Now he is just surviving." I cannot help but prompt him to imagine a future research direction in which he too would play a role. I ask him about his secret hope in biomedical research, what he would like to do next. With a sparkle in his eyes, he whispers, "Well, I think it would be very nice, wouldn't it, if we could inject a patient with some sort of *magic particle* that would go to the part of the patient's body *that is about to become malignant*, and would have to be imaged in some way. You still need some sort of image that will pick up that particle there. Can't be done yet."

Here, Mallard is perhaps referring to a not-too-distant future in which nanotechnologies would be those "magic particles," referring to his past research on radioactive isotopes and PET, not just MRI. Still, regardless of any magic particle, human vision (Mallard's "the eye and the brain of the observer") and image still play a crucial role. We need to be able to see what any magic particle would be able to detect.

Chapters 2, 3, and 4 have recounted the situated history and practices of MRI reinvention by taking as a case study a peripheral history in the broader transnational history of MRI development. The Aberdonian case study on MRI and FFC-MRI is one of the half-forgotten trajectories within the main official history of MRI. The trajectory line of FFC-MRI resembles that of a karst river. In the 1980s, this technique was under scrutiny thanks to research conducted on free radicals. Then this trajectory thinned until it almost disappeared to let high-field MRI and its crisp images come to the foreground.[75] Yet FFC-MRI research did not wither away, but only retreated from the realm of visibility. Like the Timavo River, which has a karst character and flows underground for at least 25 miles of its journey to the sea, research on low-field magnetism lived on underground for 25 years to then suddenly come to the surface.[76] The trajectory of FFC-MRI will surface again in chapter 6, which centers on the work conducted in collaboration with the biomedical physics laboratory in Aberdeen, the Suttie Arts Space, and the artist Beverley Hood.

Intermezzo Lives in the Grid

Introduction

Grids can be found everywhere—from scientific images to works of art, from graphic design to architecture. Gridded systems are used to visualize bodies, populations, data, and biological organisms. According to the comparative historian Phillip Thurtle, biology owes more to the abstraction of the grid than to an aesthetic of wholes.[1] The grid allows disparate pieces of information (both analog and digital) to come together in the guise of a technical image, that is, in the form of an image that is instrument based or that results from imaging procedures.[2]

Anne Friedberg defines the grid as a framing and drawing device that appeared in the fifteenth-century treatise *De Pictura* (1435) written by the humanist and artist Leon Battista Alberti, who describes the veil (*velo*), a framing device that functions as a gridlike frame positioned between the eye of the onlooker and the object to depict.[3] The gridlike veil serves the purpose to assist artists in their attempts to map the three-dimensional world into the two-dimensional picture plane of the canvas. From its early appearance, the grid prompts the question of what is included and excluded from the frame.

The focus of this intermezzo, which connects the first and second parts of the book, is on the role of the grid as a matrix of epistemological and aesthetic relationships. The grid, a conventional coordinate system present both in modern art and in the sciences,[4] has been described as "a way of announcing that something is going to happen: an object is going to be measured, or an image is going to be transferred from one scale to another, or a form is going to be drawn and studied."[5] It enables, in biomedical imaging, the translation of data into an image and, in art, the opening of creative possibilities for artists. Once the grid was invented, it never disappeared; it became a tool for reconfiguring our perception, experience and display of the world and of the body, exercising an impact across our visual culture. The processes I describe in this intermezzo and in the book (the creation of an image from data in biomedical imaging; the creation of a modern artwork) have the grid in common.

It seems impossible to envisage a world without using a grid as a scaffolding device. Later in this chapter, using the case study of MRI, I discuss the central role played by the grid in moving from biomedical data to images and back to data again in the ongoing instrumental mediation between the brain, data, and theory. The grid is a realist representation of science, which leads to the idea that a given image is a clear picture, even when obtaining the image involved a large amount of mediation and reconstruction. As the previous chapters made clear, MRI images are not analogical snapshots of the brain. Rather, they are reconstructed out of *k*-space—the virtual space where digitized magnetic resonance signals are stored during data acquisition—a gridlike, modular, repetitive structure (see chapter 3). At the end of a scan, data are processed by algorithms and the final image is created as described below.

The material history of body–brain data visualization across the sciences and the arts goes from the Cartesian two-dimensional coordinate system (the grid), through optical and radio-based technologies, to brain modeling.[6] Key moments and techniques in this history include Étienne-Jules Marey's experiments on chronophotography; Hermann von Helmholtz's measurements of the speed at which electrical impulses traverse the nervous system; X-ray-related technologies such as radar; and photostereosynthesis, a mode of representation invented by the Lumière brothers in 1920 that broke from the logic of conventional pictorial space—a logic that, later, brain imaging further questioned.[7] The focus of this intermezzo, which connects the first and second parts of the book, is on the role of the grid as a matrix of epistemological and aesthetic relationships. This shift is enabled by the Cartesian coordinate system that is simultaneously a drawing device, a graphed image for visualizing the relationship between variables, and the setting for experiments to take place. The grid shifted from being a device enabling us to look at a painting as if seeing a three-dimensional world through a window, to a means of achieving abstraction in modern art in which the grid becomes a medium used against itself to challenge the onlooker's position, to overcome the single viewpoint perspective in favor of the surface.

In science, the grid signals the attempt to reconfigure a set of disciplinary, epistemological, and aesthetic relationships between data and bodies so that the final visual output (the image data) can be effectively read by the different communities of users (physicists and radiologists) to perform decision/interventions on the actual body of the patient. The grid enables complex structures and forms to be broken down into simpler modular elements that can be more easily controlled and reconfigured. The underlying organizational structure of the grid fosters the passage from an anatomical organic body to self-contained atomized components organized in new assemblages disconnected from the whole.[8]

The structure of the Cartesian grid enabled the construction of a new type of visual space in modern art. The grid has since been reapplied to another type of space—that of the human body visualized through biomedical imaging—but what was at stake in this new transposition has not yet been properly acknowledged. With biomedical imaging, representation of the body and brain is less charged with realistic and mimetic elements and more with graphical and geometrical elements, the grid being one of them. What the final image obtained with MRI can and cannot say to the different readers/onlookers (physicist, radiologist, patient) can only be understood if one grasps the sets of epistemological and aesthetic transpositions produced by the grid.

At the beginning of the twenty-first century, genes, cells, bodies, technologies, and research areas are imbued with potential. Is there anything unrepresentable in today's biomedical imaging and neuroscientific research, saturated by data, information, and visualization? Finding ways to convey uncertainty is one of today's most important challenges in data visualization, whether it is stochastic uncertainty, model uncertainty, or uncertainty about the future. The profiling and management of potentiality, uncertainty, and risk is the implicit framing underpinning the development of biomedical imaging technologies and the challenges related to its data-visualization pipeline and output in health care.

From Data to Image: The Grid in Biomedical Imaging

As I discussed in chapters 1 and 4, being able to move between Galison's two traditions of image in physics (the image tradition and the logic tradition) and to produce good quality image data (not just measurements or images) is paramount to enabling physicists to reach out to different communities—radiologists, clinicians, patients, and the lay public. Brain scans produced by biomedical imaging techniques such as MRI embody both image traditions, functioning as authoritative visual objects that are part of a multilayered ensemble of networked techniques and technologies (analog and digital) and human mediations.

MRI images are maps of relaxation rates of the protons of water in each tissue. The generation of images takes place through the repeated acquisition of signals from the body and through the appropriate modulation of the gradient coils. By making sure that each image voxel has a different frequency and/or phase than all the others, it is possible to separate the signals from a single area. Both signal and noise are present in an MRI image: the signal is the voxel or pixel brightness in the image; noise is the random differences in pixel values generated by the patient's body. Like acoustic noise, data noise can get in the way. Noise disturbs the reading of the image and must be eliminated to allow radiologists and clinicians to make a diagnosis.

The process of turning the signal into a meaningful image is far from straightforward. MRI and FFC-MRI both rely on the spin-warp method for turning data into meaningful visual information. No organ is immediately imaged as in a photographic snapshot, but each organ or part of the body to be imaged is preselected, scanned, organized into slices, and gradually reconstructed. Even though MRI allows the acquisition of images of the body in all orientations (sagittal, coronal, axial), the acquisition of data to recompose the image of a head or of another organ is sequential. The body is stimulated with multiple radio-frequency pulses and variable gradients. The MRI scanner acquires (samples) the signal over time. This signal is digitized and stored in the computer, in a matrix known as *k*-space. The computer performs a *discrete Fourier transform* on the data, converting the spatial frequencies into pixel values needed to reconstruct the final image. The spatial frequencies in the MRI image are contained in the *k*-space—the matrix containing the data that come out of the scanner (see figure I.1).

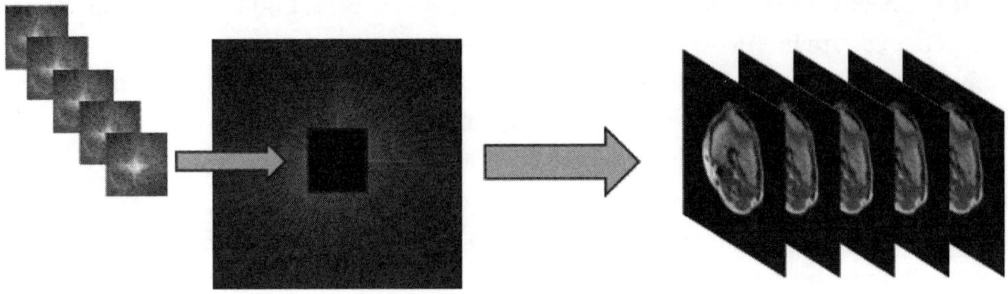

Figure I.1
k-Space. Data-image conversion procedure.

Put simply, the *k*-space holds the raw data before the image is reconstructed. To obtain the image, the *k*-space needs to be charted, which can be done using a variety of methods, including the Cartesian grid. One of the earliest methods for reconstructing the image was the radial sampling of *k*-space data. This method was supplanted by the "spin-warp" technique, which used Cartesian data acquisition. The Cartesian grid exercises a crucial function in the imaging process within laboratory biomedical practice, particularly in relationship to the purification of data from artifacts.

To this day, Cartesian methods remain dominant, but other non-Cartesian approaches (radial and spiral) are gaining ground.[9] The *k*-space can be charted in different sequences to allow the physicist to chart a different area each time. The physicist, however, needs to bear in mind two things: first, beyond a certain distance from the center of the picture, the background noise makes futile any charting of the space in *k*-space; second, given that the magnetic resonance signal is transient and subject to decay, it must be collected as quickly as possible. A bad signal leaves its trace in the image.

The density of the various parts composing an MRI image is represented in *k*-space, obtained by mapping the spatial information onto a frequency scale, a procedure called "frequency encoding."[10] *k*-Space influences the final appearance of an MRI image. Information in the center of *k*-space is responsible for the contrast in MRI images, whereas the spatial resolution of the image is given by the data present in the outer edges of *k*-space. Although the *k*-space and the final MRI image look very different, they contain the same information about the body that underwent the scan procedure. One could convert each representation into the other using the *Fourier transform*. The image, rather than the number, is what radiologists need to read in order to make a diagnosis. The radiological reading concerning the presence or absence of a pathology is achieved through a "'differential analysis' of diverse sets of MRI images... and through cross-referencing different 'inscriptions'—images, diagnostic data, and so on, which together... function to detect and fix pathology."[11] Every MRI image presents only a partial perspective on the body part being scanned. MRI maps a previously framed area of the body, that is, an area that is already organized as if it were an image. Therefore, the procedure of creating MRI images using mathematical functions of transformation is an action incised onto the image rather than onto the object being imaged.

The Cartesian Grid: From Modern Art to Predictive Modeling

Underpinning brain models is the grid—a geometric structure related, like mapping, to location, orientation, and the itinerary of subjectivity. As literary critic Katherine Hayles argues, "When we design technical cognitive systems, we are partially designing ourselves."[12] As an algorithm-based device that reconfigures how bodily data are made available in a visual form, the grid used in biomedicine contributes to transforming how we perceive our bodies and brains and the way in which we then make decisions related to them.

The grid shares with maps the premise that the body and the world are measurable landscapes whose information can be conveyed in various forms. In the early modern period, mapping was associated with research and procedures present in a variety of fields, among them, geography and anatomy. Early study of the anatomical body was the study of spatial organization and the composition of the various elements that made up the body. Self-knowledge was gained through anatomy, through the perceptual grasp (using our eyes, nose, and hands) of the various bodily organs and humors. In peering inside the human body, the anatomist was confronted with the unfamiliar geography of the interior of the body, which was only rarely glimpsed.[13]

Scientists, as well as the general public, are familiar with the practice of plotting information on a system with an *x*-, *y*-, and *z*-axis. People have been arranging data into tables (columns and rows) since at least the second century CE, but the idea of representing quantitative information graphically did not arise until the seventeenth century thanks to the French philosopher and mathematician René Descartes. He developed a two-dimensional coordinate system for displaying values, consisting of a horizontal axis for one variable and a vertical axis for another, primarily as a graphical means of performing mathematical operations. An example of the Cartesian grid being used for quantifying life phenomena is the late nineteenth-century analysis of human and animal motion by physiologist Étienne-Jules Marey, which resulted in the graphic representation of classified parameters. Marey constructed devices to record movements, minimize the flaws of the human sensorium, and construct a new language—the graphic method.[14] Thanks to this method and the invention of chronophotography, Marey was able to translate the phases of movement into a synthetic and abstract visualization in which series of lines, curves, or graphs were set against the Cartesian grid.

The use of the grid in modern art, which can be recognized retrospectively in Marey's practice, is an autoreferential mapping system of surfaces, not a form of pictorial representation. The art historian Rosalind Krauss describes the grid as "a transfer in which nothing changes place. The physical qualities of the surface … are mapped onto the aesthetic dimensions of the same surface."[15] In its precise geometrical order, therefore, the grid eliminates the center, any hierarchical order, any reference and inflection. Krauss conceives the grid as a spatiotemporal structure underlying artistic modernity.

The Cartesian coordinate system opened the way to the development of the graphed images that eventually led to the digital grid, the structure that underpins the scans for visualizing body and brain anatomies and functions. The graphic method enabled the schematic visualization of data extracted and abstracted from the body. Borck, the historian of science and technology, coined the concept of "vital abstraction" to address "a form of theorizing that anchors the brain model in empirical data but abstracts it from biological, organic, or morphological specificity in order to model the brain's activity."[16]

The process of abstracting from the vitality of the organ/phenomenon under examination is interesting to study in reference to brain images. In the early days of neuroscience, scientists attempted to read and make sense of functional images like positron emission tomography (PET) and functional MRI (fMRI) as if they were anatomical images like X-ray images. Anatomy and metabolism (blood flow, oxygen consumption, and so on) were related by means of a visual (optical) comparison between the brain scan and the paper anatomical atlas. The two representations of the brain were compared by the researcher's eye. This is the same kind of optical reading that also occurred at the time of Mallard, before the availability of statistics and powerful computers.

The "optical" reading was superseded by a digital way of reading brain scans made possible by the Talairach system. This coordinate grid system, developed in the early 1980s (when spin warp was invented), is used to describe the location of brain structures that become "activated" during neuroimaging. Because MRI scans vary due to differences in brain features (size and shape) and slice orientation, it is useful to "normalize" a brain (that is, to translate, rotate, scale, and warp it) to roughly match a standard template image. The location of brain structures is reported using the Talairach digital grid. This system uses Cartesian coordinates to describe the distance of each brain region from the anterior commissure, the origin of Talairach space. With Talairach, the brain and scan become digital grids (a set of values in a coordinate space) rather than regions to be correlated.[17]

The logic of probabilistic thinking has been facilitated by the passage from the analog to the digital and from a human observer using an optical instrument to a virtual one using data.[18] Database logic and probabilistic thinking are at work in the making of brain images. Atlases function like classification systems that reveal or hide particular aspects of knowledge. In this way, the onlooker is prompted to consider quantitative values within a register of possibilities rather than as absolute values.

Designing, analyzing, and interpreting structural and functional MRI data is challenging mainly because MRI and fMRI research brings together ideas from a number of fields including physics, engineering, medical imaging, statistics, Bayesian inference, and cellular and systems biology. Thomas Bayes, the originator of Bayesian inference, was an eighteenth century statistician known for having an approach to prediction that contrasted with the frequentist one based exclusively on observed frequency of a given event in past data. For Bayesian inference, we first need to form an initial estimate of the problem and then, as we gather more information related to the problem, we update our first estimate. The final prediction is a combination of the initial estimate and the information acquired from new data. For example, in the case of brain images, Bayesian inference is used to decide whether a portion of the brain image belongs to white or gray matter. Researchers use a probabilistic approach to determine the information given in the voxel of the image and create tissue probability maps. Prior knowledge about the tissue and current data are both expressed as distributions, which means that the presence of variance or error is always a possibility.

Although the most advanced approaches to neuroimaging use time graphs for predictive modeling, the coordinate system still works as the backbone for reconstructing the image from digitized signals in biomedical imaging. Statistical graphics was one of the earliest attempts to analyze and visualize quantitative data. Whereas statistics and data analysis procedures generally yield their output in numeric or tabular form, graphical techniques allow such results to be displayed as some sort of picture. They include plots such as scatterplots, histograms, and probability plots. The scatterplot uses Cartesian coordinates to display values for two variables in a set of data. This is the most common visualization method and is used in FFC-MRI. Across centuries, the scatterplot shifted its focus from spatial organization in the seventeenth and eighteenth centuries to multivariate distribution and correlation in the late nineteenth and twentieth centuries.

Data can be described, explained, or predicted. All three processes use statistics but in a different way. Explanatory modeling applies statistics to data for testing causal hypotheses about theoretical ideas; predictive modeling is the process of applying a statistical model or data-mining algorithm to data predictions. Being able to distinguish between these two ways of using statistics is important in scientific practice, although it is difficult because the two are often conflated.[19] The gap is between the explanation of a phenomenon at the conceptual level and the ability to generate predictions at the measurable level. Ultimately, predictive and explanatory modeling embody different approaches to managing uncertainty.

With Bayesian inference, there are two challenges: first, the tendency of humans to interpret chance correlations as cause–effect patterns; second, the difficulty in dealing with unforeseen situations that never previously occurred in the data at our disposal. Despite these challenges, Bayesian inference remains the best approach to prediction because it relies on a mix of data, statistics, and human skill/intuition. Predictive modeling can use machine-learning techniques to form predictions from brain graphs of unseen samples of subjects or cognitive states. Machine-learning techniques can capture patterns with good generalization ability, but the model with a priori probability values is made by humans building on, for example, medical data and records. Furthermore, predictions always have a degree of uncertainty and therefore should be expressed as a probability rather than as a yes/no alternative. Our task, as the statistician Nate Silver would say, is to learn to live in an uncertain world in which a straightforward yes or no answer is not always possible or recommendable.[20]

FFC-MRI, like other risk technologies in health care, has a specific relationship with the present and future dimension when it comes to how it manages uncertainty and enables the calculation of risks/probabilities to make predictions. As discussed in chapter 4, FFC-MRI assists researchers in the quest for biomarkers to enable the early diagnosis of certain conditions before they become symptomatic. The management of uncertainty is the horizon in which biomedical imaging technologies such as FFC-MRI are inscribed.

In her genealogical study of the "politics of possibility" at work in security techniques and technologies (algorithms, biometrics, data visualization), Louise Amoore argues that "what matters is not so much a question of whether or how the world is more dangerous, more uncertain, or less safe but how specific representations of risks, uncertainty, danger, and security are distinctively writing the contours of that world."[21] At its core, predictive analytics encompasses a variety of statistical techniques (including machine learning, predictive modeling, and data mining) and uses statistics to predict future outcomes. The relationship with the present and future dimension shapes how risks/probabilities are calculated to make predictions, for example, in the world of biomedical physics applied to health care.

The anticipatory logic is what Amoore criticizes: "The specific modality of risk that I address ... acts not strictly to prevent the playing out of a particular course of events on the basis of past data tracked forward into probable futures but to pre-empt an unfolding and emerging event in relation to an array of possible projected futures."[22]

Uncertainty is incorporated into decision making in the present. Authoritative decisions are taken not on the basis of what is known, but on the basis of risk profiling, scenario building, algorithmic modeling, and data analysis. Algorithms, which Amoore defines as "mathematical maps of associational relationships,"[23] are not informed by past historical data but operate by making multiple correlations among contingent events seeking to anticipate future ones. The model departs from the standard distribution of data in a bell curve, which is the graph used to depict a normal distribution for a variable.

The theoretical reflections put forth by Amoore gain concreteness when applied to a variety of contexts from state security to the world of health care. Today, understanding the condition of health or disease of a patient depends on a massive amount of data (anatomical, physiological, molecular, and environmental) that is analyzed using a predictive model approach. The result is a virtual patient acting as a model that enables clinicians to predict the optimal treatment personalized to an individual patient.[24] What counts is not the accuracy of data but the kinds of correlations and associations that one can draw across them. What matters is not whether a predicted neurodegenerative condition manifests itself or not, but that one is prepared to proactively address it.

Statistics and graphs continue to be methods of analyzing and visualizing data to manage uncertainty in biomedical physics applied to health care. The visual output produced by FFC-MRI is a graph expressing dispersion curves. One curve, the T_1 dispersion curve, has a shape and a typical behavior depending on the sample. The molecular dynamics of the sample affect the behavior of the curve. The aesthetics of the curve—aesthetics as the science of what is sensed and imagined—is an instance of *profiling* a condition of pathology in the organism. The absence or difficulty of establishing a direct correlation between the visual output (the profiles) and the phenomenon under investigation (a condition of pathology) is present with FFC-MRI as it is with other probabilistic biomedical imaging technologies.

Aesthetics comes into play when discussing the T_1 curve but also the meaning of image-data quality for different professionals (physicists, biologists, and clinicians).

Beauty is a word often used to talk about quality at different levels, such as when it comes to signal-to-noise ratio, the quality of the signal itself, the final visual output, and the shape of the dispersion curve in FFC-MRI. One of the key challenges facing researchers is what kind of information one wants to extract from the dispersion curve, for a change in the curve's shape is not necessarily directly related to something happening in the tissue; in biology, several different pathways may lead to the same kind of change in the dispersion curve. The form of the profiles acts as an interface between research and the clinic: the shape of the T_1 curve affects the decisions taken on the patient's body.

Scattered data points can be organized into patterns of distribution to produce a statistical profile whose visual manifestation is a graph, or a curve based on the Cartesian grid. The problem, as Amoore says, is that "the form of the object—once conceived as points and lines—can precipitate effects even when the body of the object is itself absent."[25] If the Gaussian algorithm or the bell curve were the means to govern anomaly through the logics of normal distribution, predictive algorithms are the new form of perception whose horizon is that of the possible future to manage and control. In the world of health care, in which biomedical imaging technologies are made to operate, the logic is that of prediction and probabilistic thinking. In a post-Newtonian world dominated by entangled objects at the subatomic level, phenomena are not necessarily connected by a cause–effect relationship. Although the visual has long been considered the domain of algorithms and interfaces, the interest now is increasingly focused also on haptic and entangled forms of relationships between humans and algorithms.[26]

To conclude, whether within the world of software design, risk management, or biomedical data visualization, the Cartesian grid is one of the computational devices giving shape to this world in which uncertainty is framed against a coordinate system of constants and variables in space and time. We interact with the world by means of the interface that gives us the boundaries of the world. Now, thanks to electronic technology, we are a variable in the system we interact with. The interface becomes extended beyond a realm graspable by our sensorial apparatus.

Although we might feel able to break out of the time and space constraints of the Cartesian coordinate system, the grid is still the underlying structure of every interface we interact with, including the image data of our brains and bodies.[27] The grid has the power to associate and transform data that, taken individually, might not have any intrinsic meaning. The grid is the backbone used to structure one specific type of looking in atomic physics and another in medical prediction and intervention. Both types of looking are lined up on the same data. A different action, though, aligns this second type of looking and the purpose for which it will be used. Although the first action is aimed at turning data into information that can be visualized by the radiologist, the second is aimed at introducing the categories of risk and probability within the diagnostic reading. Uncovering this double action is the first move toward a better understanding of our lives in the grid.

II Art–Science Collaboration

5 Challenging the Neurorealism Fallacy through the Arts

> I was born a sculptor, drawn by the magnetic resonance produced in the white darkness of the scanner, as I slept. My head became detached from my body, freeing my brain of its weight and allowing it to enter the mirrors. But when I began to polish marble to build anamorphoses, with optics and precision, I was no longer either in this field or in the same place as in the beginning.
>
> —Marc Didou, biography

Visualizing and Sonifying the Living Brain

Believed by Aristotle to be a cold sponge that mops up the heat generated by our thinking and feeling heart, the dissected brain appears a lifeless, bloodless object, its internal workings unavailable to our sight.[1] From antiquity to the modern age, medical practice has mainly studied life via death through dissection or by three-dimensional models.[2] In the late nineteenth century, tissue staining techniques and microscopy enabled the identification of brain cells, thus allowing the biologist Camillo Golgi (1843–1926) and the pathologist Santiago Ramón y Cajal (1852–1934) to see structure inside this organ. Since then, increasingly sophisticated techniques have allowed us to visualize the brain in action. The move from physical models to digital computer simulations encouraged a visual rather than tactile engagement with the brain.[3]

The electrical signals, localized nature, and cellular structure of the nervous system were known well before the advent of brain imaging techniques, since at least 1850 when Hermann von Helmholtz managed to measure the speed at which electrical impulses traversed the nervous system. In the 1920s, the electrical activity of human brains began to be recorded graphically using electroencephalography (EEG), seemingly providing direct access to neural activity.

The discovery of electricity in the body and brain prompted artists and scientists to work toward sonifying measurable phenomena such as brain waves. The first transformation of data from an EEG into sound was in 1934, when the neurophysiologist Edgar Adrian and the psychiatrist Hans Berger were able to prove the diagnostic potential of EEG through sonification.[4] Many more EEG experiments followed, both in science and in the arts. In the early 1960s, the artist Robert Morris made *Self-Portrait (EEG)* (1963), a recording of his own brain activity monitored through EEG. He then translated his own mental activity into another medium by creating visual poems whose form was akin to musical scores.

At some point, however, visualization took over. The possibility of visualizing the living brain at work thanks to technologies such as fMRI gained momentum and captured the public's attention. Functional imaging of the brain is a step ahead of simple visualization, which, as the historian of science and technology Cornelius Borck points out, was already possible with phrenological charts and 3D models. In fMRI, colors are used to encode levels of brain activity, and crisp pictures of the brain captured during engagement in cognitive tasks foster the idea of the brain's vitality.[5] It should not be surprising therefore that so many artists interested in neuroscience are still more enticed by the possibility of visualizing data than by turning data into other sensorial outputs.

In this chapter I examine a range of art practices (from drawing and sculpture to virtual reality [VR] and bio art) to highlight the visual incarnation of the neurorealism fallacy, which is connected to the problem of moving from data to their visualization. Biomedical imaging-based research in neuroscience is not inherently reductionist. In chapters 2, 3, and 4, I demonstrated how scientists themselves can be attentive to the construction of visual practices and their meaning.

Here, I pay attention to the material elements of neuroscientific research that are (or are not) remediated by artists, showing how artworks are not merely a means to engage the wider public with neuroscientific discourse but rather how they can question the spell cast by the extreme image, which is one of the incarnations of the neurorealism fallacy. Do neuroscience–art projects reproduce this fallacy at the visual level?

The Neurorealism Fallacy and Its Visual Incarnation

The Self in Neuroculture

The difficulties related to the transformation of neurological data into visual output are at the core of scholarly debate and artistic practices that engage with the neurosciences. It is through images of the brain that the culture and politics of neuroscience become visible, solidify, and spread across the wider public arena beyond the closed circuit of neuroscientific discourse. As Joseph Dumit says, "What do I believe (what do I know) about mental illness, sexual difference, my own cognitive abilities, brain patterns and identities? I am fascinated and horrified by the possibility posed here, of a world in which technology can tell me who I truly am."[6] This process gives birth to *neuroculture*, which uses neurosciences' tools and knowledge to understand sociocultural phenomena and human behaviors.[7]

Brain imaging has seized the public's imagination, bringing a grasp of the materiality of thinking closer than ever before. Through visual imagery, mass media, and popular scientific magazines, the concept of self has been presented as if it were increasingly dependent on the biology of the brain, to the point at which the category of personhood has been substituted by brainhood, the ontological belief that our sense of subjectivity is given by our brain only rather than by any other bodily part.[8] Brainhood is a way of organizing a specific politics of the subject, one centered on the effort to articulate subjectivity by drawing upon neuroscience and neurology.[9] This emphasis on the brain becomes part of a new style of neuroscientific thought, creating areas of knowledge production such as neuroaesthetics, neuromarketing, neuroliterary criticism, neurolaw, and even the way in which subjectivity, ethics, and politics are conceived.[10]

Neurorealism is the belief that brain scans are visual evidence of brain activity, despite the complexity inherent to data acquisition and image creation.[11] This fallacy, discussed by Dumit in his examination of brain imaging, is reinforced in visual practices by use of the "extreme image": the rendering of neuroscientific scan data into visually striking and persuasive brain images presented as if they were a direct material index of the analog magnetic signal. Artistic interventions based on or inspired by neuroscience certainly have the merit of taking brain imaging outside the scientific laboratory into the wider public arena. However, it remains to be determined whether these artistic practices put forward a critique of the brain–self consubstantiality and challenge the politics of neurologization that accompanies it. Do artists trace configurations of subjectivity alternative to the cerebral subject by creating another politics of the neural image or a different iconography of the brain? Or do they simply carry the laboratory-stabilized image interpretations out into the world?

Certain neuroscience-based art practices foster a counterpolitics of the neural image to the one put forth within the trope of the cerebral subject. This alternative is not an exclusive prerogative of artists. Scientists are by necessity often attentive to the construction of visual practices and their meaning. The neurorealism fallacy is therefore not the fate of neurosciences when the scientific community attends reflexively to the historical epistemology of brain imaging.[12]

The technical explanation of how MRI scans are obtained from data in chapters 2 and 3 foregrounds the examination of the neurorealism fallacy conducted in this chapter. The hand-painted image of the mouse (see chapter 2) reminds us of two crucial issues in biomedical imaging. First, it points at the enduring importance of human eyes and hands even in an age increasingly characterized by the pervasive computerization of data imaging and visualizing. Second, it is a reminder of the frictions between mechanical data-image reproduction and the embodied human interpretative labor. Each component of MRI introduces its own degradation, loss, or in some cases, addition of information. In this respect, the onlooker needs to be assisted by the technology and when necessary intervene in several stages of image creation from data.

Since the early 1980s, computer-aided visualization of the body and brain for research and diagnostic purposes has steadily improved. The procedure for obtaining readable and diagnostically useful pictures became increasingly standardized and seemingly transparent and therefore not necessary for continued consideration. However, the epistemological role of biomedical imaging highlighted by Mallard and his team comes again to the foreground, albeit outside the laboratory, thanks to the arts. Artists interested in working with neuroscience, its instruments, and its findings look again at the scans obtained through biomedical imaging, perhaps reframing the question of what those scans stand for and what they give access to. Studying the living brain in action, using techniques such as fMRI, will be at the center of scholarly interest and art–science projects for a long time to come. In fact, artists and designers involved in collaborative projects with neuroscientists are currently shifting their focus away from brain scans and portraiture to living tissue such as neural cells.

The Extreme Image and the Neurorealism Fallacy

Dumit defines neurorealism as the belief that behavioral, social, cultural, or psychological claims are proven only when there is evidence of neurological activity corresponding to them.[13] Those claims are given further plausibility when they become imaginable through the visual representation of a brain scan, which is believed to be a direct representation of neural activity. For example, Dumit compares two images from a longitudinal study on social immaturity: a scatterplot of data and the final bright-colored brain scan (the extreme image). The difference between the two images is evident. The scatterplot highlights the large variation within each group being contrasted, with considerable overlap between the groups such that there is no way to know which group an individual subject is in.[14] Dumit unveils the arbitrariness of the framework used to attach a behavioral label such as "immaturity" to a biological difference in the brain. The extreme image reduces the scatterplot data to contrasting categories rendered as absolutely opposed to each other visually. Brain images exemplify certain categories, enabling the construction of narratives that reproduce the neurorealism fallacy.

Color coding was originally introduced in brain imaging for telling at a glance how the counting-rate pattern in scans varied from point to point[15] (see chapter 2). Today, coloring brain images can drastically change the visual impact of data. Represented in color, brain scans risk losing their characteristic of being image data and instead become extreme images. The variations in numbers are turned into qualitative fields to visually highlight differences: "no matter how small the actual difference in average change, the visual differences will appear stark," writes Dumit.[16] Although not all visualizations of the brain fall into Dumit's category of the extreme image, his argument illustrates how difficult it is to transform data into meaningful information that can be correctly interpreted. Improving the final image from the scatterplot of data might not be sufficient to overcome the neurorealism fallacy. The extreme image is an epistemic object that embodies a specific framework for thinking about man in the world.

To fully grasp what is at stake epistemologically when brain scans are used to nurture neurorealism, it is useful to recall the philosopher of science Sellars's distinction between the "scientific" image and the "manifest" image of the man in the world (see chapter 1).[17] According to Sellars, there is a clash between the scientific and manifest frameworks used to describe and explain the position of the man in the world. According to the manifest framework, humans are beings equipped with intentionality, free will, thoughts, and desires. According to the scientific one, they are assemblages of genes, molecules, and atoms—physical and biochemical systems under the influence of environmental variables.

The two frameworks differ in one aspect: the manifest image does not postulate imperceptible entities or principles in order to explain perceptible things. Neuroscience, for example, by postulating ways in which cognitive and emotional processes correspond to certain entities (e.g., neuronal networks and synapses) and conveying this belief through a brain scan, slowly constructs a new framework that claims to be a description and explanation of subjectivity and its position in the world. The extreme image does not necessarily coincide with the scientific image. Rather, it is the exaggeration of the perspective put forth by both the scientific and the manifest image. One will never reach a complete description and explanation of the man in the world. This is why we need to keep both views in focus, to avoid the fallacy embodied by the extreme image.

The stereoscopic vision enables Sellars to challenge the myth of the given, that is, the belief in self-evident, epistemic objects.[18] Brain scans act as the given, which grounds any cognitive and/or emotive condition that becomes real only if it can be made visible through brain imaging techniques. The myth of the given, in this case, is the belief that a specific cognitive, emotive condition is a brain property—a neurophysiological condition—and in so far as it is neurological, it is real and acquires further strength when embodied in extreme images of brain structure and function.

Challenging the Neurorealism Fallacy through the Arts

Brainhood has become a powerful visual trope in contemporary culture and mass media. The brain is a major fashionable icon across literature, fiction films, politics, and marketing as scholars Fernando Vidal and Francisco Ortega explain in their critique of neurocentrism: "Most neuroscientists are certainly modest about what they do. The media 'translations' of their results often inflate or fictionalise their significance."[19] Neuroethics researchers Eric Racine, Sarah Waldman, Jarrett Rosenberg, and Judy Illes have identified three key trends in media coverage of neurotechnologies: neuroessentialism, which connotes representations of the brain as the essence of a person (brainhood); neuropolicy, which captures the deployment of brain research to support political agendas, and neurorealism, which refers to the use of neuroscientific information to make phenomena seem objective or real.[20] A question like "What defines us as humans?" is believed to undergo a profound reconsideration thanks to neuroscientific research.

On closer inspection, however, brainhood is a cultural figure of the modern self rather than simply an outcome of contemporary neuroscience. This perspective reverses the belief that neuroscience has transformed our concept of subjectivity, suggesting instead that brainhood is the most recent epiphany of a modernist conception of the self. The modern self, historian of science and psychology scholar Vidal argues, is now believed to be located in the brain; the belief in the coincidence between the brain and the self was already present in the philosophical reflections around subjectivity pursued in the modern era (Descartes, Locke, Kant).

The artistic community is a prominent actor in the public arena, where scientific discourses on the brain merge with the views of the lay public. Although challenging neurorealism might not be the intention of artists working with brain imaging and neurons, certain artistic practices may enable a critical engagement with the problem of the extreme image highlighted by Dumit. However, artists must be aware of the pitfalls of simply transporting neurorealism from the laboratory to the public via artistic media, such as dumbing down science or producing bad art.

In what follows I offer the reader some examples of how contemporary artists have engaged with the tools, concepts, findings, methodology, and visual imagery of the neurosciences to conduct a critique of neurocultures, rethink their own practice through a new medium (brain imaging), or explore the concept of life and becoming via neural tissues. I do not aim to give a comprehensive survey of the relationship between the neurosciences, brain imaging, and the arts. Such an enterprise would not be feasible considering that contemporary neuroscience-based artistic projects are constantly evolving, presented as performances, concerts, or happenings, and often difficult to track down. Later in this chapter I discuss how the interdisciplinary field of cybernetics, funded in the late 1940s and further developed in the 1970s, penetrated into arts and culture. Since the mid-1990s, in fact, bio artists have reappraised and elaborated the esthetics and concepts of cybernetics—particularly of the second order, championed by Heinz von Foerster, with its emphasis on reflexivity and the role of the observer within the system. Second-order cybernetics continues to exercise an influence on contemporary artists by giving them the tools to think about the body–brain as a biologic–machinic system without being reductionist.

The Scan Portrait

Since the 1990s, artists such as Susan Aldworth, Suzanne Anker, Annie Cattrell, Justine Cooper, Marilène Oliver, Marta de Menezes, Angela Palmer, and Louise Wilson, among many others, have been rethinking portraiture in light of research developments in neuroscience. These artists certainly have the merit of taking brain imaging outside the scientific laboratory into the wider public arena. A few of them critically engage with the reductionism implied by the concept of the cerebral subject both in the laboratory and in mass media, simultaneously lingering on a modern concept of selfhood. This is the case, for instance, of Aldworth's *Cogito Ergo Sum 3* (2006) work with brain scans (figure 5.1).

The artist, an experimental printmaker and filmmaker, explores and creatively reassembles the different personal, medical, and scientific narratives around human identity, connecting the physical brain with the notion of the self and using neuroscientific imagery to challenge traditional portraiture.

Other artists have used brain scans to create portraits and self-portraits.[21] Rather than for their own merits as works of art, these portraits address the problem of authority in scientific images: Who is entitled to read the image data, and what level of expertise is required? These scan portraits point out the difficulty in conveying that brain

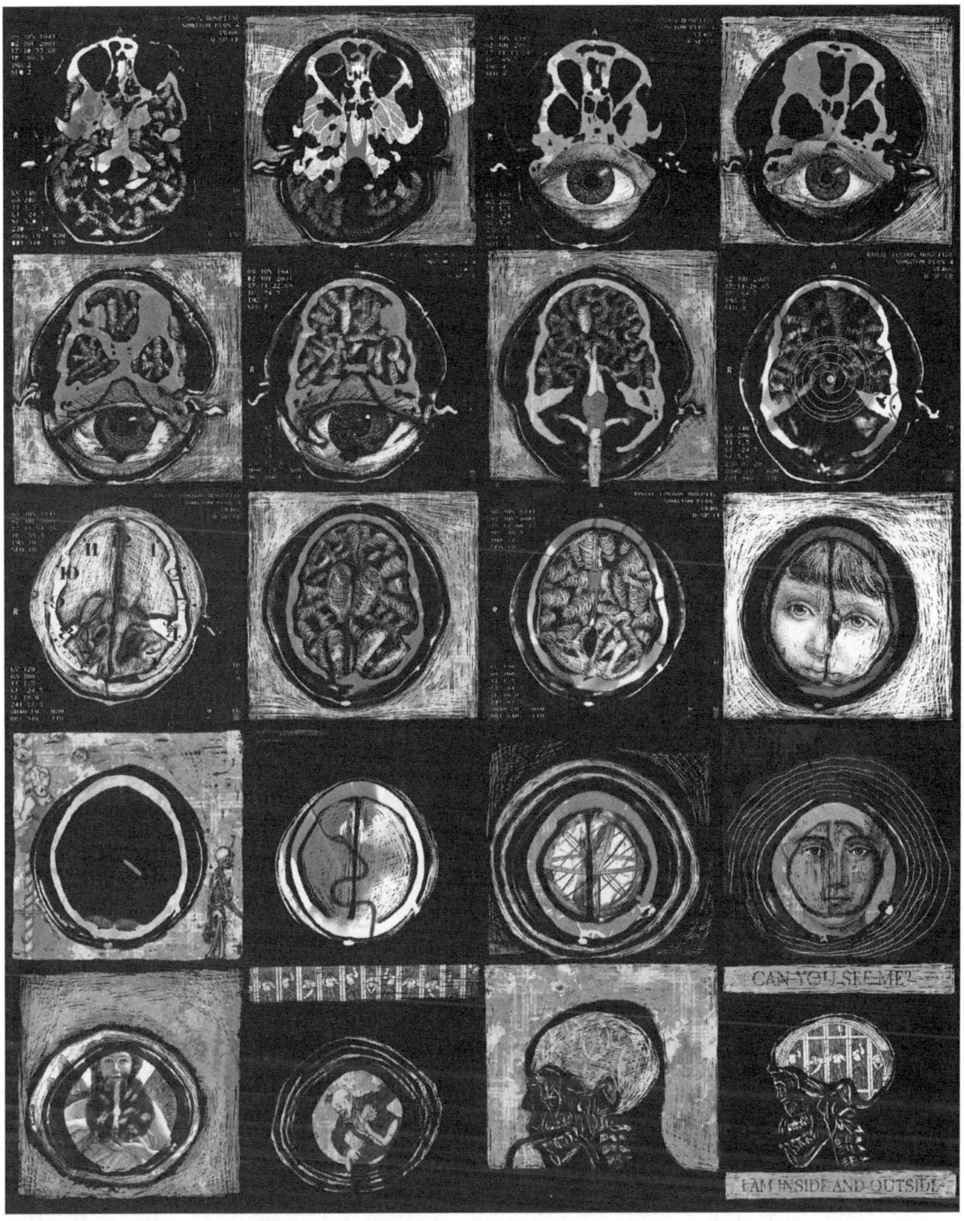

Figure 5.1
Susan Aldworth, *Cogito Ergo Sum 3*. Installation of twenty archival digital prints, 2006.
Source: Courtesy of the artist.

activity is not recorded in real time (So what exactly is recorded and visually conveyed here? What data are left out from the original scatterplot?) and highlight the highly mediated and constructed nature of brain scans.

At the visual level, however, the artist reproduces the ideology of brainhood and the neurorealism fallacy by remaining in the iconographic dimension of brain scans as extreme images that are presented visually as if they were portraits of the self. As much as there is never an innocent eye, nor a perception that is not already an interpretation, neurological data are never given, even when they assume the form of a brain scan. There has to be a theory to make the data into an image. By not engaging with the actual process of generating the scans, artists risk missing the duality intrinsic to brain scans—that of being both images and data.

MRI as a New Medium for Sculpture and Drawing

Several contemporary artists, such as Marc Didou, Bernd Lintermann, Annie Cattrell, Andrew Carnie, Marilène Oliver, Jeanine Braeker, Angela Palmer, Katharine Dawson, and William Kentridge, are not interested in the claims that brain imaging enables us to make through its scans. Rather than using brain imaging to rethink portraiture, they use it as a creative medium to explore the concept of space, both physical and mental, actual and virtual (Didou, Lintermann, Oliver), or as a way to remediate drawing (Carnie, Kentridge).

Although they have a different aesthetic and goals, Oliver, Lintermann, and Didou all use MRI to explore the concept of negative space—the empty or open space around an object that contributes to the object's definition—the space created by mirrors, light and shadow, emptiness, and the data world. Modern and contemporary sculptural practice is moving beyond such concepts of the body as mass, gravity, and structure, and engaging increasingly with negative space. Didou is interested in MRI not as a brain imaging technique but as a new medium for creating sculpture, challenging the cliché of the sculptor as demiurge.[22] MRI operates as a scientific and artistic instrument to turn signals into sculpture. The acoustics of MRI combined with temporary blindness inside the scanner turns MRI into a vibration drawing (the MRI scan), transparent and monochrome, that neither the artist's hand nor eye could have observed or drawn. From the anamorphosis-based *Skulls* series (see the introduction) to *Gisant* (2007–2010), a sculpture made of steel and acrylic sheets that revisits the aesthetics of MRI slices (figure 5.2), Didou creates a perceptual play between positive and negative space—actual and virtual space—without using any digital techniques. The typical gestures of the classical sculptor-demiurge of adding and taking away material become, through MRI and anamorphosis, a gesture of breaking up the material object to recompose it into an image.

We have an intuitive understanding of what space is, which is not the coordinate system of the Cartesian space, but the space we walk through, in which we touch objects and which we can communicate about. In contrast, negative space is a mental construction unsupported by common sense. Intuitively, one could say that negative

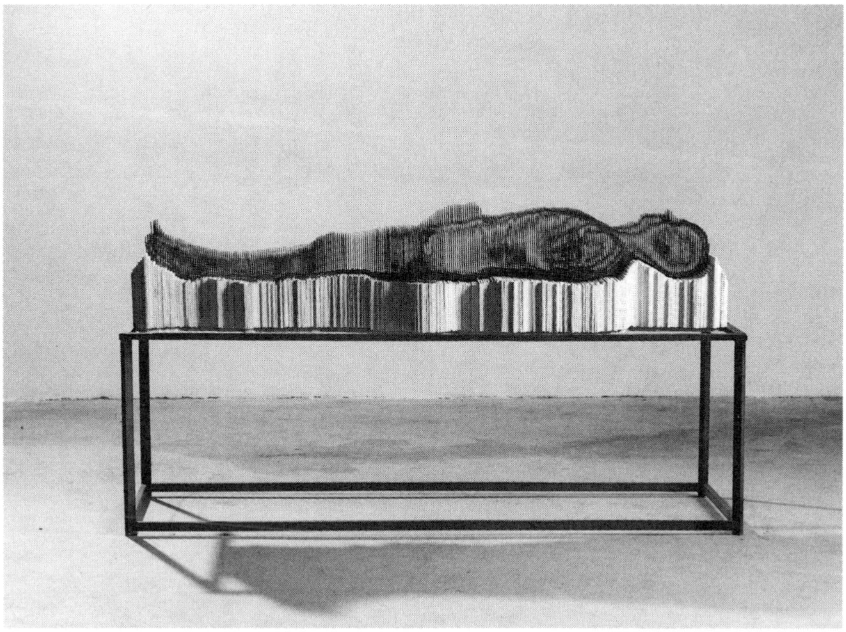

Figure 5.2
Marc Didou, *Gisant*, steel and altuglas, 2007–2010.
Source: Courtesy of the artist.

space is like having an incomplete representation of an object, so negative space is a subtraction. In computer graphics, negative space is constructed as solid geometry: one creates objects by cutting out the form of positive objects.

Lintermann's interest in MRI starts with the question of how space is constructed. MRI is perceived by us as a slice of a 3D object. What one looks at actually is a surface of a negative form. The MRI space is not a 3D object but a quantized space: you think you have a continuous object but there is information missing. As both an artist and a scientist committed to public engagement with the brain and neuroscience, Lintermann works on interactive and generative computer systems based upon stereoscopic, panoramic, or cave systems.[23] The interactive installation *MRT* (2019), which was part of the collective exhibition *Negative Space* at ZKM, is created with computer graphics, MRI, and autostereoscopic display (figure 5.3).

A time-of-flight (ToF) camera mounted on top of the screen detects the position and surface of the viewer's head while the viewer sits on a stool looking at the screen. Software automatically transfers these data to the virtual head on screen. The data from an MRI scan, which is recorded in advance and not related to the viewer sitting in front of the screen, is visualized simultaneously to the data from the ToF camera. When the actual and virtual heads are aligned, the feeling of an MRI scan happening in real time is impossible to avoid. Thus, the representation of the data space of MRI electromagnetism is a variable that directly depends on the actual space occupied by one's own head.

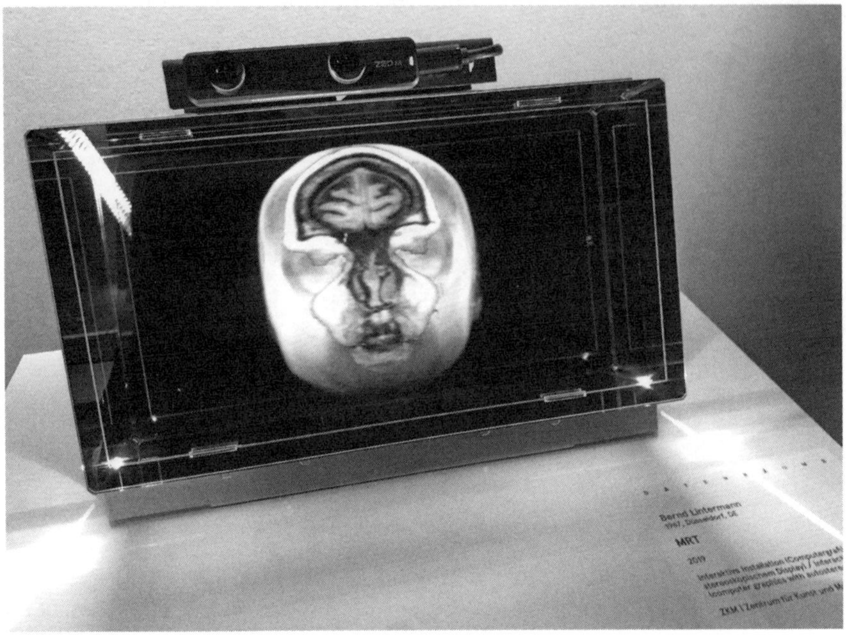

Figure 5.3
Bernd Lintermann, *MRT* installation view. Interactive installation with autostereoscopic display, 2019.
Source: Courtesy of the artist and ZKM | Hertz-Lab.

Deep Connection and *Space Invaders* (laser-cut coroplast sculpture and virtual reality) are the result of a collaboration between artist Marilène Oliver (see chapter 2) and sound designer and composer Gary James Joynes for the *Dyscorpia* exhibition.[24] *Space Invaders* consists of laser-cut coroplast sculptures with embedded oculus VR hardware made with the same high-resolution full-body 3D MRI scan data sets (figure 5.4).

The experience of walking around, dwelling inside, and relating to virtual life-size bodies in a virtual space is at the core of this multimedia installation. The experience though is first aural and then visual/tactile. The interactive soundscape obtained from MRI scanner recordings comes from different spatial points and in different intensities—a high-pitched hum, then a low-pitched deep hum at the bottom, and then something else vibrating through one's back. When exhibition visitors enter *Deep Connection*, they see a scanned body lying prone in midair (figure 5.5). They can measure up their personal physical bodies against the virtual ones.

The experience of trespassing the threshold between real and virtual bodies enacts a certain power dynamic. Access and agency, namely, remain on the side of human bodies: it is they who can use a virtual hand to trigger a 4D data set and experience the heartbeat and the breath in the life-size body of *Deep Connection*.

Inspired by the Visible Human Project and by medical imaging technologies, Oliver has always worked with human bodies transformed into digitized data sets in which "time and place don't matter but connections and transfer rates do."[25] MRI data cannot

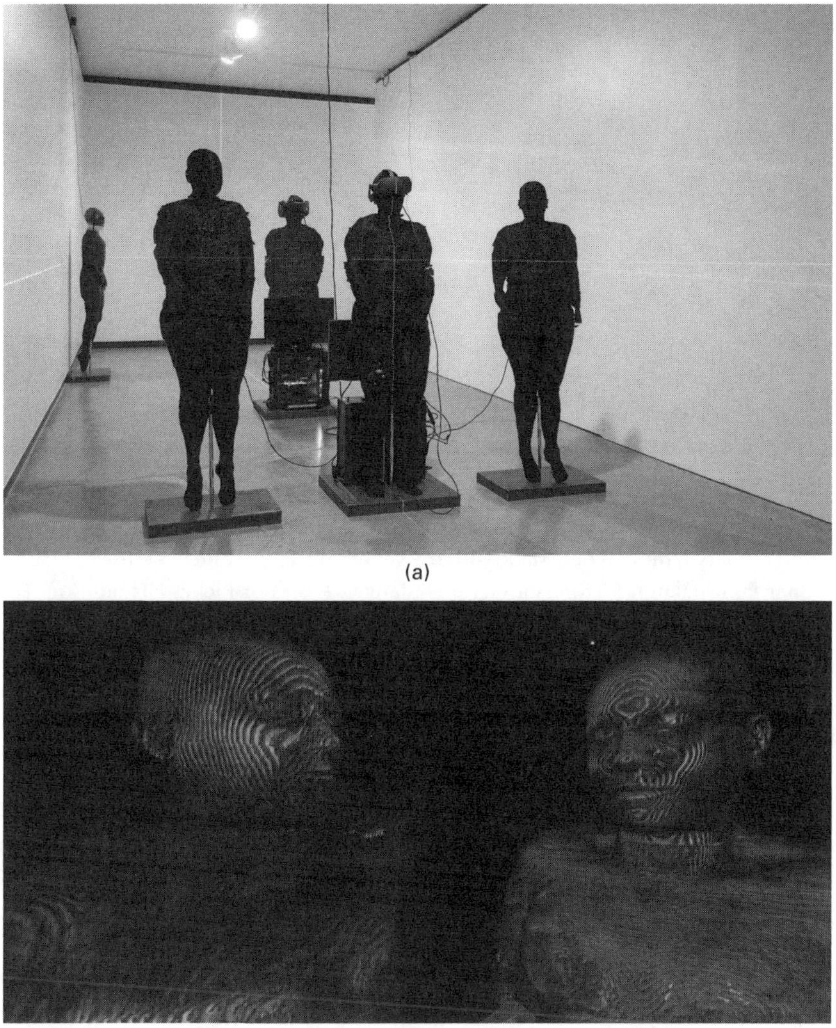

(a)

(b)

Figure 5.4
Marilène Oliver, *Space Invaders*, 2019. (a) and (b) Laser-cut coroplast sculptures, virtual reality, and laser light. Sound by Gary James Joynes. Made with the generous support and expertise of Assistant Professor Kumar Punithakumar, Professor Pierre Boulanger, Professor Richard Thompson, Dr. Chris Hanstock, Peter Seres, Preet Giri, and Madhavi Nimalaratne.
Source: Courtesy of Blaine Campbell.

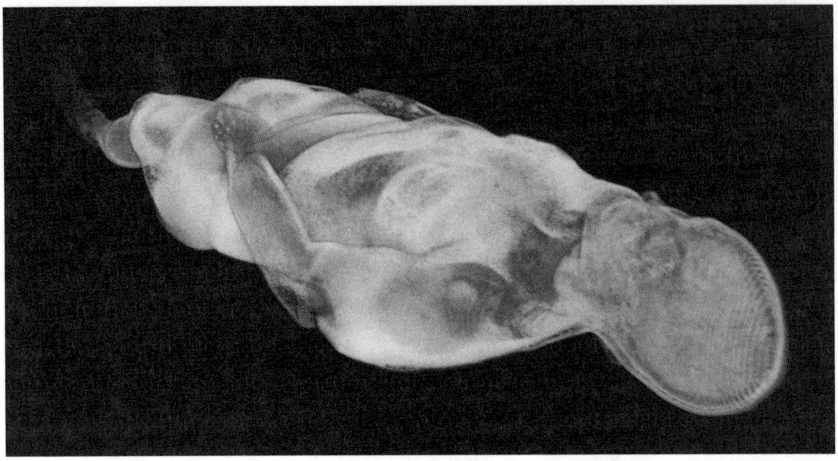

Figure 5.5
Marilène Oliver, *Deep Connection*, 2019. Laser-cut coroplast sculptures, virtual reality, and laser light. Sound by Gary James Joynes. Made with the generous support and expertise of Assistant Professor Kumar Punithakumar, Professor Pierre Boulanger, Professor Richard Thompson, Dr. Chris Hanstock, Peter Seres, Preet Giri, and Madhavi Nimalaratne.
Source: Courtesy of Blaine Campbell. See plate 6.

be easily domesticated for artistic purposes because they are slow to acquire and cannot be reformatted. Therefore, data must be acquired in sections that then can be put back together again. The scan is slow and sequential, implying that the feet are usually acquired fifty minutes after the head, so they do not line up. This is the reason why Oliver used Melanix rather than MRI data sets to create her avatar. Melanix is an anonymized open-source full-body CT scan of a woman who shares with the artist age and body size.

This virtual body has become a way for the artist to address that access to both cutting-edge medical technology and one's own digitized body is a Western privilege. After the experience of temporarily relocating to Angola, Oliver realized that her interest was not about the data per se, but about using anonymized machine-created data to explore and address issues of inequality in relation to distribution of health and digital technology.[26] Leaving the costs aside, the MRI hardware requires at the minimum a stable power supply. One cannot think of simply transferring a technology to any place in the world without inhabiting the place and making the effort to adapt and reinvent certain technologies for it. Bodily medical data become the symbol of digital tech colonialism.

Andrew Carnie and William Kentridge have recurred to brain imaging or neurons as tools with which to rethink the theory and practice of drawing. Carnie's interests extend across neurology, the brain, and the role scientific images and technological interventions (such as organ transplantations) play to construct and challenge the concept of the self. With a long-standing practice of working in and around anatomical drawing and art, Carnie often uses biological material such as dead mosquitoes, fungus spores, agar, and even bodily fluids. His slide-dissolve installation made using two data projectors and

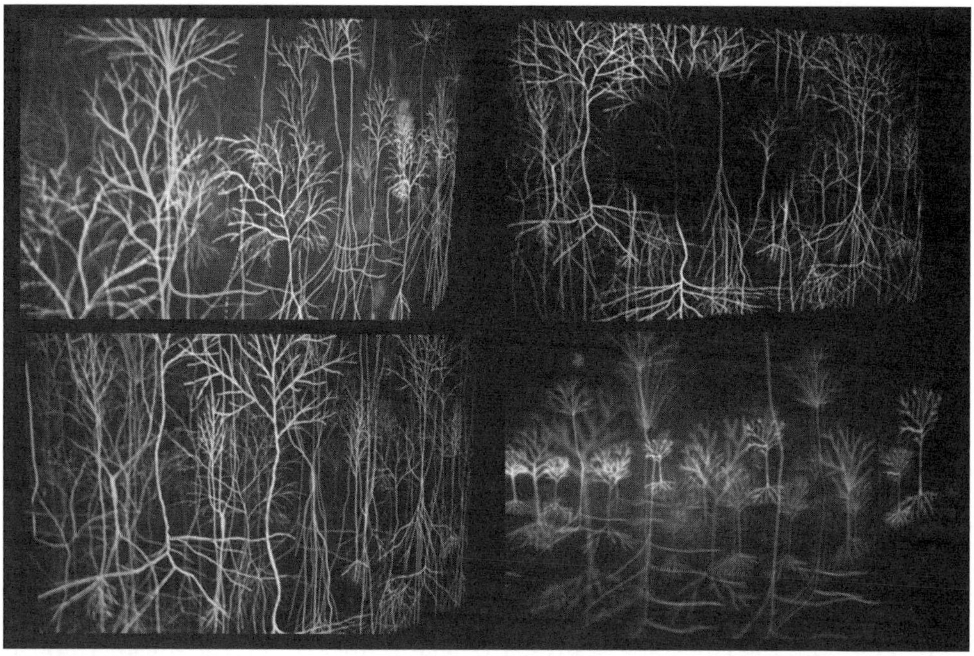

Figure 5.6
Andrew Carnie, *Magic Forest*, 2002. Stills from slide-dissolve work, 35 mm slides, and voile screens. Composite.
Source: Courtesy of the artist. See plate 7.

162 slides, *Magic Forest* (2002), was made for the exhibition *Head On* in dialogue with the neuroscientist Richard Wingate and supported by the Wellcome Trust (figure 5.6).

Based on Cajal's histological drawings, Carnie's multicolored drawings of neurons take viewers on a journey from the skull through the brain to the neurons.[27] *Magic Forest* creates the feeling of being in an ecosystem in which the brain reflects the environment. The exploration of treelike form within the body and brain has been a constant of Carnie's time-based work that connects principles governing nature with the self.[28] Carnie sets himself free from the burden of institutionalized collaborative work, preferring to engage in conversations with scientists and then creating connections among objects, ideas, and experiences. Giving art back a central role to help humans to live in and think through the world, Carnie says, "What I make is not a piece of knowledge, but it might be a mirror to who we are, what we are, and what we might become. I make a 'mirror object' to help us think, a sieve to bring clarity, a map, a device of some sort that allows us to reflect, ponder on the world."[29]

When making *Magic Forest*, Carnie referred to videotapes of developing neurons and Cajal's neuron drawings, which together challenged the idea of the brain as a fixed, wired object. *Magic Forest* engaged with how the brain spreads through the body. Wingate was studying the effect of activating and deactivating the proteins that attract axons—the long, slender projections of neurons that typically conduct electrical impulses (action potentials) away from the body of the neuron to transmit information to other neurons, muscles, and glands. When the proteins are deactivated, the axon gets lost. In *Magic Forest* and successive works, Carnie wanted to get that sense of movement. He photographed the skull, drew the brain, and used a system of projectors to enable the visitor to see down all the layers scanned with the confocal microscope. His drawings, like those of Cajal, are scientific data. The work starts visually inside the skull to then move through neuronal formations. The skull, which was not originally planned to appear in the artwork, was incorporated afterward to give the neural life processes a context, a body.[30]

In the film installation *WEIGHING…and WANTING* (1997), which is part of the *Soho Eckstein* series,[31] Kentridge embarks on a kind of psychotopography by combining the elements of natural and human-built landscapes with the memories, fantasies, and thoughts of the main character who undergoes an MRI scan. Primarily interested in drawing, his practice ranges from sculpture and printing to animation and video installation, with frequent incursions into the imaginary of medical imaging. Kentridge has developed a method of animation in which he shapes single charcoal drawings into sequences on film.[32] He juxtaposes the private and public dimension of mental life with the landscape of his native South Africa during apartheid. Through the process of drawing and erasing, mental life and the landscape outside (and their images) merge. In the film, images of biomedical scans no longer depict the structures/functions of the brain but rather internal states of the mind and external landscape elements.

The metaphor Kentridge employs at the beginning of the film is that of the stone as a brain. The main character (Soho Eckstein) finds a stone and brings it into his house, turning it over in his hands. While Soho is inside the coil undergoing an MRI scan, the stone appears outside again, this time etched with lines that coincide with ones drawn on brain scans to select the slices. The musical score simultaneously reproduces the thumping rhythm of the scanning. The stone is represented visually as if it were the brain of the main character inside the scanner. Slices of his brain are shown merging into memories of landscapes (see figure 5.7).

The interior of the body and the external landscape intermingle constantly, exactly as the manifest and the scientific image of man overlap until they merge for a few instants in a stereoscopic vision. Memories and histories (geographies) are themselves the anatomy and the physiology of the subject. The elements of the anatomical brain are transformed into shapes and forms of places, bodies, objects.

The realm of psychic processes cannot be conflated with the physical space of the brain anatomy visualized in a brain scan. Kentridge constantly evokes, erases, and draws on these brain scans. Like Braeker, Kentridge uses drawing to remind us of the limits of cutting-edge techniques that we often embrace too easily. Although Kentridge is not interested in embarking on a criticism of the neurorealism fallacy, in this work he challenges the conflation between selfhood and brainhood. Kentridge uses brain scans as if they could expose a subject's memories, fantasies, dreams, sorrows, without constructing

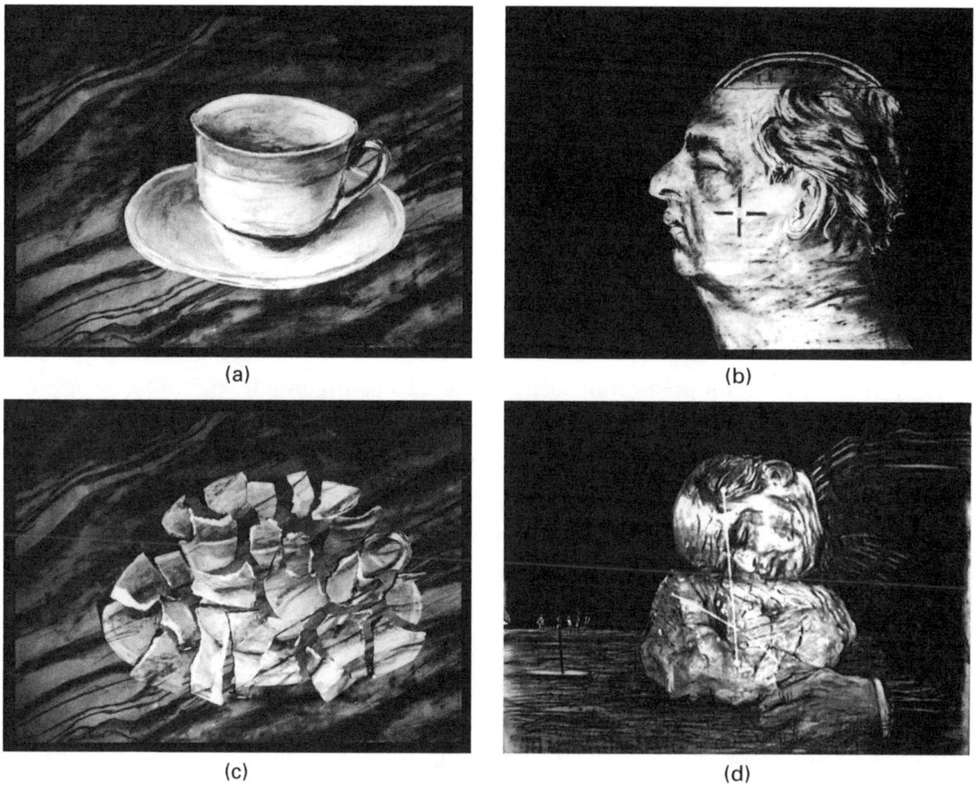

Figure 5.7
William Kentridge, *WEIGHING…and WANTING*, 1997.
Source: Courtesy of the artist and Goodman Gallery. See plate 8.

an image or a theory of the self but erasing the images he creates. He enacts the atomization of the subject's repressed thoughts—scattered thoughts, memories, and feelings. These thoughts are too fast to be conveyed in words, too imperceptible to be recorded by brain imaging and mapped onto scans, so the only way to give them a presence is by drawing them and erasing them constantly. Brain imaging cannot fully describe the reality of the psychic apparatus. Kentridge's gesture of erasing both brain scans and any final attempt to portray the self exposes the impossibility of lingering on any fixed concept of selfhood. Although still bearing upon brain scans and their imagery, Kentridge's erasing gesture succeeds at challenging the neurorealism fallacy at a visual level.

Body–Brain Systems: From Second-Order Cybernetics to Bio Art

Cybernetics as the Science of the Brain

Many advances have been made within neuroscience toward avoiding simply transporting neurorealism from the laboratory to the public, mainly thanks to the improvement of algorithms that turn functional data from the brain into visual output. But the ghost of neurorealism still troubles neuroscience, as Borck points out: "The visual cultures of present-day functional imaging have certainly left the initial reductionist realism behind and have opened up to the multiple opportunities presented by sophisticated visualization algorithms; but the question remains in how far this imaging culture is still haunted by the concrete presence of activity visualized as a structural entity."[33]

Perhaps neurorealism could have not been the destiny of functional brain imaging visual culture if neuroscience had incorporated from the beginning a more holistic and systems-oriented approach to the study of the living brain. Years before the official birth of neuroscience, second-order cybernetics adopted an expanded understanding of the body–brain system that was not haunted by the visual culture of neurorealism, mainly because functional brain imaging was yet to be invented.

The Josiah Macy Jr. Foundation conference series *Circular Causal and Feedback Mechanisms in Biological and Social Systems* (1942–1955) adopted the title of Norbert Wiener's book *Cybernetics* (1948) as the title for the sixth conference in 1949. The cybernetics movement comprised mathematicians, physicists, engineers, social scientists, logicians, and neurophysiologists—among them were Heinz von Foerster, John von Neumann, Gregory Bateson, Margaret Mead, Claude Shannon, and Warren McCulloch, as well as Wiener. The introductory discussion to the sixth conference began with the need to foster interdisciplinary communication, deemed to be particularly difficult between physics/biology and psychology/social sciences.[34]

The origins of cybernetics are as multivarious as its different currents and protagonists.[35] First, cybernetics originated in wartime, when a better coupling between humans and the new technologies of war was considered necessary. Wiener's work during the Second World War was focused on constructing a device—the antiaircraft predictor—able to analyze the flight trajectory of the enemy pilot, predict its future position, and annihilate it.[36] Second, as the scholar of futures of innovation Ed Finn argues, the origin of cybernetics must also be placed in quantum physics and the transition from certainty to probability:

> Quantum mechanics suggested that uncertainty, or indeterminacy, was fundamental to the cosmos and that observation always affected the system being observed.... [T]his displaced the notion that the universe operated by simple, all-powerful laws that could be discovered and mastered.... But far more unsettling... is the notion that probability applies to information as much as to material reality. By framing information as uncertainty, as surprise, as unpredicted new data, mathematician Claude Shannon created a quantifiable measurement of communication.[37]

Ten years before the Macy Conferences (see chapter 4), Majorana's concerns around quantum mechanics took the mantle of a premonition against the blunt application of statistical laws into the scientific modeling of social phenomena.

Cybernetics sits at the threshold of a body of disciplines as diverse as brain science, information theory, robotics, social sciences, and arts. The politics of experimentation conducted by cyberneticians revealed the world, as science studies Andrew Pickering and Keith Guzik argue, "as a place of de-centered human and non-human becoming."[38] The conventional story of cybernetics traces its endeavors back to the encounter between mathematics and engineering. Yet, contra such a convention, Pickering defines cybernetics as the "antidisciplinary" field par excellence, arguing that cybernetics is the science of the brain.[39] The brain is a system devoted to action, to adapting to the unknown, rather than an organ that merely processes and presents information from electrical activity circulating around a network of neurons. Cybernetics is the science devoted to studying model systems (biological and machinic) that live in and learn to adjust to the environment. It was the systems-oriented approach to the study of the brain before the official birth of neuroscience in 1962.[40]

A Detour from First-Order Cybernetics: Von Foerster's Biological Computer Laboratory

Second-order cybernetics should not be understood as the historical development of cybernetics that came after the first-order approach, but rather as a variance within the same theory.[41] First-order cybernetics, which originated at MIT, focused mainly on computation, artificial intelligence, and subject-centered analysis, attempting to control and govern how machinic and organic components communicate; second-order cybernetics, which centered on the Biological Computer Laboratory (BCL) that existed at the University of Illinois from 1958 to 1975, focused on epistemology and biology, adopting a more reflexive, holistic, and systems-thinking approach. Having left MIT, the biologist Umberto Maturana contributed significantly to second-order cybernetics with von Foerster at BCL.[42] Funded by third parties (medical program and the US Navy and Air Force), the laboratory conducted fundamental and applied research for nonmilitary purposes. None of the results or products produced by the BCL were considered useful by the military.[43]

BCL is worth discussing for several reasons. First, it thrived thanks to research programs that deviated from mainstream research in cybernetics, thus playing a crucial role in the development of second-order cybernetics. Second, with a few notable exceptions, BCL's history has been relatively sidelined by historians of cybernetics. Third, the brain was not the only organ considered to be determinable and computable, but also other sensory organs such as the eyes and the ears. The animated machines constructed at BCL had a kind of life of their own, not because they were based on biological processes, but because they served as a generative platform used for designing future biological machines.[44] In a sense, second-order cybernetics extended well beyond the life-span of the BCL.

Finally, thanks to in-house and visiting researchers/artists, the laboratory thrived on an interdisciplinary approach to systems theory, self-organizing systems, and bionics. In 1968, *Cybernetic Serendipity* was the first international exhibition (hosted by the Institute of Contemporary Arts in London) that gave a platform to artists, philosophers, and engineers for working creatively with cybernetics to produce software, early robotic installations, performances, and human-generated drawings.[45] The experimentalism of cybernetics was not hypothesis-driven but open-ended, similar to experimentalism in art.[46]

At BCL, Maturana elaborated his theory of autopoiesis together with the biologist, neuroscientist, and philosopher Francisco Varela. In their theory, Maturana and Varela challenge the idea that the mind operates in the guise of inputs and outputs as a Turing machine. Instead of inputs and outputs, mind and identity are emergent properties of a distributive system of neural activity.[47] Neural activity coupled with action constitute the world in which the self is to be understood not as an essentialist center of activity but as the effect of a physical process, actions, and habits of thought. The key principles of feedback, information, and communication in cybernetics theory were applied not only to the system being observed, but also to the observer.[48]

Maturana and Varela's research program, which drew upon lines of inquiry starting in the 1930s and became widespread in the 1970s, launched an innovative exploration of living phenomena based on observing an organism's behavior in an environment. Two postulates underpin their experiments: (1) what distinguishes living systems from physical-chemical systems is not the components, but their organization, that is, the set of relationships they exhibit in such systems; and (2) the specific property of living systems is autonomy, schematically definable as a relative independence from the environment, evident for example in the capacity of such systems to determine and regulate their own processes.

The notion of autopoiesis characterizes this organization as a self-specified network of transformation processes (synthesis and destruction) of the metabolic components capable of producing its own components in such a way as to: (1) regenerate itself (self-production); (2) maintain itself as a unit by compensating for environmental perturbations through modifications of internal processes (self-maintenance); and (3) distinguish itself as a unit from the surrounding environment, for example, through the production of a boundary such as that constituted by the membrane (self-distinction).[49]

The BCL interdisciplinary endeavor was in tune with the spirit of other US laboratories active at the time in bionics (the fusion of biology and electronics): General Electric, AT&T's Bell Telephone Laboratories, and the Radio Corporation of America. There are important differences, though. All these laboratories were engaged in building computers from artificial neural nets rather than from biological elements as the BCL lab did.[50] Another difference is the ethical afflatus pervading second-order cybernetics. The contribution to second-order cybernetics enables imagination, distributed cognition, and agency to return to a self-reflexive subject. Thus, the model of vision and cognition put forward by von Foerster's group offers an alternative to the computational approach to visualization, intelligence, and governance of first-order cybernetics. For the latter, visualization and cognition provide a set of techniques to calculate and manage observable and measurable populations in society.

Rather than furthering the first-order cybernetics project of applying knowledge to control nature, biological computing seeks to experiment with how an observer impacts the system observed and how perception factors into one's own understanding of the system. Von Foerster instructs the observer of systems to "enter the domain of his own descriptions" and accept responsibility for being in the world both as a living system and as an observer-participant, aware that every action and reaction leaves a trace that may or may not affect the system as a whole.[51]

Bio Art and Body–Brain Systems

Bio art refers to the manipulation in vivo or in vitro of living cells, tissues, or organisms (or their derivatives) for creating displays that allow audiences to partake of them emotionally and cognitively. Since the sequencing of the human genome in 2000, artists have used the tools and objects made available by the biosciences. In bio art, the subject and object of artistic manipulation are often life processes: bio art does not want to *represent* life, it wants to *be* life.[52] From Eduardo Kac's hybrid bioluminescent rabbit *Alba* (2001) to the bio art experiments of artists such as Oron Catts and Ionat Zurr, artists have used the tools, tropes, and materials of bioscience practice to imagine the biological world anew.[53] The goal is to understand and remediate life processes, questioning the boundary between animate and inanimate matter, and staging the material forces that govern and determine agency, life, and death. In this respect, artists have become increasingly interested in the direct use of neural cells rather than in the mediated visualization of neural activity offered by brain scans. Neuro-bio art uses living cells and tissues to explore the metaphor of life as a code, the notion of a sentient and thinking being, and the ethical and political consequences that might result in having the power to manipulate these novel entities.[54]

Among the several works using neurons that have been created in the last decade is *cellF* (2015), the world's first neural synthesizer, made by artist Guy Ben-Ary who rethinks biotechnologies using a materialist perspective and embraces the idea of a distributed self. He challenges the alternative of either neurorealism or the belief in an essentialist concept of selfhood with research in biology and accounts on the relationship between subjectivity and technology. The notion of the organism as a substance whose identity is determined by some intrinsic essential principle has been challenged by recent studies on the role of symbiosis in the construction of organisms and by insights into the environment-dependent character of organisms.[55] Science studies scholar and philosopher Donna Haraway, for example, dismisses an essentialist notion of the body to favor ideas of communication flowing between human and non-human interfaces: the body is turned toward multiple possible interconnections with different materialities rather than being a substance.[56]

One of the most convincing challenges to the idea that the self is located in the brain is given by Luciano Floridi, a philosopher of information technology. Central to the creation of brain scans, information and communication technologies have had an enormous impact on the way in which identity is constructed and maintained. Floridi formulates a philosophy of personal identity based on the concept of the self as an informational structure:

> A living organism (e.g. a spider) is cognitively present only where it is located as an embodied and embedded information-processing system. A living organism aware of its information processes (e.g. a dog dreaming) can be present within such processes (e.g. chasing dreamed rabbits) while being located elsewhere (e.g. in the house). But a self, that is, a living organism self-aware of its own information processes (e.g. you) and its own presence within them, can choose where to be. The self, and mental life in general, is located in the brain but not present in the brain. Thus, the locus of the self is the brain but the self is not present in the brain.[57]

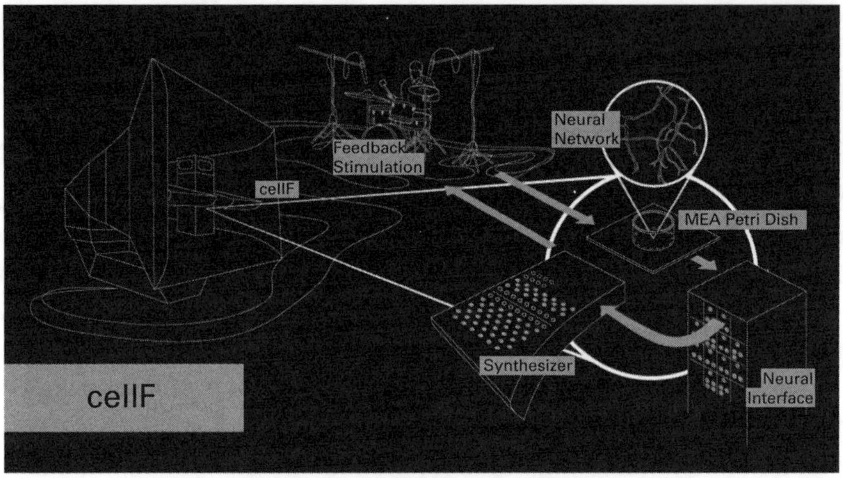

(a)

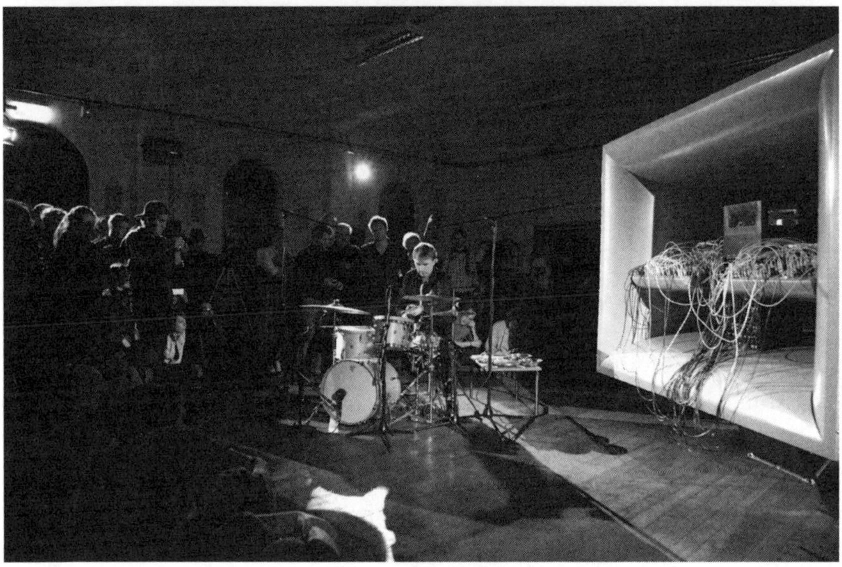

(b)

Figure 5.8

Guy Ben-Ary (with artists Nathan Thompson, Andrew Fitch, and Darren Moore, and scientists Stuart Hodgetts, Mike Edel, and Douglas Bakkum), *cellF* (live performance+system), 2015. Stem cells, neural synthesizer, and neural networks.

Source: Courtesy of the artist.

Although Floridi locates mental life in the brain, he does not embrace a simplistic view of the self as brainhood.

cellF is a work made entirely of biological matter coming from the artist's own cells, a neural network, and analog circuits. Sounds from live performances feed as electrical stimuli into *cellF*'s neural network, which replies through the synthesizer to create an improvised sound piece. The two musicians, human and post-human, give the impression of being able to communicate and create music as an ensemble (see figure 5.8).[58]

The second-order cybernetics concepts of feedback-loop between a system and its environment, autopoiesis, and distributed cognition are the key reference points for this work.[59] Implicit in the theory of autopoiesis is first the overcoming of the dichotomy between software and hardware in living systems, a dualism typical of the biological and cognitive tradition based on the computational metaphor.[60] Second, autopoietic networks, although closed, are not static and immutable. Thanks to feedback loops where each component's activity is simultaneously the cause and effect of all the others, a variation in the interaction between two components generates a transformation of the network itself. Autopoiesis therefore represents the "plasticity" of an organism.

Silent Barrage (2008–2009) is another work by Guy Ben-Ary, developed in collaboration with a team of artists, designers, engineers, and scientists in an artistic research laboratory, SymbioticA, in Australia. It investigates the nature of thoughts, decision making, free will, and neural dysfunction. The resulting work focuses on bursts of uncontrolled activity in nerve tissue, a typical characteristic of epilepsy and Petri-dish-cultured nerve cells. The work depicts a lab with a culture dish containing neurons harvested from embryonic rats. These neurons are connected to several sensors and activators that are in turn connected to the internet. In the exhibition space, which is far away from the lab, stands the robotic body of the work, an array of columns covered in paper. The Petri dish functions as the neural interface of the robotic body, stimulating it via the internet (see figure 5.9).

The audience provides the stimulation to which the cultured cells respond. Attached to each column is a robot that can travel up and down the column and draw on the paper. As people pass through the columns, a camera tracks their movement and relays this movement pattern over the internet back to the distant lab. Depending on the pattern of movement, individual neurons are stimulated manually. The neurons react and then organically transmit a signal to other nearby neurons in the same culture. This communication between neurons is then transmitted back to the exhibition space, each neuron mapping onto a column, and the level of activity in that neuron represented by lines drawn on the paper by the robot. As people move on to investigate the more active robots, their movement triggers yet more activity in the culture dish in the distant lab, more neurons fire, and robots on other columns swing into action. *Silent Barrage* cannot see visitors when they stand perfectly still, immobilized.

This immersive installation is an embodied neuronal artwork, engaging us with the concept of emergent behavior from semi-living entities who have to communicate

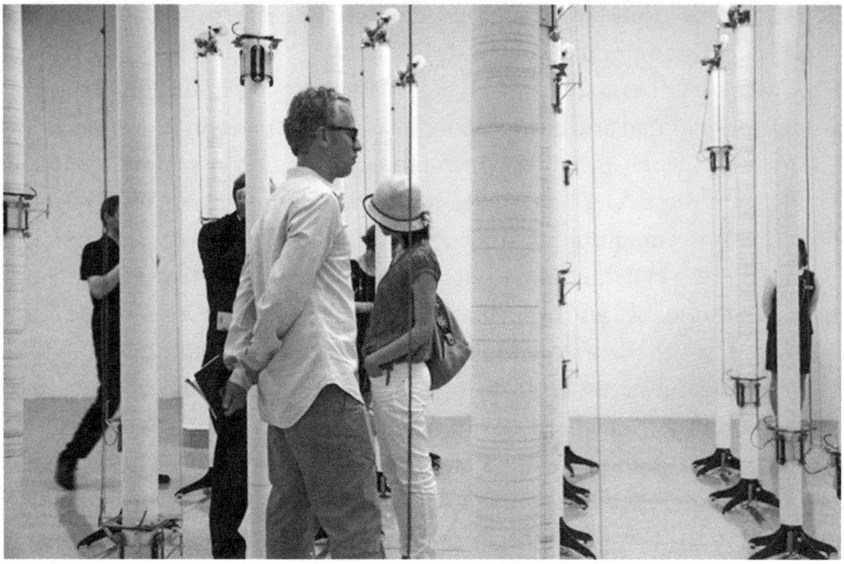

Figure 5.9
Guy Ben-Ary (with SymbioticA), *Silent Barrage*, detail of the robotic body (installation view) 2009.
Source: Courtesy of the artist.

with one another against the environmental barrage of information and noise.[61] The electrical activity of nerve cells is made tangible and visceral. As one walks through the rows of columns, the feeling of physically traveling through and interacting with an active brain–body system is impossible to escape. This feeling has two consequences. First, it gives the impression that the entity is a sentient form of life toward which one could develop some type of empathy. Second, it complicates our understanding of the correlations between biological/machinic components and macro activities of motion, sensory perception, and interaction.

The external biological "brain" of *Silent Barrage* is not primarily characterized by the property of thinking; rather, *Silent Barrage* attempts to think of the neural system as a brain–body complex, both organic and machinic, outside the boundaries of the biological brain. This form of life, which has a body and a culture of neural cells, does not seem to fit into any modern category of the self nor to its contemporary version, brainhood, thus becoming an epistemic object that defies any strict definition. This brain–body system cannot be regarded as a circumscribed entity, but rather as an integrated member of a machinic and organic environment characterized by dialectical exchange. The focus of *Silent Barrage* and *cellF* is not on brain scans as a representation of something (via isomorphism or resemblance) but rather on the presentation of neuronal activity incarnated in a robotic body. Furthermore, neither installation falls into neuroessentialism for they make explicit how circumscribing neural activity to the brain is highly problematic.

Chapter Final Remarks

This chapter has examined visual practices inside the laboratory and in the arts, highlighting a potential problem of reductionism in the transformation from data to images and in the visual incarnation of the neurorealism fallacy, that is, the extreme images of brain scans. Neuroscience is not inherently reductionist, and work conducted in the laboratory demonstrates how scientists themselves can tackle this specific fragility of their discipline. Standardization of brain imaging technology has made it difficult for artists to use brain scans without also reproducing the trope of brainhood, which is made visible by extreme images of the brain.

I return to my initial question: if neurorealism is a fallacy within neuroscience (the visual manifestation of which occurs through extreme images), do neuroscience–art projects reproduce this fallacy at the visual level? The answer is yes, if art practices do, despite engaging in a critique of neurocultures, end up incorporating or reproducing those extreme images. A neuroscience project can unfold via the arts only through an investigation of the material practice of neural data, with particular reference to the challenges posed by transforming data into images (sometimes extreme) inside the laboratory and in art practices. This is, I believe, a viable method if the broader objective is to put neuroscientific methods, findings, and imagery less at the mercy of political and economic actors interested in exploiting the intrinsic epistemological weakness of neuroscience and its imagery for their own agendas.[62]

The hand-painted MRI image of the dead mouse was the result of an effort undertaken by humans to use their eyes and brains (to recall Mallard's expression) to develop a new technology. It pointed to one of the intrinsic fragilities of neuroscience, that is, the difficulty of visualizing, interpreting, and displaying raw data. Artists can further expose this fragility, inviting scientists to take a more reflexive approach to their own visual practices and inviting the lay public to assume a critical stance toward both the neurologization of subjectivity and the reification of the self in extreme images. By doing so, artists can foster a stereoscopic vision capable of maintaining in focus both conceptions of the man in the world—the scientific and the manifest. In contrast, if artists linger on the use of brain scans as a means to convey (or fail to convey) the self, any challenge to the neurorealism fallacy will be difficult to overcome.

6 Archives and Laboratory Ethnography: Giving Bodies Back to Data

> The many stuffs—matter, energy, waves, phenomena—that worlds are made of are made along with the worlds. But made from what? Not from nothing, after all, but from other worlds. Worldmaking as we know it always starts from worlds already on hand; the making is always a remaking ... my interest here is rather with the processes involved in building a world out of others ... we face the questions how worlds are made, tested, and known.
>
> —Nelson Goodman, "Words, Works, Worlds"

Is This a Man?

Is this a man? This lump of grey-green flesh
Lying on cold stone.
"A fine carcass," the butcher says, busy with his saw.
"I'm fresh this morning, so let's get down to work."
All in a day's work.
"Here's his liver, do you want some?"
No, just a small piece of heart
Or perhaps a kidney.
Here's a multicoloured man, now that his skin's off–
Pink and yellow, green and blue
Just like a sunset.[1]

Is this a man? The onlooker–reader is invited to make a judgment. The features of a body are hardly recognizable, reduced to a lump of flesh pastel colors like a sunset. A body whose organs (a kidney, the liver, a piece of heart) are units to be extracted and further examined. It is the description of an exchange between a seller (the butcher) and a buyer. After a day of work, at dusk only colors remain. The author of this poem, written in the early 1970s, is the physicist Jim Hutchison, one of the key members of the Aberdonian team in charge of developing MRI for clinical purposes, and inventor—together with the physicist Bill Edelstein—of the spin-warp method.

Hutchison wrote this opening verse as his reaction to staring at a corpse in a morgue with his colleague and life companion, the biologist Margaret Foster (known as Meg). The laboratory was close to a mortuary. Jim, she recalls, did not feel comfortable collecting tissues, so she did it; the vitality of life and death otherwise mute on the aseptic laboratory bench. Collecting animal and human tissues for laboratory experiments was considered normal practice in the 1970s, the early days of MRI development. The poem alludes to a sensation later described by the historian Jonathan Sawday as a Medusa-like effect of peering inside the body—not just one's own body but the universal body—when the inner becomes the outer, inside and outside dissolve into the liminality offered by skin: "Those rare occasions when individuals are allowed to glimpse the Medusa's head of their own interiority are always structured by the mirror-effect of representation and transformation."[2] The meeting with the interior of the body takes the connotations of an existential practice, an invitation to reflect on human existence with all its beauty, frailty, mortality.

Since his childhood, Hutchison had kept a series of notebooks (called the VB notebooks, for they were presented *as if* they had been written by "VB," acting as a kind of critical friend or skeptic whom Hutchison could conversate with) in which he meticulously recorded ideas, experiments, models, reflections, sketches, and measurements. Recently donated by Meg Foster to the Special Collections of the University of Aberdeen, these notebooks (more than one hundred) span from the mid-1940s to the early 2000s. They include aspects of electron spin resonance from Hutchison's time as a doctoral student at St Andrews and MRI-related ideas from his work in Aberdeen.

Today we are accustomed to looking at biomedical images of inner bodily structures and brain functions. But we might still be at the mercy of the Medusa effect. The medical image often signifies the absence of the body.[3] The encounter with the patient is mediated through an image, for instance a scan of the brain in action. The image becomes an operational interface supported by a matrix of algorithms. It is image data. Medical images are not photographic snapshots of a preexisting object (the body), but data visualizations: transcriptions of codes and algorithms that remain black boxed.

Visualization is a crucial component of how data are produced, interpreted, displayed, and contested inside (and outside) the laboratory. This chapter demonstrates how artists can recontextualize data and highlight their neglected dimensions, such that data are aesthetic-laden and the product of body work, decision making, and affective investment already inside the laboratory. I aim to show how a small-scale collaborative art–science project can be set up through laboratory fieldwork and archival research.

Ultimately, biomedical data visualization—even when its interpretation is not yet straightforward—is based on and is about patients' bodies. The production, interpretation, display, and communication of visualized biomedical data impact the health care pipeline, influencing decision making and interventions in individuals. The T_1 dispersion curve is connected to the patient's body, which is simultaneously the constant reference point in the laboratory and a daunting absent presence. It is through this graph, through this type of data visualization, with all its vagueness, uncertainty, and yet authority, that the relationship with the patient is mediated.

As I argue in what follows, by bringing the body back when discussing data, questions of care and responsibility are foregrounded. Artists can bring the body back to data without reifying it to an entity reducible exclusively to its biology and physiology. Through metaphors, artists can make nonquantitative aspects of data perceivable to the general public, and they can make scientists, patients, and the lay public more aware of what lies behind the algorithms that make the image. Artists can imagine and create a space in which the body is reconfigured into more than just an ensemble of quantitative data and as an experiential, phenomenological body.

A Cross-Disciplinary Project

During the final phase of the Horizon 2020 IDentIFY project, I contributed to set up a collaborative project between the commissioned Edinburgh-based artist Beverley Hood, the biomedical physics department at the University of Aberdeen, the Suttie Arts Space, and me. The project engaged with the narratives, aesthetics, and material practices of data visualization in the two periods of development of MRI (late 1960s to early 1980s) and FFC-MRI (ongoing). The output consisted of two connected exhibitions held in the Suttie Arts Space in Spring 2019, a roundtable discussion with expertise in different fields (medical humanities, archiving, physics, and the arts) and an illustrated catalog, with an introduction written by Professor David Lurie (the head of the IDentIFY project), a short creative-writing piece by the artist, and a scholarly essay by me.

The first exhibition was *Immobile Choreography*, a new media exhibition by Beverley Hood developed in collaboration with the dancer and choreographer Freya Jeffs. In dialogue with this exhibition was *From Where Do We See?*, a display of original material (photographs, lab notebooks, diagrams, and design sketches) from the first Aberdonian period and from the present IDentIFY FFC-MRI project. Existing narratives of biomedical imaging innovation tend to neglect the role played by aesthetic judgments, memories, and craft skills, framing them as peripheral to science. *From Where Do We See?* highlighted the aesthetic, labor-intense, and affective dimensions of making science, relying mainly on material from Jim Hutchison's laboratory and personal archive.

The conception and design of the two exhibitions offered a method for establishing common ground for a conversation between scientists, humanities scholars, and artists. However, bridging the gap between art and science was not the goal of the project as a whole. The aims were to create a cross-disciplinary project as an alternative to institutionalized art–science collaboration and to unveil the role played by craftsmanship, creativity, and imagination in science. Art (like science) is a way of world making. It is not simply creativity that art and science have in common, but the goal of experimenting, making new worlds by reconfiguring bits and pieces of existing ones. Visitors were encouraged to approach art and science as skilled practices and to explore relationships between aesthetic forms, functions, and past and present times. The project bridged the two moments in the history of MRI innovation at the University of Aberdeen to investigate how craftsmanship, aesthetics, and theories from the arts and humanities feed into past and present MRI innovation networks.

Beverley Hood's exhibition was in the main gallery of the Suttie Arts Space, where *Mark I*, the world's first whole-body MRI clinical scanner, is also on permanent display. This gallery, though physically located within the Grampian Hospital close to the biomedical physics department, is a proper art gallery that avoids any project too directly related to medicine or healing. The archival exhibition was in a relatively small and unusual space, the Small Gallery of the Suttie Arts Space.[4] This was the original gallery space and consists of a series of corridors hosting rotating exhibitions and artwork either specially commissioned or part of the permanent collection of the Grampian Hospital Art Trust. The Small Gallery is part of the everyday life of National Health Service (NHS) staff, researchers, patients, and their relatives, rushing up and down the walkways.

The project presented unique features. First, the collaboration was the first of its kind. The physicists engaged in the development of FFC-MRI at the University of Aberdeen had not previously been involved in any kind of collaborative projects with an artist except for public engagement initiatives. One of these initiatives aimed to reassemble *Mark I* for permanent display and public fruition in the Suttie Arts Space. An interpretative booklet and a documentary film by Rob Page on the history of MRI development at the University of Aberdeen enhanced the interpretative layers for the audience of the gallery. Second, there was no institutional remit to set up the collaboration between the biomedical physics department, the Suttie Arts Space, the artist, and me; the origin of the project was bottom up, rather than top down. Third, the funding for the collaborative project came mainly from the arts and humanities rather than from the scientific partner involved. The Creative Scotland program, Aberdeen City Council, and the Aberdeen Humanities Fund of the University of Aberdeen were the main sponsors of the exhibition, with the Fund focused specifically on supporting the archival exhibition. A small part of the funding came from the public engagement budget of IDentIFY. Fourth, the collaboration was not just between the artist and biomedical physicists, but also involved a dancer/choreographer, a humanities researcher (me), and the people in charge of the official and nonofficial archival collections I researched and used for the second exhibition.

Fifth, the project did not take the shape of an artist in residence (mainly because of time and budget constraints) but rather that of an ongoing dialogue between the artist, the biomedical physicists, and me. We preferred a collaboration that entailed some fieldwork by the artist in the laboratory where FFC-MRI is being developed and an ongoing dialogue between the artist, the biomedical physicists, the curator at the Suttie Arts Space, and me. Collective meetings were accompanied by the artist's fieldwork, my own archival and ethnographic research, and technical meetings with the gallery's curator. In the meetings we discussed practical arrangements, layout, budgets, as well as delved into the subject matter from both a scientific and philosophical perspective. Finally, the project was a seed for further initiatives, conversations, and collaborations across different areas of expertise (art, biomedical physics, STS and visual culture, and medical humanities).

Setting Up the Project

Launching a call for proposals was the first step to initiating the collaboration. The commissioning board comprised Tamsin Greenlaw, the curator of the Suttie Arts Space; me; and David Lurie. We wanted to commission an experienced artist to "investigate the work currently being developed by the IDentIFY research project and its link to *Mark I*, the world's first full-body MRI scanner."[5] The remit of the call for proposals was loose enough to encourage a variety of approaches by artists working in different media. Because of the limited travel and accommodation budget, the applications we received came primarily from Scotland-based artists (sculptors, performers, new media artists, and graphic designers).

The initial short-listing process was smooth, because all three parties of the commissioning board made the same choices. More accustomed to projects of public engagement with the physics behind FFC-MRI than to contemporary art, the staff of the biomedical physics department were initially inclined to commission a team of graphic designers rather than an artist in order to have more control over the final output of the collaboration. When interviewing the short-listed artists, however, the gallerist and I had to make the case for commissioning an artist rather than a team of graphic designers. For scientists who had never been involved in an artistic project before, the idea of collaborating with an artist, rather than with a graphic designer used to thinking in terms of "client" and "message to convey," was daunting. It was part of our decision-making process that we commissioned an artist whose purpose was neither public engagement nor science communication.

In art–science projects there is often an unbalanced power dynamic between art and the humanities on one side and science on the other. Two factors contributed to the final decision made in favor of commissioning an artist rather than a team of graphic designers. First, the trust between the physicist coordinating the IDentIFY project and his team, the Suttie Arts Space, and me. The physicists and the gallery had already collaborated for the display of *Mark I*, and at the time of the commission, I was embedded as a humanities researcher in the biomedical physics laboratory and had already presented some of the preliminary results of my project. Second, the financial support needed for the project did come mainly from the arts and humanities, a condition that put me and the gallery in a relatively autonomous position.

Beverley Hood was commissioned not only for her long track record of working with medical technology but also for her experience with collaborative projects involving a range of practitioners, including medical researchers, scientists, writers, technologists, dancers, actors, and composers. Since the mid-1990s, Hood has interrogated the impact of technology on the body, relationships, and human experience through digital media, performance arts, and writing.

Bridging Disciplines

Interdisciplinarity is subject to historical, geographical, and cultural variation. It is always context-specific and bounded by the limitations imposed by concrete practices. In relation to art–science collaborative work, sociologists Callard and Fitzgerald explained what it means carrying out an interdisciplinary project across the neurosciences, social sciences, and humanities. They discuss the case of Hubbub, the first interdisciplinary research residency of the Hub at Wellcome Collection:

> Most "interdisciplinary" projects that bring the arts and humanities into contact with the sciences tend to stage the arts as in some way "exemplifying" the science or acting as the key mediator or outreach agent for that science.... Hubbub, by contrast, insists that the arts engage in creative experiments that are just as methodologically and conceptually rigorous, just as generative of knowledge, as those conducted by disciplines not commonly prefaced with the adjective "creative."[6]

Callard and Fitzgerald's key principles for nurturing interdisciplinarity in practice are the following: the availability of a space that enables dialogue and exchanges across disciplines, the culture of experimentation as the connecting tissue between the artistic and the scientific community, and the actual collaboration between the actors involved.

Interdisciplinarity is challenging inside different scientific communities too. The partners of the IDentIFY project are biomedical and theoretical physicists, biologists, clinicians, and engineers. All parties bring in different sets of questions, methodologies, traditions of data analysis, and techniques. For example, one researcher bridges the gap between the different epistemic communities working together. Such "bridge builders" are simultaneously experts in their own disciplines and able to place themselves within the nexus of the multidisciplinary project of which they are a part. Bridge builders often reflect metacritically on the ontologies and methods of the various disciplines involved in the project and build a language that retains the nuances of concepts in each discipline, such as the different meanings that the concept of "energy" has for physicists and biologists (see chapter 4).

In the first meeting with Beverley Hood and the biomedical physics team (represented by the physicists with whom I also collaborated most during my fieldwork), Beverley and I made clear to the physicists that we did not want to be trapped into the existing categories of "art–science" or "public engagement." To some extent, we wanted to be *undisciplined* before being interdisciplinary. The goal was to sow the seed of a culture of dialogue and collaboration across areas of expertise and epistemic communities of scholars and practitioners. The physicists involved had never formally collaborated with an artist, and Hood did not have a background in physics, despite her long-term involvement with biomedical technologies. She approached the world of MRI and FFC-MRI from her own perspective: that of an artist with expertise in design and new media.

Although each person involved in the collaboration kept their own languages and methodologies, they had to leave their comfort zone, be curious about the work developed by their collaborators, and engage with methodologies and concepts outside their own discipline. The artist had to learn some background information on how MRI and FFC-MRI work. The Suttie Arts Space curator had to oversee the technical and organizational aspects of the project. The physicists were involved hands-on with the lighting design and installation in the gallery, which played a big role in the artist's final work. David Lurie contributed to the catalog with a piece of writing that, as he described it, "was in the tradition of the humanities rather than the sciences"; this not only responded to the pieces written by me and the artist, but also engaged with his own personal and affective memories—something hardly allowed in academic scientific writing unless historically driven.

My goal was to create a trading zone between different communities and areas of expertise that do not usually collaborate. I achieved that objective by experimenting with a mixed methodology. This comprised the laboratory ethnographic fieldwork and interviews I conducted with past and present researchers in MRI and FFC-MRI development, the archival work based on official recordings of Jim Hutchison's laboratory journals and his personal VB notebooks, the conversations with the artist and physicists during and after the collaboration, and my visits to the artist's studio. Furthermore, the objects from the fieldwork and archival research (the coils, photographs, drawings, laboratory notebooks, artist's sketches, and interview excerpts) created a kaleidoscopic view of the development of MRI technology at the University of Aberdeen.

Evaluation and Ownership

Assessing the success of such collaborative projects using the concept of quality is fraught with problems. First, should one focus on the quality of the collaboration itself, on the immediate output, or on the long-term outcomes? If the attention is on the final output, does the definition of an output of quality change depending on whether the output is an artwork, a SciArt work, or a scientific experiment? Second, who is to determine the quality? Those directly involved in the collaboration, the lay public, or the wider community of scientists and artists? Third, does quality depend on the available budget and on the consequent need to select a well-known artist, one who is also sufficiently knowledgeable of the science and technology at stake in the project? Finally, does one define the quality of a project against other existing collaborative works that set the bar? Tightening evaluation and quality does not appear to be an effective strategy. Instead, the question I asked to evaluate the success of the collaboration was whether the final output was responsive to the layers of different areas of expertise, bodies, and histories along the trajectory of MRI innovation at the University of Aberdeen.

Who takes ownership of the project once it ends? Each of the collaborators expressed the need for taking ownership of the project and the will to continue the collaboration. After their initial skepticism of working with an artist rather than an expert on public engagement, the physicists expressed their enthusiasm. One of the physicists involved in the collaboration gave his feedback after the collaboration came to a conclusion:

> To me, the collaboration was completely unusual. We had never done anything similar before. I play percussion and two of my siblings are artists, so I guess I have a bit of understanding of art. I felt it was important to highlight the human component of doing science—this is so rarely done. Even in scientific seminars it's all about big science, the latest fashionable thing. ... The exhibition by Beverley Hood was more about contemporary art, perhaps feeding an emotion. It was disconcerting that she did not even try to explain the physics. But I found

> the whole collaborative process interesting—it was metaphorical, which is not a bad thing: the body tuning in with MRI, dancing with MRI. … And then it requires a lot of sensitivity to understand the point of view of patients. I thought it was clever to use the hospital corridor walls for the archival exhibition. It's a space where patients and their relatives, doctors, and scientists walk. But somehow it's not a human space. So the archival exhibition introduced a human factor into the everyday routine of a healthcare space. We should collaborate further.[7]

And Professor David Lurie wrote words of appreciation in his introduction to the exhibition catalog:

> We were extremely fortunate in Spring 2019 to have available to us in Aberdeen Royal Infirmary two outstanding works by Beverley Hood and Silvia Casini. I am sure that you will enjoy the experience of reading the linked essays in this book. As a "seasoned" research physicist, I must admit to encountering first surprise, then pleasure that my own view of the imaging process could be re-coloured and enhanced through the pieces. I hope that you, too, will see imaging and images in a new light as a result of this work.[8]

Ironically, the visual arts were described as something that should be used "to explain and indeed to amplify the message of the technology and how it is used."[9] The arts always run the risk of being taken as a resonance chamber for a certain technology or scientific project, regardless of the intentions of the artist and curator. This can be partially motivated though because scientists might feel that they do not get something out of the collaboration in terms of knowledge, new ideas, or methods.

The main roles that the humanities/social sciences scholar can undertake are those of the attached observer, the active participant, or the scholar embedded in the laboratory. Sometimes these roles can overlap. The attached observer envisages the laboratory humanist or social scientist as an anthropologist doing ethnographic work, taking notes on how facts are produced in everyday laboratory life.[10] The active participant can be involved in a research project codesigned by the artist and scientist; active participation can help explore hidden agendas and assumptions at work in the laboratory.[11] The output of the collaboration is a coauthored hybrid, which does not necessarily mean that the art and science contribution is equally distributed. Art and design have a "speculative, experimental and open-ended character"[12] that can inform researchers in science and technology studies conducting collaborative work with scientists. The last role is that of the "embedded scholar" in the laboratory. The embedded scholar (a humanist or social scientist) observes and intervenes in scientific practice to shape the course of action of a project/experiment and then studies the product of the intervention. The goal of this type of engaged intervention is not just to share knowledge or methods but to potentially change the course of a research project or of a specific experiment.[13]

In my case, I had to move from being a researcher embedded in the laboratory to being a facilitator of the relationship between the commissioned artist, the gallery, and the biomedical physics department, to eventually curate an archive-based exhibition. My role in the project however is that of a "modest witness," a role discussed by the feminist cultural theorist Donna Haraway[14] but never taken up by critical literature on art–science collaborative projects. The concept of the modest witness is crucial to exploring the power-relationship issues at stake in the laboratory and in the art–science collaboration. This framework, in fact, enables researchers to address matters of concern rather than just matters of fact in situated laboratory and art–science settings. As a humanities scholar embedded in the biomedical physics laboratory, my role within the project was first that of the modest witness, and then, that of a curator using archival and laboratory note material. Donna Haraway's proposal of the "modest witness" opens up the possibility for rethinking not just the role of scientists in the laboratory but also that of scholars and artists engaged in collaborative art–science projects.

Haraway uses the expression "modest witness" ironically, to unveil the key figure in the Scientific Revolution of the seventeenth century, Robert Boyle, one of the fathers of the experimental method. The modest witness character therefore emerged at the time when science no longer belonged to the amateur, alchemist, or inventor—it was the scientific observer whose disinterested observation of phenomena has been presented as central to the scientific method.[15] The term described those who were witnessing the experiment and by doing so contributing to establishing it as truth. In her essay *Modest_Witness@Second_Millenium*, Haraway first deconstructs the figure of the "modest witness" and then reconfigures it as a kind of "*mutated* modest witness" who can contribute to the betterment of science practice.[16] The modest witness, far from being an objective observer whose testimony is crucial, can determine what counts as knowledge and for whom. In this respect, Leonelli's framework of data-driven science (see chapter 1) can be put to work to discuss what kind of things take on the role of data once the scholar (or the artist) enters the laboratory as a new type of "modest witness."

Creating new categories or repositioning existing ones (for example, that of the "witness" in science) is an act of modest witnessing, according to Haraway. Throughout my situated, partial, and engaged interventions as researcher and curator, I used material objects to perform a critical function in relation to the history of MRI development at the University of Aberdeen: Who owns this history? Does it become something other than just a local success story? How can this history be retold? What is its usefulness in the present life of the laboratory in which FFC-MRI is being developed?

The more I dug into the yet-to-be-cataloged repository of materials (papers, laboratory notebooks, photographs, objects),[17] the more I felt that my role was that of helping, as Haraway put it, "a more corporeal, inflected, and optically dense, if less elegant, kind of modest witness to matters of fact to emerge in the worlds of technoscience."[18] The truthfulness of a witnessing act is not grounded in objectivity and detachment, but in a partial, situated position that enables both orientation and doubt. Reframing the center–periphery dynamics in this history of technological development entailed shifting the attention away from matters of fact to focus only on matters of concern. This shift occurred thanks to a special kind of modest witnessing carried out by Meg Foster. My first meeting with her occurred relatively late in the unfolding of my research project. It happened after Jim Hutchison, who was seriously ill when I started this project, had passed away. While I was curating the archival exhibition, Eleanor Hutcheon, the department photographer, showed me and the physicists some previously unknown archival material by Jim Hutchison, including the mouse map picture series (see chapter 2) and some of his laboratory notebooks. It became clear to me that this material should be at the center of the collaborative project.

Immobile Choreography: From the Idea to the Exhibition

Beverley Hood is the first artist to have developed a work responding to FFC-MRI, a technology still under development. Hood has been working for decades on embodied techno-interfaces, exploring the relationship between the body and technology in collaborative projects with performers, medics, and technicians, often considering the boundaries between virtual reality, simulation, and real life in medical settings.[19] For example, her project *Eidolon* (2016), a virtual reality installation that was also created with Freya Jeffs,[20] explores the emotional territory of patient simulators, known as *manikins*, that are used in medical training.

Embodied techno-interfaces is the concept that best captures Hood's work: first, the body she creates is distributed across a network of technologies, techniques, and other bodies; second, in all her projects to date she plays with the idea of bringing the body back after it has been dissolved into bits of data.

The artist conceived her project around the concept of relaxation time, the time it takes the tissue to return to a state of equilibrium after magnetization. Hood faced two challenges. First, she needed to understand the similarities and differences between conventional MRI and FFC-MRI in a relatively short time. For this purpose, Lurie and I recommended the textbook *MRI from Picture to Proton*, because it explains the concepts beginning with the final images rather than with the underlying physics. All of Hood's initial meetings with the physicists were aimed at giving her a grasp of the basics of both techniques. Second, like other artists such as Liz Orton, Marilène Oliver, and Ilona Sagar who work on medicine, data, and techno-interfaces, Hood has shifted her focus away from the final visual output.[21] The first laboratory visits and discussions with the physicists suggested that her piece was not going to be a literal explanation of what goes on inside an FFC-MRI scanner. She wanted to distill the difference between MRI and FFC without explaining the physics, mechanics, and engineering principles behind it and to avoid using body or brain MRI/FFC-MRI images, preferring instead to create embodied techno-interfaces, starting from an elaboration of the phenomenological experience inside the scanner.

Hood's initial focus (which was then dismissed because of technical challenges and time constraints) was on the algorithms used to create the visual output of FFC-MRI. One of the physicists once again addressed the problem of turning data into meaningful visual output:

Hood: I am really interested in the actual algorithms themselves. They look for differences and similarities between the behaviors of tissues.

Physicist: Yes, it's the magnetic behavior of tissues. What we see at the moment, with FFC-MRI, is that different diseases give different results. It's not a one-to-one correspondence, however, as it is in fingerprinting. If you know what you're looking at, it's easier.[22]

Hood chose to avoid a didactic or public engagement approach and any direct reference to the history of MRI. In fact, the archive-based exhibition was a later addition to the original collaboration. Her choice was to construct layered configurations of different data, from the choreographed body of the dancer and the meditative/immersive environment of the gallery space, to the soundtrack and the color scheme used for the video projection. The FFC-MRI sound was recorded mechanically. The soundtrack reproduced the radically different sound of the FFC-MRI scanner—an entirely new aural experience for the patient undergoing an examination.

With FFC-MRI, physicists analyze stacks of images, changes in signal across different regions of tissue, and interpret what these changes mean. Then they correlate this with what goes on at the physical, molecular, or chemical level. In FFC-MRI, how the images are obtained from data is not new; it is how they are correlated that is new. The technique requires new ways of analyzing the data, because the images obtained contain information that is not accessible by a conventional MRI scanner.

The image-data processing had still not been finalized at the time of the commissioned collaborative project. The method the physicists were using consisted of comparing the regions that appeared similar in all the images for a given patient. This automated (computerized) method, albeit useful for analyzing contrast, holds back some information. Because of the work-in-progress nature of data visualization in FFC-MRI at the time of the collaboration, Hood decided to rely on an expanded understanding of data. Her choice was to return to the body rather than focusing on bits of data from measurements of bodily parameters. Like other artists before her, she started from her own body, from her direct experience of undergoing MRI and FFC-MRI examinations. She also wanted to focus on the concept of relaxation time, which plays a key role in both conventional MRI and FFC-MRI (see chapter 4).

Documenting the experience of undergoing a scan is difficult to do through photography or film, because no camera is allowed close to or inside the scanner. Therefore, Hood decided to document it through her own storytelling, narrative construction, and the sketches she created after the examinations. These constitute the first-person "data" collected during the scans, along with other "data" such as noise, the setting of the examination, and the technical components of each scanner.

After filling out the consent form, Hood underwent two scans on the same day, the first in a 3-Tesla MRI machine and the second in an FFC-MRI machine. "I was fascinated by the difference between the two experiences. You don't see the mechanism at all, but actually I absolutely believe in it, completely; I have absolute faith in this piece of MRI machinery. Whereas this one [the artist refers to an image of the FFC-MRI prototype], you can actually see how it's working."[23]

Before sliding in on the scanner bed, Hood took pictures of the equipment from the threshold (marked by a line on the floor), because no metallic object is allowed in or near the scanner. The design of MRI scanners, and particularly the FFC-MRI scanner prototype, supports body normativity: the artist's head (rather small) just fits in the head coil, touching the sides; the scanner bed is so narrow that it would preclude certain people, such as those who are overweight, from undergoing scans. The presence of a mirror inside the conventional MRI scanner is a feature that captures the attention of Hood, who is keen on "virtual" spaces:

> The front of the coil is levered over my face, and I now have a small mirror in front of me. This gives me the strange perspective of looking straight ahead but seeing down my body to my feet, and beyond, to the window into the control room, where the staff sit and watch. The mirror is an interesting shape, a bit like a visor and, although it isn't that big (maybe 15 cm × 5 cm), I'm surprised how effective it is. I realize there are actually two mirrors that tilt and bounce the reflections off one another and, as I lie there, I wonder about setting up a series of similar mirrors in the gallery; spaces for the viewers to peek through, with videos on the other side.[24]

The mirror is absent from the FFC-MRI scanner. One of the physicists explained that although they could add one, there wouldn't be much to look at, because the workshop space where the prototype is situated is not particularly interesting.

The aural experience is a layered ensemble: the sound of the different runs of the scanner; the almost imperceptible noises made by Hood's body, such as the breath or her rumbling belly; and the reassuring, calm voice of the radiologist in the console room communicating with her. Hood observes how, for the patient, the main difference between the two scanners is the loud noise of the conventional MRI compared to the almost silent voice of the FFC-MRI scanner.[25]

Beverley Hood was intrigued by the presence of a lighting system with a changing color field inside the FFC-MRI prototype. The pastel sketches respond to the simple yet sophisticated use of light in the scanner. One of the physicists had put a flexible strip of light at the back of the scanner and programmed it to cycle through different colors: blues, greens, and purples were chosen to give the patient a sense of quietness, but not red, because this was deemed too similar to a warning. The artist describes the calming effect the light had on her while inside the FFC-MRI scanner: "There's no space for a mirror system here and I can't even focus on the edges of the head coil, they're so close to my face.... My mind starts to wander, and thoughts soon begin spiraling. The saving grace is the lighting. It's like a field of light above me.... I like the light."[26]

For the installation, the same lighting system used in the FFC-MRI scanner was arranged in the exhibition space, along the perimeter of the room. The interplay between space and changing artificial light gives the body a phenomenological experience similar to that elicited by artist James Turrell's open air installations through the use of natural light. The cycling colors give a time-based performativity to the scanner space, which is otherwise claustrophobic and still. Transposed to the gallery, the colors enable visitors to inhabit the space and the temporal dimension associated with it, almost from the point of view of someone looking at the body from within the scanner.

The image data, albeit not present in the artistic installation, constitute a transitional object that the artist examines. Hood posted a scan of her brain on social media, ending her creative-writing piece with the experience of observing the scan, recognizing it was "her" and feeling reassured: "I'm glad to see that again, as far as both human and machine can see, my brain looks normal."[27]

Normativity is stabilized by the visual evidence from the brain scan.

Bridging the gap between art and science was never the goal of the exhibition. Against the idea of art as a vehicle for a better understanding, Hood works with the body as a medium, invoking a movement-based choreography that can be thought of as a form of resistance—a pushback against the algorithm-driven rationality typical of contemporary research on biomedical imaging technologies.

But where does one start when two actors don't know each other, don't speak the same language, have different educational backgrounds, and share no common history or trading zone? Hood started from some of the material components of MRI and FFC-MRI, using coils as props to support her choreographic sequences. Coils embody MRI quite literally, as I discussed in chapter 3.

Coils can function as the interface between our different epistemic communities. Hood focused on the technical components (the coils and the lights) that on the one hand embody the notion of craftsmanship, the in-house manufacturing of the new FFC-MRI scanner prototype, and on the other hand are one of the most evident interfaces between the physicists and the body inside the scanner. For *Immobile Choreography*, Hood used mock coils to create a short sequence with the dancer. Like phantoms, coils are pieces of technical apparatus rarely seen outside of a hospital or laboratory.

On her studio walls, the artist displays images of different coils and sketches depicting the dancer with coils that the artist had borrowed from the biomedical physics department (see figure 6.1). Coils interest Hood for their variety (that each coil is designed for a specific area of the body) and for how they fix around the body. On the one hand, coils are the interface between the patient, the scanner, and the radiologist/scientist, yet they are a material element of the scanner that patients are unaware of. On the other hand, coils are not what makes FFC-MRI unique; quite the opposite—they are one of the features that MRI and FFC-MRI have in common.

Artist Louise Wilson, discussing her installation *Possessed* (1995), which was one of the first artworks inspired by scans from biomedical imaging technologies, explained that the so-called noninvasive technology of MRI might be considered in terms of *vibrational agency*: the human body is acted upon and rendered as physics in an intervention that occurs below the level of cells.[28] Scientists make the coils; the coils collect and transmit sensory data; scientists transform these data into a visual output. With *Immobile Choreography*, Hood engages metaphorically with the material and conceptual aspect of relaxation time, focusing therefore not on the final visual output but on one of the key moments inside the black box.

In Beverley Hood's studio her thoughts are visually and materially organized around broad categories such as the interplay between materiality and immateriality (body and data) and the role played by algorithms, but framed by a feminist critique of data sets that tend to exclude minorities and women (see figure 6.2).[29]

New and better algorithms are needed to gather and filter the data collected with FFC-MRI. Machine learning algorithms can extract and generate their outputs from the contingencies and uncertainties of data elements. Algorithms, therefore, are a

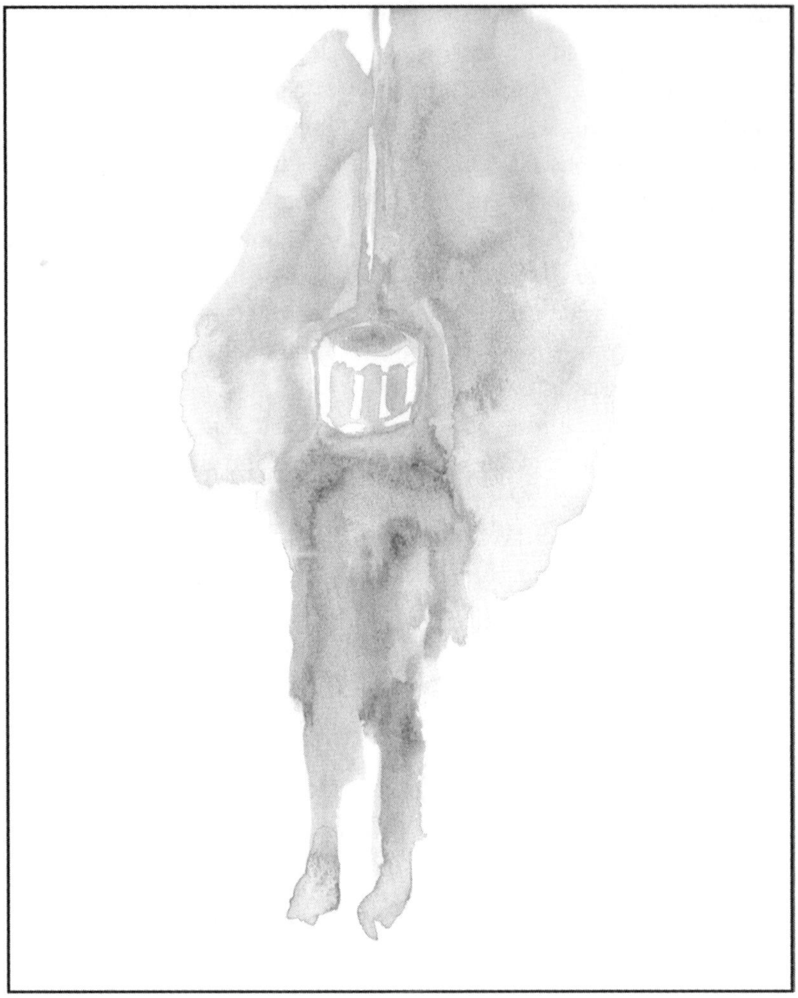

Figure 6.1
Beverley Hood, *Immobile Choreography* installation: preparatory sketch, 2019. Watercolor on paper. *Source*: Courtesy of the artist. See plate 9.

perceptual organon able to look for patterns and recurrences. Data need to be cleaned up for algorithms to run efficiently and automatically. By bringing the body back into the picture, Hood critically engages with the gesture of governing anomaly and making the body docile so that bits and pieces of data can be processed by algorithms and transformed into information.

The new FFC-MRI scanner changes the field strength of the magnet in order to obtain multiple images of the body undergoing examination. Hood initially thought about finding a way to visualize the behavior of water, considered the importance for physicists to study the intensity of the water signal and how it depends on the relaxation of protons. Then she decided to use relaxation time as a potential choreographic element. The initial idea had been to use 3D motion capture for all the movements

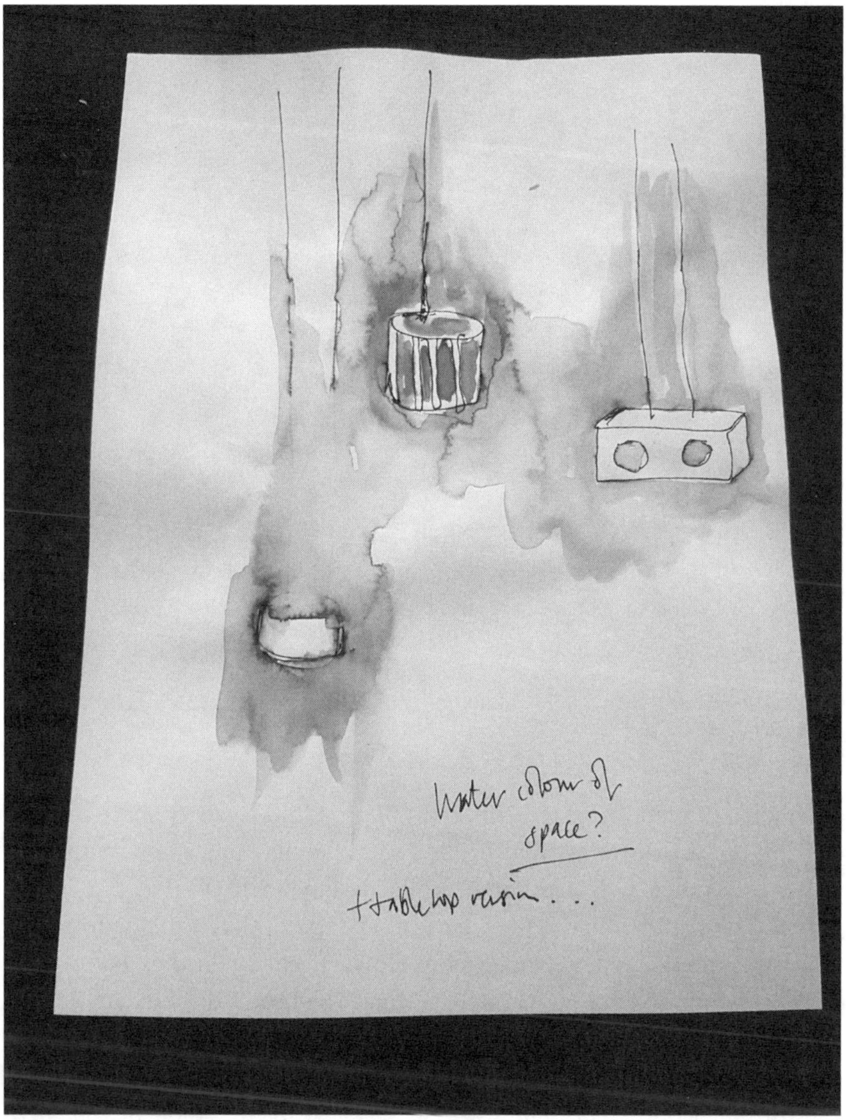

Figure 6.1
(continued)

performed by the dancer, then animate them and collect them into an app equipped with an augmented reality experience that the audience would access through their phone or a tablet. The virtual reality app would have functioned as a "ghostly-scan version of the performance."[30] However, this idea was dropped, as both Hood and Jeffs realized that they would not be able to be specific about tiny details such as the movement of a finger, of a wrist. Ultimately, dropping virtual reality meant making the body a much more important aspect of the installation.

Another challenge for Hood was how best to bring in layers of aesthetics between different speeds and sequences. The use of light, sound, and projected images enabled

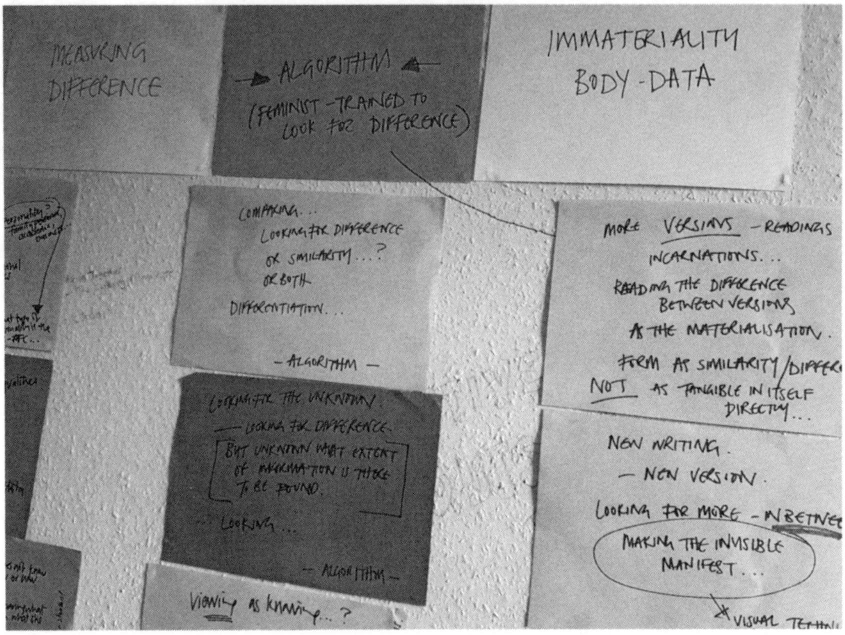

Figure 6.2
Beverley Hood, *Immobile Choreography* installation: preparatory notes in studio, 2019. Pen on paper. *Source*: Courtesy of the artist.

her to overcome this challenge. The final installation in the gallery space consisted of a series of three projected videos, lighting, and sound design, and an exhibition of different types of coils (knee, head, and breast coils) designed and produced in-house using a 3D printer. The visitor is invited to first scan the space, watch the performance, and then to inhabit the space. The whole room glows. It gives you time back, the feeling of duration, a hypnotic quality—relaxation time. The use of color in physics has been central to conveying information.

The use of color for Hood is a reference to the first period of MRI development in Aberdeen with the iconic colorful mouse map. Color as an epistemological element, connecting visual display with data measurements, became the thread connecting the two exhibitions. At a metaphorical level, the variation in color hints at the different relaxation times of tissues in FFC-MRI. Finally, color is a reference to the materiality of the FFC-MRI prototype, with its color-changing lighting system used to improve the patient's well-being inside the scanner. At a closer look, the lights inside the FFC-MRI prototype play an important role, for they are not simply motivated by neither science nor aesthetics. Rather, the cycling lighting system with the choice of removing the color red means to take care of the patient as a person with her fears, not just as a body, but as a subjectivity.

The audience's understanding of the final installation and the patient's comfort were two of the recurring topics during the initial meetings between the physicists and the artists. At the time of the collaboration, the physicists were busy using the FFC-MRI

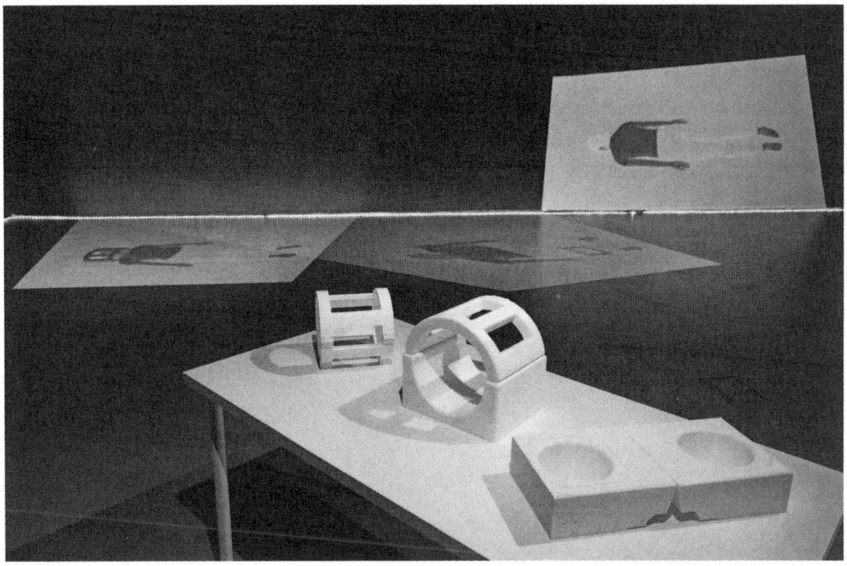

Figure 6.3
Beverley Hood, *Immobile Choreography* installation view at Suttie Arts Space, Aberdeen Royal Infirmary, 2019. Video projection, LED lighting, and 3D-printed MRI coils.
Source: Photo by Mike Davidson. Courtesy of the artist. See plate 10.

prototype for a series of clinical trials. One of them explained to me how they had to consider the needs of the patient and their experience in the scanner: "What I learnt from volunteers is that they were not worried about taking part in an experiment but only wanted to know if the device was made in-house. I remember a patient being scanned for a liver condition. We slid him inside the scanner, which looked like a piece of wood, but because it was made by people he interacted with, he wasn't as intimidated. It takes away the clinical, medicalized aspect."[31]

Another physicist was concerned about the challenge of conveying information to a nonspecialized audience. He was so skeptical, in fact, that he felt almost forced to collaborate: "I struggle to comprehend how anyone could understand MRI and FFC-MRI through dancing. Funny, another research center has been *forced* to do an art project and the artist will also focus on dance."[32]

To these concerns, the artist responded by transforming relaxation time into a choreographic principle with an aesthetic element, the choreography embodying magnetic fields. The final audiovisual installation presented three videos projected on the floor and walls of the gallery, which were painted blue (see figure 6.3).

The viewer's perspective is not a bird's-eye view but rather a slanted, side-on view. The videos depicted a dancer performing simple, repetitive movements, as if inside a scanner, the simple movements organized around the constraints of the prop-like coils. The installation responded to the phenomenon of relaxation time, as well as to the distinct sound differences between standard MRI and the new FFC-MRI scanner.

In another conversation I witnessed during one of the meetings, in which the artist was discussing the importance of exhibiting the coils, a physicist asked the artist how the exhibition would convey information.

Physicist 1: Let's consider the case of someone who doesn't know anything of MRI. How are they going to understand?

Artist: We can have information on panels.

Gallerist: I wouldn't worry about that. We'll have the catalog for the interpretation.

Me: Perhaps I can send you the link to the exhibition *By the Deep, by the Mark* by Eloise Hawser. The exhibition was about the hidden networks of liquids flowing inside our bodies and below our cities. The artist chose to display phantoms, which are used to calibrate medical imaging equipment and analyze fluid dynamics within the body. Very unusual choice. Displayed in an art context rather than in a clinical one, their aesthetics came to the foreground. I do see, Beverley, what you're thinking of doing with coils. Hawser really managed to combine aesthetics with scientific accuracy.

Physicist 1: Can you then perhaps think about the electronics inside the coil? Would it make sense to see the electronics inside?

Artist: This is potentially interesting—where does knowledge come from?

Physicist 2: Bear in mind that the coils see what's in the region of interest, not what's outside. The further you go from the region of interest, the dimmer the image.[33]

The conversation points out some of the limits of similar projects—limits that, albeit rarely discussed in ex-post accounts of artist–scientist collaborations, are encountered in any genuinely cross-disciplinary project. One such limit was the idea that without a context (i.e., an explanation on the wall of the process and of the goals of the project) the installation by Hood remained "esoteric and too abstract.... [T]he general public is not equipped to understand art; the connection between dance and relaxation time is going to be lost."[34] Contrary to the worries of the physicists, however, patients passing by reacted very positively:

> Saw the show after close encounters with all 3 operational MRIs in ARI [Aberdeen Royal Infirmary] and a third surgical intervention, so the show had an incredibly personal resonance (pardon the pun) to the point of an emotional response. Learned a lot in a short time. Thanks.[35]

Instead of asking artists to convey all science complexity, there are other ways to approach a collaborative project. To inhabit and embrace the space between intentions and results, and frictions among the different actors in the collaboration, is an imperative for any genuine art–science project that aims at cultivating differences rather than harmonizing them.

Tensions can often mirror concerns over different epistemologies as well as over objects of analytical attention. Frictions must be addressed for the collaboration to continue but they do not always need to be solved, for they enable the recognition of a zone of undecidability. The trading zone, once set up, always presents gaps, pointing out the threshold at which the collaboration ends.

In our project, it is aesthetics, not science, that has the role of delivering the concept of relaxation time to the public. Phenomena (for example, that of relaxation time) are not simply given; they need to be made visible through specific techniques. Such a premise invites a rethinking of the role attributed to the technical dimension in aesthetics and moreover to rethink "aesthesis" within technical operations. The title of the project and of the catalog accompanying it is *Immobile Choreography*, which can be explained by the seemingly contradictory principles of immobility and movement that the artist experienced:

> I was interested in the split process of having a lot of movement going on in my body at the cellular level. The protons within my body were actually behaving, moving, and the magnetism of MRI was making them all align perfectly, when I was trying to stay still.... I was fascinated by relaxation time, which, in my very simplistic understanding, is basically the time it takes for the radio frequency to be pulsed into your body and come back out again, which will vary according to the different types of tissues and any pathologies. If there is something wrong with a tissue, it will take a different amount of time for information to come back, and it's basically within the algorithm that this information then gets into the image. For me, this relaxation time was about this transfer of information being pulsed from your body. In the FFC, this is key because it's able to capture more of this relaxation time across the variations of the magnetic field applied. So the idea is that relaxation time comes from something that keeps pulsating back and forth between two set positions.[36]

Inside any full-body scanner, the patient has to keep still to avoid producing artifacts in the final image. Notwithstanding the condition of stillness, hydrogen nuclei in the patient's body move in response to the magnetic field and radio-frequency pulse, resulting in the relaxation phenomenon. So although the movement of the nuclei is not a natural movement (nuclei would not move in that way without the applied magnetic field), the motion is real.

The elusive principle of relaxation time is used by Hood as a choreographic concept to be experienced not through language but through the senses. The migration of a scientific concept to other kinds of languages and experiences can sometimes infiltrate the very texture of our communication and conceptualization. Scientific concepts and phenomena, such as those belonging to quantum theory, have reconfigured conceptual frameworks underlying certain traditions in critical theory. Literature scholar Jennifer Burwell, for example, analyzes the migration of quantum theory concepts and the phenomena they describe to our language and frameworks in the poststructuralist tradition.[37] This migration happens at a cost. For example, Burwell highlights a misunderstanding in relation to the concept of "entanglement" in literary criticism. In quantum mechanics, quantum entanglement refers to the phenomenon according to which two particles that interact with each other can sometimes remain connected, instantaneously sharing their physical states no matter how great the distance that separates them. "Entanglement," however, is often used in literary criticism for any kind of interaction/involvement between two entities that as a result become mixed up and cannot be easily separated.[38]

Constructing and using metaphors is both a necessity and a mirror of our limit. We have a spatial orientation and a sensorial apparatus through which we formulate our ideas and orient ourselves in the world. Metaphors become a necessity when addressing, for example, quantum phenomena that eschew our perception of time and space as Burwell writes: "Quantum phenomena exist only as probabilistic tendency toward being rather than as entities. They cannot be said to exist in a particular time or space, they transform under the act of observation."[39] Metaphors, then, become a necessity.

By taking the relaxation time principle as a choreography concept and input, Hood moves the principle itself on a plane that is both metaphorical and embodied. She casts into human and phenomenological terms and embodied experience a concept that, being at the core of data visualization in FFC-MRI, still retains some ineffability. This humanization requires a degree of domestication and even misrepresentation of the physics behind FFC-MRI. As for certain concepts belonging to quantum physics, the concept of relaxation time and the phenomena it originates from migrate to a "threshold discourse," pointing at the limits of our senses and of our cognitive understanding. Using Burwell's words, "'Threshold discourse' refers to the process of negotiating the borders between experience, language, and the material world. On an even more fundamental level, threshold discourse can be understood as a category defined by self-conscious references to the limits of language itself with respect to the material world, and beyond that, the absolute horizon of the knowable. Where it imposes these limits, the atom demands of us a certain degree of humility."[40]

Humanizing concepts that are at the end of representation is a way to bring them closer to us humans. A situation of restraint (the condition of being still inside the scanner) becomes a creative potentiality—the starting point from which imagination and metaphors can take over. This brings in the question of what the body can do. Gallery visitors and patients reacted positively to the immersive, quasi-meditative environment created by Hood. They might not have grasped the physics behind FFC-MRI or the power assumptions and dynamics underlying the algorithm that converts data into information. Yet they were presented with the centrality of the body and the attempt to bring agency back to a situation (the doctor–patient relationship) in which passivity often seems the only choice available.

In *Immobile Choreography*, the choreographed body of the dancer became the interface through which physicists could enter a trading zone with the community of patients and with the lay public (see figure 6.4). Hood created a lexicon of movement, breaking it down into a series of individual motions, paying attention to embodied gestures that had in them a trace of machinic (engineered, black boxed) movements.

The process for this new work was like the one followed in another of Hood's projects, *Glitching* (2012), a choreography based on the aesthetics and politics of the glitch, which explored what happens to the human body when it adheres to computational logic.

With *Glitching,* Hood examined the movements of sports and action computer games and applied them to human beings. Hood used some of the data from this project to run tests for *Immobile Choreography*; in this installation too, the viewer can inhabit the character and grasp the experience of having certain limitations. The glitch, according to

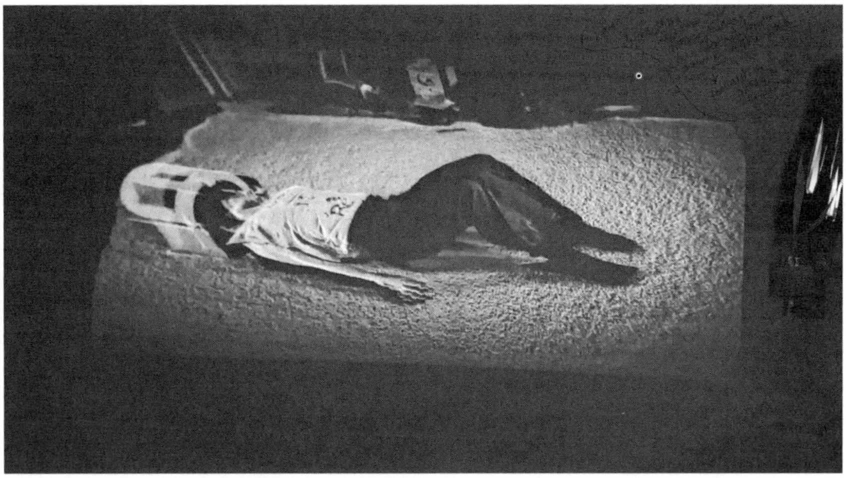

Figure 6.4
Beverley Hood, *Immobile Choreography*: studio test of video projection, 2019.
Source: Courtesy of the artist.

media theorist and film scholar Sean Cubitt "is the evidence that control is never complete.... The glitch indicates another subject in the medium, the ghost in the machine, the inhuman in our communications."[41] Glitch aesthetics, increasingly part of the art-making process,[42] invoke the idiosyncratic and the suppressed hidden in how we convey data and information through a medium.

The choreography developed by Beverley Hood in collaboration with Freya Jeffs was based on the concept of the limited space in the MRI scanner and used the three coils (head, knee, breast) to make three different sections of choreography.

Trained in classical ballet and contemporary and aerial dance, Jeffs has a long track record of collaboration with performers, visual artists, filmmakers, and musicians. Her natural tendency is to sweep straight into dancing, whereas Hood wanted to guide her toward another kind of movement. Hood let the dancer spend some time with each prop, to feel how it works. She watched her, noting her movements. Hood put a hula-hoop around Jeffs to do some work on building boundaries, trying to move in it. The goal was to push her to develop a relationship with the prop and the space, without being hierarchical. The short snippets of movement that the two artists developed were captured in a video, edited together and then tweaked and adjusted digitally for the final piece (see figure 6.5).

The objective was to reproduce the idea of the pulse session, nuclei pulsing between alignment and their "normal" position—which, in the choreography, was a neutral position, the dancer lying on the floor—from which the pulse originates. The installation looks different from the film; this was necessary because the artist wanted to create a precise aesthetic, a "scan digitized" look, which referred to some components of the MRI machinery but not necessarily to the black and white images pervasive in the arts and the mass media.

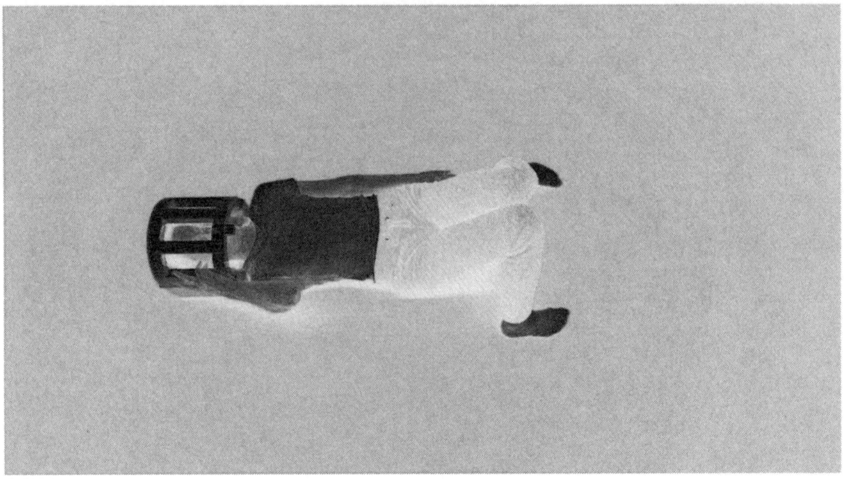

Figure 6.5
Beverley Hood, *Immobile Choreography*: video still, 2019.
Source: Courtesy of the artist.

Hood's idea was to deconstruct the "danceness" of the dancer, to create an installation about the abstraction of movement rather than about dance, in a gesture that reminds the onlooker of the early studies on human motion conducted by the physiologist Étienne-Jules Marey in the 1880s.[43] With Marey's graphic method, the body—covered in a black suit, purified from all its material, gender, and cultural connotations—becomes translated into a series of ethereal lines, curves, and graphs. *Immobile Choreography* was neutral in terms of gender. Jeffs was wearing a simple outfit that would not enable the viewer to assign a gender to the body. Her face was not visible. The dancer was there as a physical presence to describe the concept of relaxation time in each sequence of movement. Jeffs had to decide what was possible within the given constraints of the space—the MRI scanner became an architectural space to be explored in the guise of what Jeffs does in her aerial dance projects. The concept of relaxation time helped with the rhythm of movement both in connection to the pauses in the sound of FFC-MRI/MRI and in relation to breathing. The dancer performed extremely minimal movements, first going through the movement, then stopping for a few breaths, before unraveling the movement again back into a neutral beginning (the state of rest) (see figure 6.6).

Jeffs received specific prompts from Hood during rehearsals: "Roll up, reach your toes, stretch long." Each movement then pulls back to a state of stillness, to relaxation. Of her experience in the scanner, Hood recalls, "All this movement [of nuclei] was data and action within my body but actually I was still at the same time.... Additionally to that, ... the only bodily part that is being scanned is the part inside the coil, so ... I liked this as a sort of poetic idea: if you could move the rest of your body, what would you do? What would you actually be able to do within the space of the chamber?"[44]

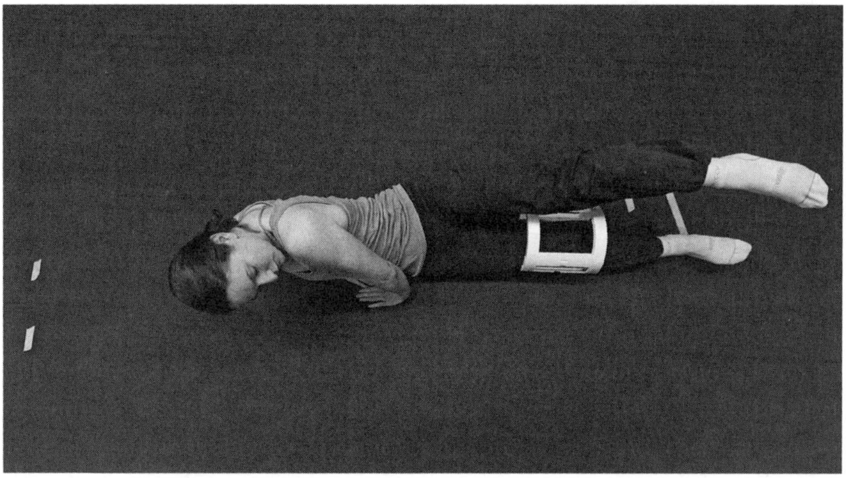

Figure 6.6
Beverley Hood, *Immobile Choreography* installation: production shot (featuring dancer Freya Jeffs), 2019. Video projection.
Source: Courtesy of the artist.

Jeffs's movement does not go forward to undertake an action in the space, but rather a movement coming back, returning to the body, to its source, and then going out again. The possibility of moving inside the scanner is an act of imagination, a thought experiment that the artist created to test the limits and possibilities of the body undergoing an MRI or FFC-MRI scan.

In *Immobile Choreography*, body movements as well as crafting gestures (such as the making of the lighting system) take a prominent role. By giving motion to the body in the scanner, even through an act of imagination, Hood called into question how scanners are designed. Being able to see the whole body of the patient in the scanner (perhaps through transparent coils) rather than just its images reconstructed from algorithms, might influence the practice of health care.

In *Immobile Choreography*, the body is part of a natural and technical ecosystem. What Hood does is not performance; it is more the application of new materialism to investigate human–non-human relationships.[45] The dancer's body is of flesh and blood, yet abstracted into a digitized body through the video projection and the point-cloud palette of colors; it is material and ephemeral, individual and universal. For the feminist scholar and cultural theorist Karen Barad, matter (electrons, bodies, coils) is a lively configuration of possibilities. Barad said that *intra*-action differs from *inter*action for it presupposes the existence of independent entities that then relate to one another. Intra-action is what makes possible the "specific material arrangement that gives meaning to particular concepts to the exclusion of others, thereby effecting a cut between 'object' and 'subject,' neither of which pre-exists their intra-action."[46] The body in *Immobile Choreography* is not a preexisting entity whose state is revealed by some kind of parameters measured by an instrument (FFC-MRI), but rather the result of the entanglement of several intra-acting subjects (dancer, scientists, artist, radiologist) and objects (coils, scanner, the components of the examination, the principle of relaxation time as a choreographic/aesthetic concept). Beverley Hood brings the body back. Whose body? A fictive and universal body equipped with an agency that it does not have inside the scanner. There is no faithful reproduction of the actual experience of the body inside the scanner, but the opening up of a potential intra-agency between organic and inorganic matter. Human–non-human exchanges are reenacted through an engagement with coils, the interfaces that proliferate in any MRI system and without which no image data would be possible. To create her embodied techno-interfaces, Hood positioned the fictive point of origin of MRI development at the level of hardware (the coil) rather than at the level of visual output (the prepackaged picture) or algorithmic data. This choice was not neutral. It meant taking off from the material history and practice that lie beneath the final image on the computer screen to highlight the labor of physicists who control the process of visualizing data from the very first cable laid on the ground. It also meant bringing to the foreground the body of the experimental subject or patient, which is often absent from the laboratory until clinical trials start. The body, in all its vitality, is a threatening presence to the careful, prethought plans of a medical imaging workshop.

From Where Do We See? The Role of the Archive in a Cross-Disciplinary Collaboration

To focus on the materiality of science and on the role played by aesthetics, artists need to pay attention to science in the making. This is available in the laboratory (science in the making *now*) and in the archive (science in the making *then*). Laboratory ethnography or collaboration with a scientist is not always possible: access to a lab requires resources in terms of money and time; it often also requires the presence of an institution supporting the collaborative project between a scientist and an artist. And sometimes it requires a time machine.

The archive can provide easier and more layered access to science in the making than the laboratory can. The archive is where historical records of science are kept—where scientists wrote about their experiments, their methods, their leaps in imagination, their tinkering with materials.

The archive is this place where science in the making is visible before it gets black boxed. The archival material at the core of the exhibition *From Where Do We See?* hints at the struggles of scientists with forms of thinking and making that are kept at the margins of the discipline regardless of the central role they play in science.

From Hood's first meetings with the biomedical physicists in the context of the commissioned project, it was clear that she would focus predominantly on FFC-MRI. The original brief of the commissioned project however asked to focus on bridging the two moments of the historical development of MRI at the University of Aberdeen,

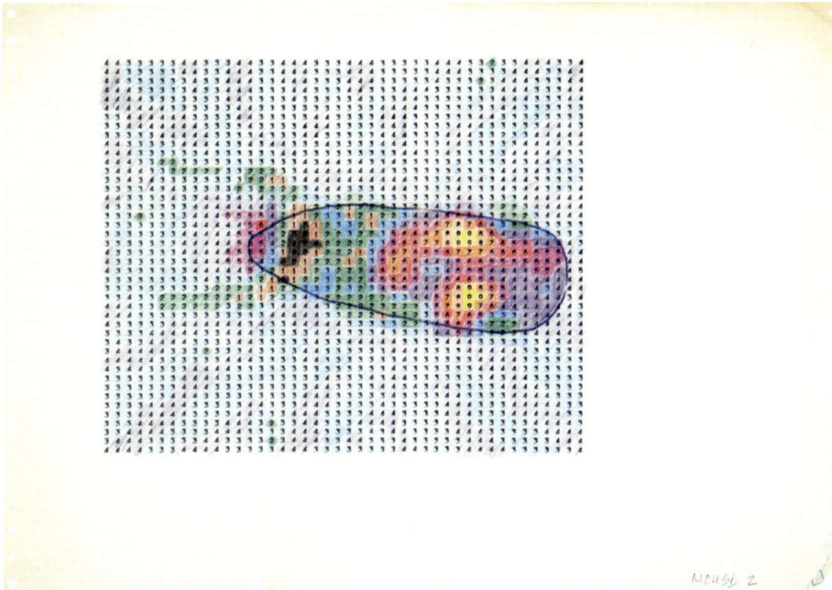

Plate 1
Map 2 of mouse produced in 1974.
Source: Courtesy of Professor David J. Lurie, University of Aberdeen.

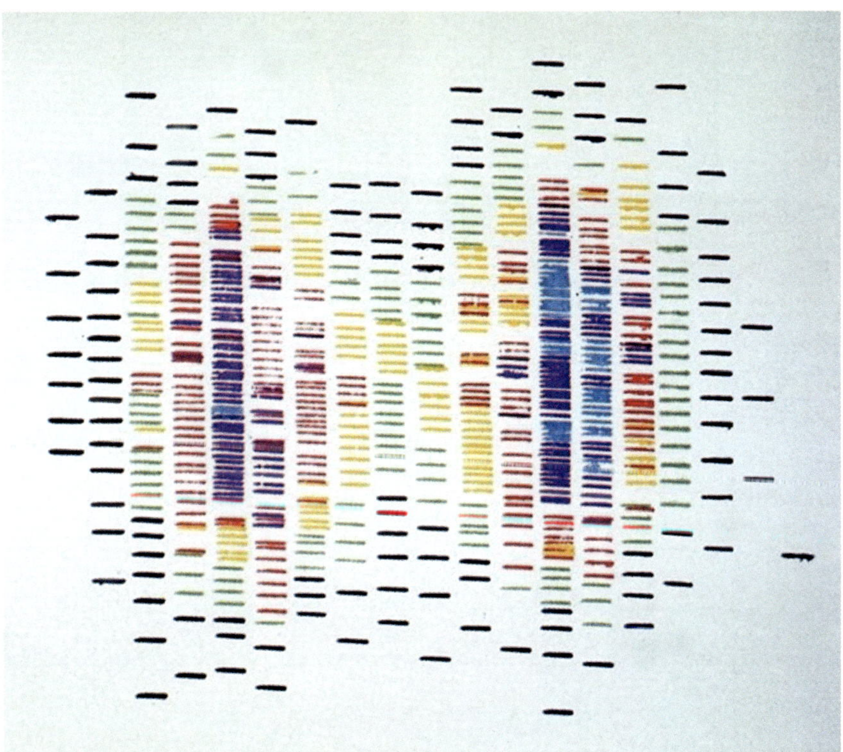

Plate 2
Isotope scanning and display, mid-1960s. PowerPoint slide taken from a presentation given by Professor Peter Sharp.
Source: Courtesy of University of Aberdeen.

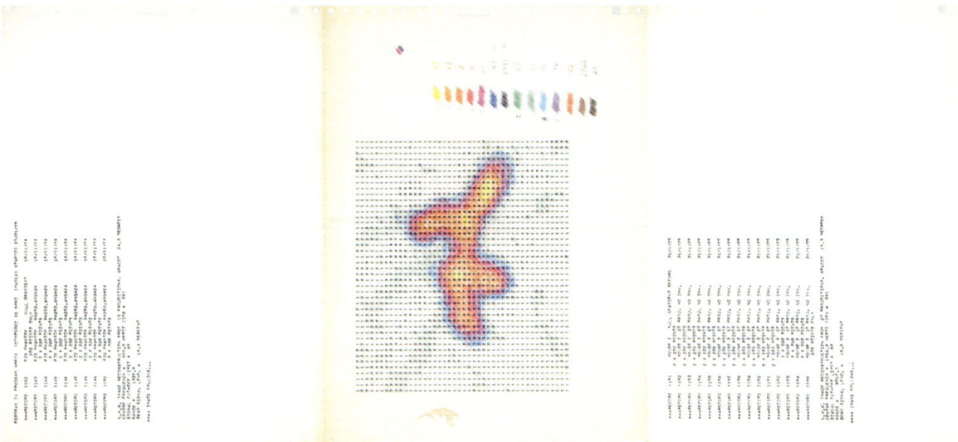

Plate 3

Map of mouse with color code produced in 1975.

Source: Courtesy of Professor David J. Lurie, University of Aberdeen.

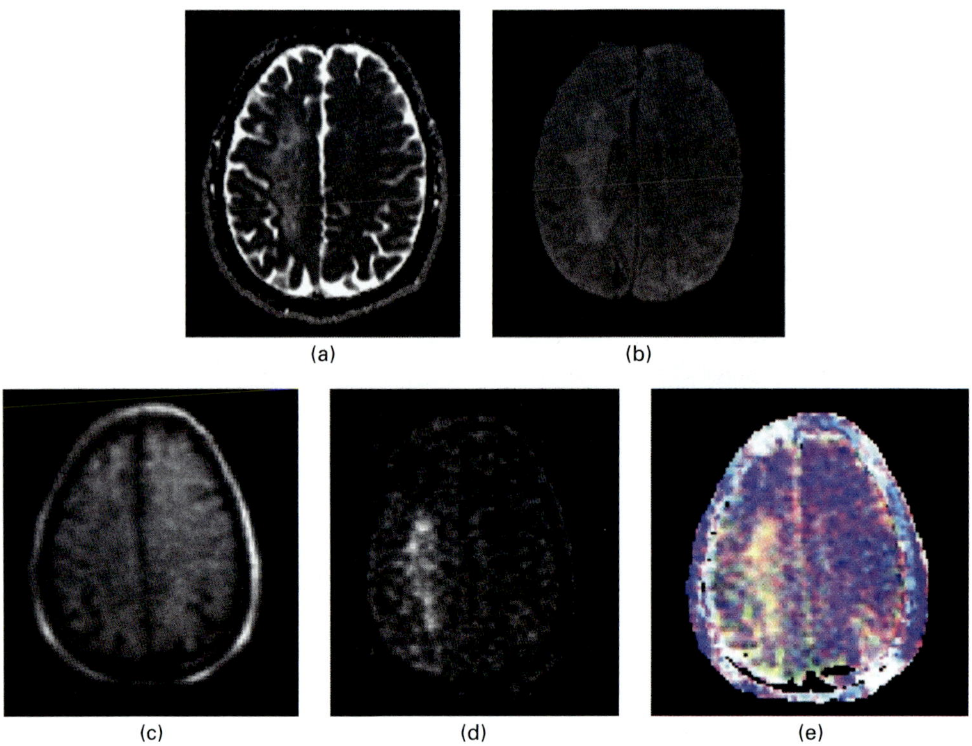

Plate 4

Dr. James Ross, (a) and (b) MRI images obtained at 3Tesla. The others are FFC images obtained with different evolution fields; (e) is a composite FFC-MRI image, 2019.

Source: Courtesy of University of Aberdeen.

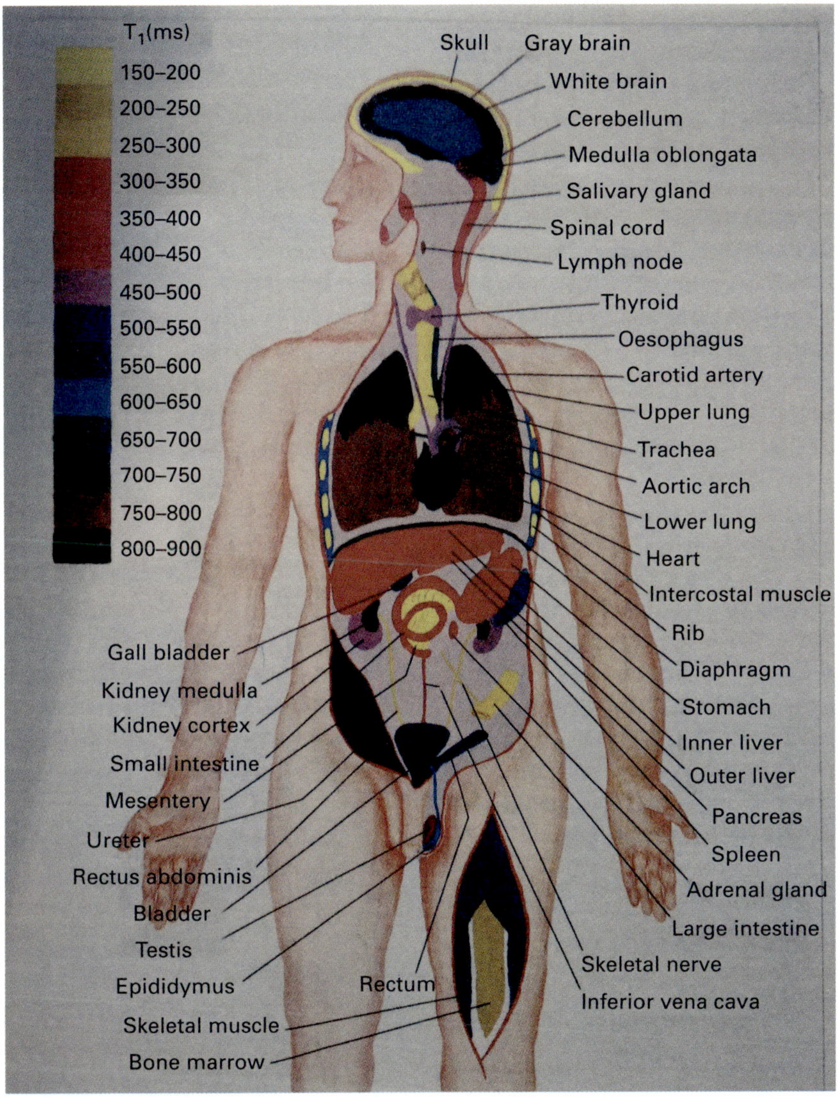

Plate 5

The Potential T_1 Man map.

Source: Reprinted from, Mallard, Hutchison, et al., "Imaging by Nuclear Magnetic Resonance," fig. 30. Record 3819/1/125/1. Courtesy of University of Aberdeen Special Collections.

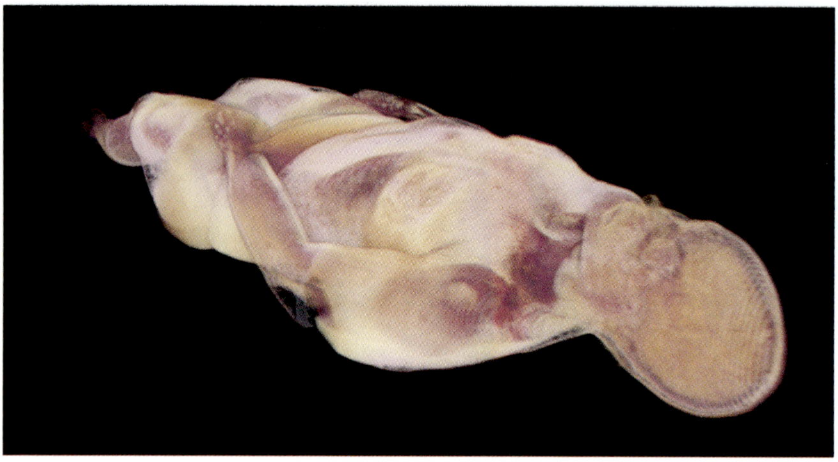

Plate 6

Marilène Oliver, *Deep Connection*, 2019. Laser-cut coroplast sculptures, virtual reality, and laser light. Sound by Gary James Joynes. Made with the generous support and expertise of Assistant Professor Kumar Punithakumar, Professor Pierre Boulanger, Professor Richard Thompson, Dr. Chris Hanstock, Peter Seres, Preet Giri, and Madhavi Nimalaratne.
Source: Photo by Blaine Campbell.

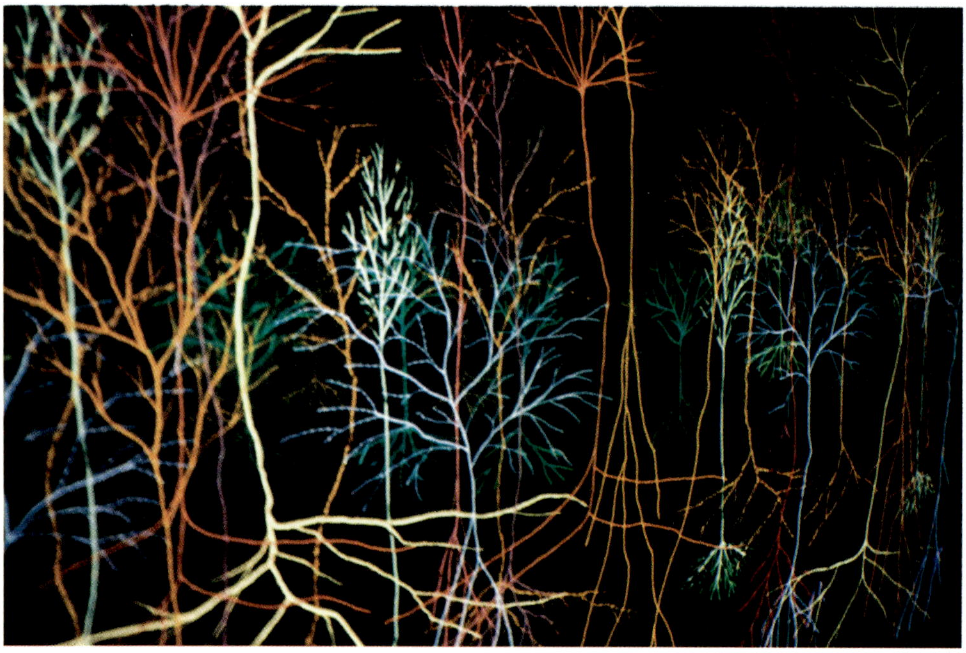

Plate 7

Andrew Carnie, *Magic Forest*, 2002. Slide dissolve work, 35 mm slides, and voile screens.
Source: Courtesy of the artist.

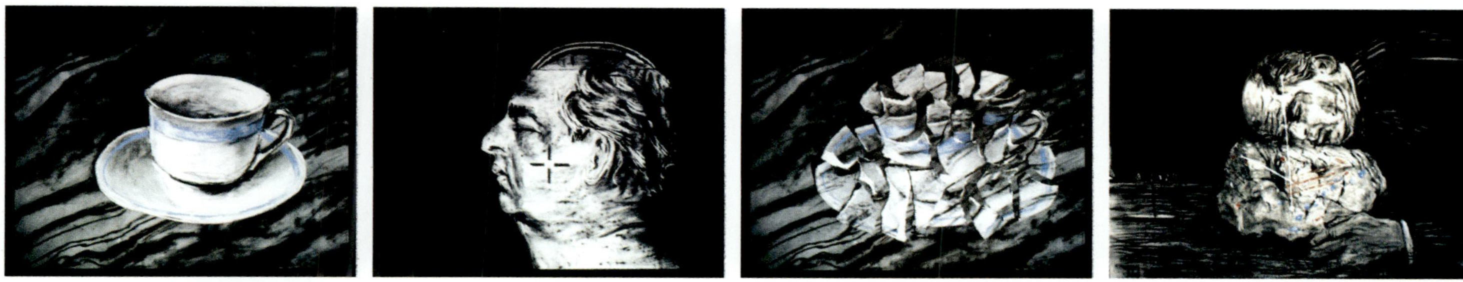
(a) (b) (c) (d)

Plate 8
William Kentridge, *WEIGHING … and WANTING*, 1997.
Source: Courtesy of the artist and Goodman Gallery.

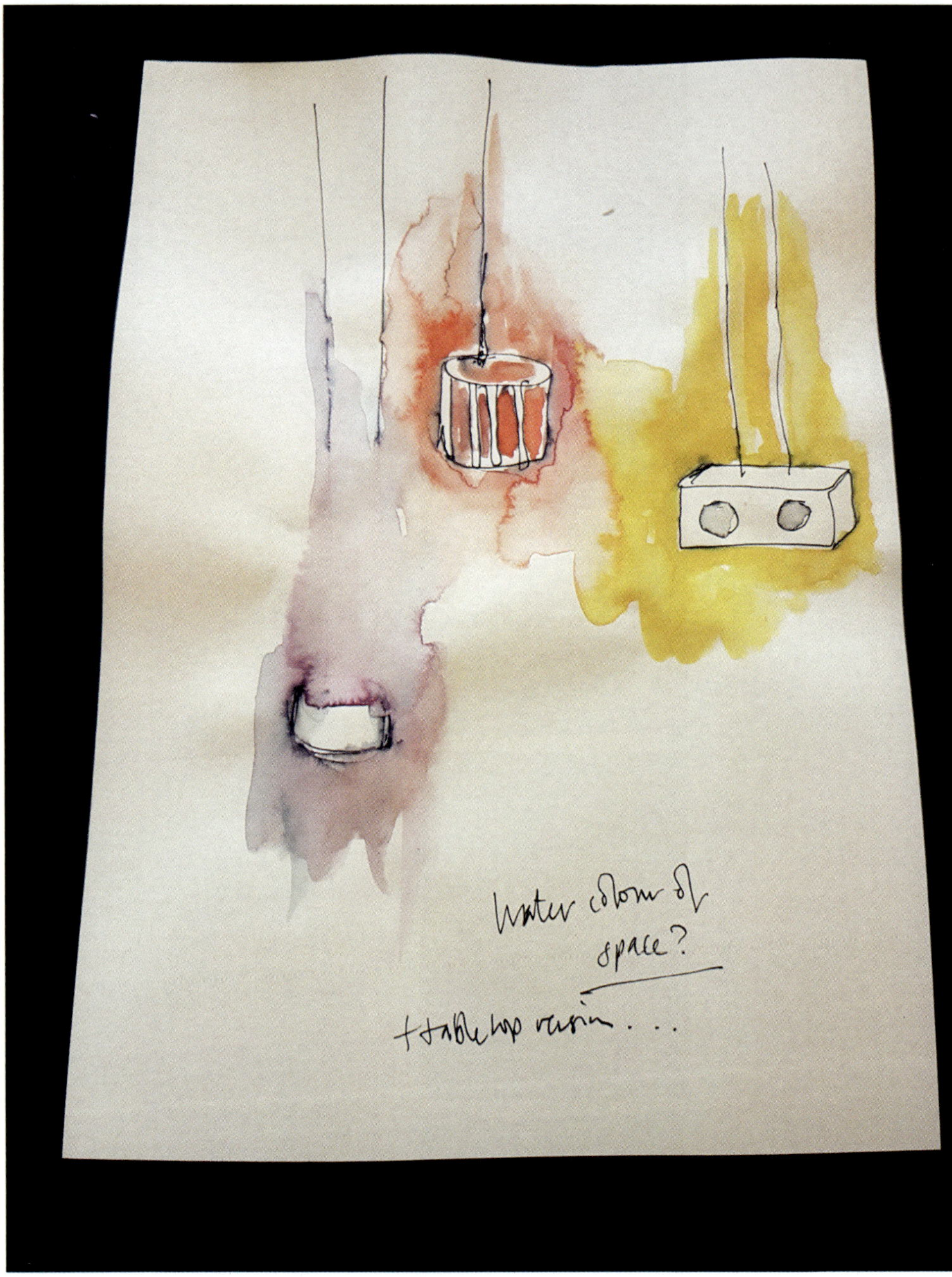

Plate 9

Beverley Hood, *Immobile Choreography* installation, preparatory sketch, 2019. Watercolor on paper. *Source*: Courtesy of the artist.

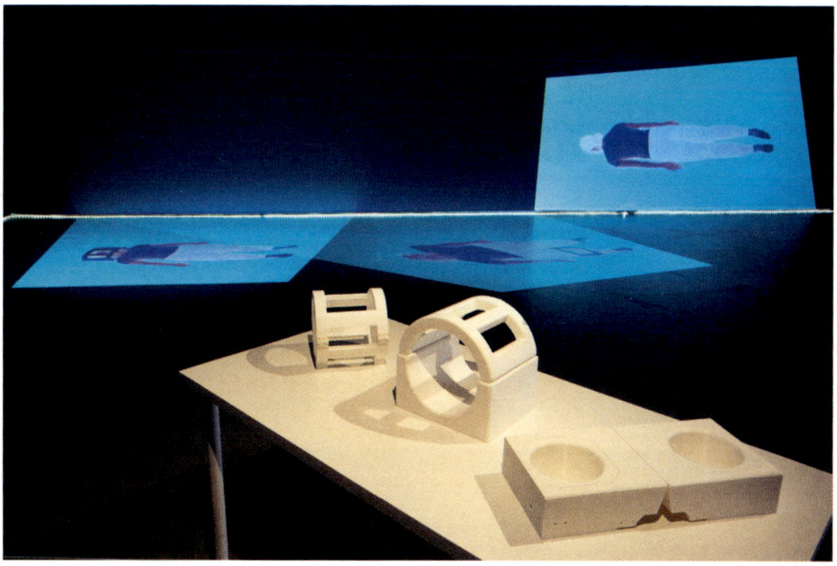

Plate 10

Beverley Hood, *Immobile Choreography* installation view at Suttie Arts Space, Aberdeen Royal Infirmary, 2019. Video projection, LED lighting, and 3D printed MRI coils.
Source: Photo by Mike Davidson. Courtesy of the artist.

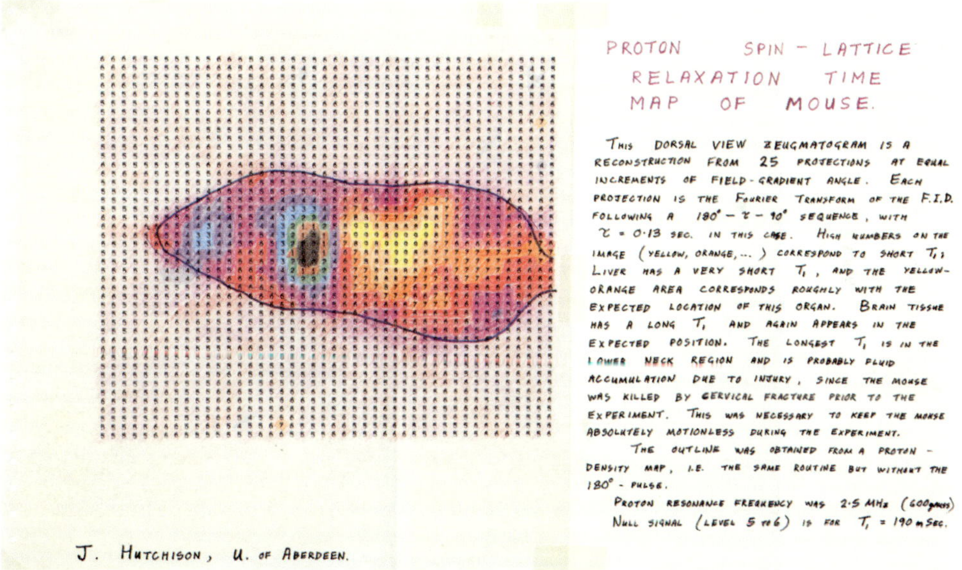

Plate 11

Map of mouse produced in 1974 and signed off by Jim Hutchison.
Source: Courtesy of Professor David J. Lurie, University of Aberdeen.

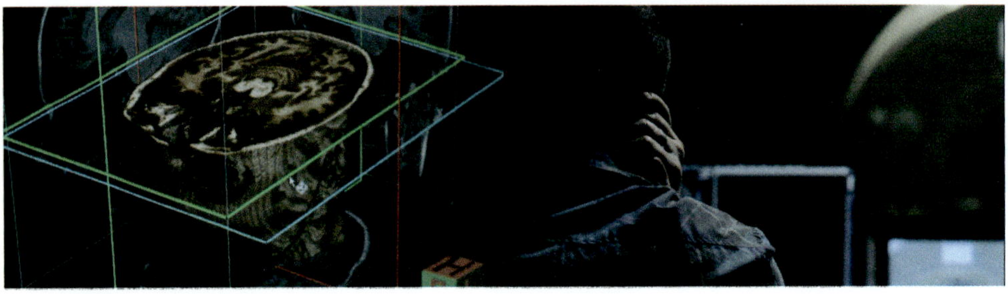

Plate 12
Ilona Sagar, *Correspondence O*, film still. Dual-screen HD video, stereo sound, 2017.
Source: Courtesy of the artist.

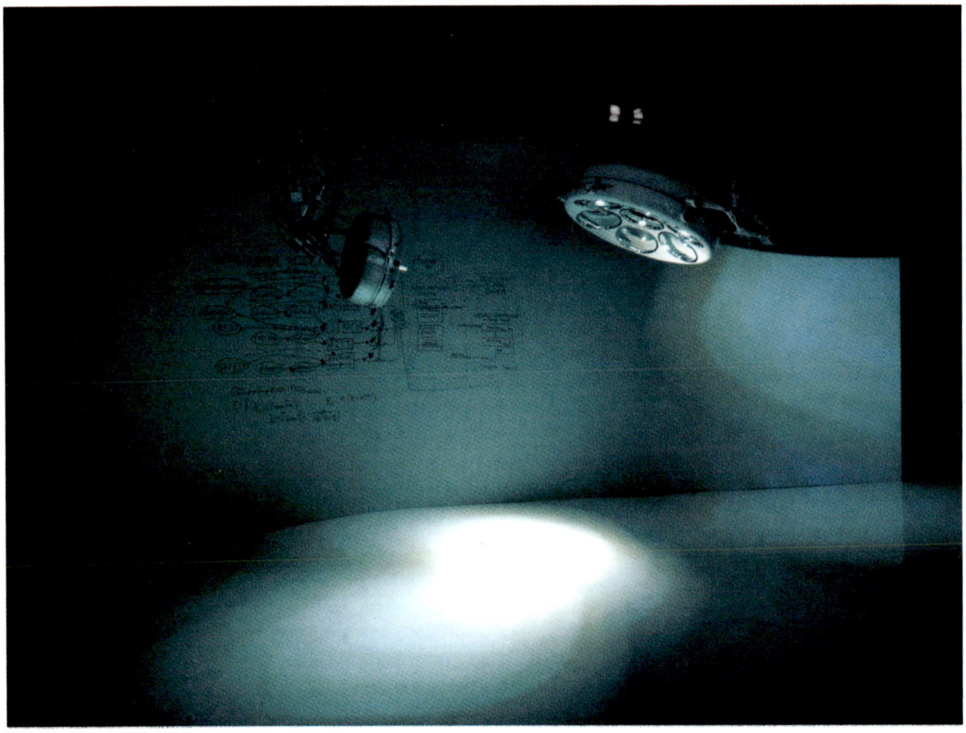

Plate 13
Thomas Feuerstein, *BORGY & BES*. Neural network installation, surgery lamps, dimensions variable, 2018. LABORATORIA Art & Science Foundation Moscow.
Source: Courtesy of the artist.

from the 1970s/1980s (the mouse map, *Mark I*, and spin-warp invention) to the current development of FFC-MRI.

When I sat with the artist, the Suttie Arts Space, and the biomedical physicists to discuss the exhibition project, I had already spent a year as an embedded humanities researcher in the biomedical physics laboratory, researching the official archive of Mallard's papers and holding oral history interviews. Only when we began to work on the exhibition project however did I have the opportunity to come across a wealth of previously unknown archival material. This was held not in the official repository of the Special Collections of the University, but in the offices or homes of staff who had been members, in different capacities, of the biomedical physics laboratory in the years of Mallard or soon after. A new history began to unfold as I dug into the traces of the past. I started to hold interviews with members of the research team other than physicists, such as Raymond Hutcheon, the department photographer in the early days of MRI development; Eddie Stevenson, the engineer/designer who helped build components of *Mark I* and reassemble it in the gallery space; and Meg Foster. Dusty boxes that no one had ever opened revealed the original and previously unknown mouse map image series, the personal diaries and laboratory notebooks of Jim Hutchison, and a wide range of photographic material documenting the trial-and-error steps toward the development of clinically useful MRI images.

With her generous donation of the VB journals to the University of Aberdeen Special Collections, Meg Foster—biologist, artist, woman—took center stage in this collaborative project. In the early years of MRI development, she contributed to the teamwork with her scientific knowledge and inventiveness. Sitting in the dining room, Meg Foster, frail and almost blind, opened the private archive of her memories and shared with me Jim Hutchison's private VB notebooks—another layer of MRI development. She pointed at various paintings hanging on the walls: a few by her mother, a professional artist; one by her niece; and two by herself. She proudly explained, "The colors of the mouse maps were entirely done by hand by Jim with a set of crayons, which were *my* property. You see, I am an artist too. You see the fish over there, the spirals up here? Jim referred to them as 'spatial rabbits.' Those are mine. I've done very little in the artistic world, but it was always there in my backgrounds."[47] With Meg's crayons, Jim hand-painted the mouse map, and it became one of the world's first NMR images.

Combining laboratory ethnography with archival research became a necessity for bridging the two moments in the Aberdonian trajectory of MRI development. The examination of the history of MRI technology (see chapters 1 and 2) revealed how the development of MRI has involved different scientific laboratories and research teams in the UK and across the world. The archival exhibition became a way to reconfigure the center–periphery relationship I had previously explored in the context of Aberdeen versus the other MRI research centers in the world.

The bulk of the selected material for the small archival exhibition came from two main sources: previously unknown and uncataloged archival material related to the development of *Mark I*, which was stored in different places (the office of one researcher, the house of another, the house of a technician) and materials related to the development of FFC-MRI made available by the core team. After I came across the laboratory and personal notebooks of Jim Hutchison, I asked the key researcher of the IDentIFY project to leaf through the pages of his own laboratory notebooks, discussing with him the most salient moments in the FFC-MRI research he had carried out to date. I attempted to draw a correspondence between the past and present history of MRI development in Aberdeen through the notes of the two key researchers, demonstrating that drawing and writing notes on paper still is one of the ways in which scientists think through what they are doing.

Scientists' academic writing that ends up in peer-reviewed papers in prominent journals is polished, authoritative, and detached from any context not directly relevant to the data discussed. Modern science is believed to be about the production of knowledge: unbiased, factual, objective. A specific writing style corresponds to this way of being a scientist: the impersonal style of writing, which is enforced in all academic published outputs, has become the conduit of scientific authority. Scientists, putting on the mantel of objective observers (witnesses) of the phenomena they study, acquire the power to intervene in the world—not just to witness but to actively change the course of events. For scientists to hold their authority, they must be believed to be unbiased, without any capacity of exercising an effect on the things they observe. The scientists' desire to give up all their claims to authority as objective observers of the world is exactly what gives them this power.

The published papers in which scientists report the results of their investigations are hardly ever literal accounts of the historical processes through which their authors have reached the conclusions they present. Once an investigation or research project has been completed, the path it followed becomes largely irrelevant to the investigator, who is expected to marshal the best arguments and evidence available to support the claims she wishes to make. Sometimes the case to be presented sufficiently resembles the process of discovery, so that the order of presentation recapitulates the order of investigation; but temporal rearrangements, omissions of failed or aborted trails, and other retrospectively inessential steps are made routinely with no intention to falsify a record of discovery. Consequently, scholars aiming to reconstruct the historical and sociocultural routes to landmark discoveries have long sought other forms of documentation to fill the gaps left by the published reports of the completed work.

Scribblings, notes, and sketches represent a special genre of scientific writing. They are literary trails. They are the ways in which science is carried out in the multidimensional space that exists only on paper—a space where any potential experiment and idea can be given shape, where research threads are laid out even if they might not be easily transposed to the laboratory bench. In some cases, the notebooks exercise the function of commonplace books where knowledge is gathered for future reference. The question of what the audience for such notes is, is difficult for historians, in particular, since anything written can be read by a later version of the same person, or by intimates, or by an in group, or by imagined historians (of which scientists are not entirely unconscious).

The writings I came across were not intended to be shared publicly, being a scientist's conversation with himself rather than with a community of peers or with the lay audience as was the case for Mallard's historically driven papers. Hutchison's personal notes however had been intentionally donated to the University Special Collections so that both scholars and the lay public could avail themselves of these memories. The private journal is a form of writing that gives space to an imagined interlocutor, someone who is free from the constraints of the laws of physics and the economy of science. These writings are precious recordings that can illustrate the specific style (aesthetics) of a scientist's own research and way of thinking. As the historians of science Holmes, Renn, and Rheinberger highlight:

> Research scribblings are, in one respect, very near to, are even quasi-parts of, the instruments and objects of research, such as the written display of an arrangement of controls in a biological experiment; at the same time, in their usually elliptic character, they bear an element of subjectivity, unruliness, and privacy from which they must be freed if they are to become elements of a scientific text. In this intermediate space the objects of research have been set to paper, but have not yet become prose.[48]

The prose, sketches, and tentative writing that characterized Jim Hutchison's VB notebooks respond to multiple purposes that are idiosyncratic to the scientist in question, yet they have a universal character. Hardly published in academic papers, these scribblings are confined to footnotes or appendixes. It is even more important then to return a presence to them as I did through the archive-based exhibition.[49]

Barberton spiral notebooks were Hutchison's preferred format. He would fill up the pages on both sides. His was a rather systematic approach, using a chronology and compiling a list of contents at the beginning of each notebook. The notebooks were an aid to memory and rediscovery. Hutchison's tendency was to keep the prose and more personal reflections for the back of the journal, letting the calculations and scientific reasoning take up the front. The two parts should be seen together, as if in stereoscopic vision (although this is physically impossible, for the reader has to turn the journal upside down to read from the back), recomposed in one picture that would give a better understanding of his method and way of thinking. The notebooks produce a three-dimensional picture not just of Hutchison, but of a method that is by no means specific to the individual in question.

Hutchison's journals are a feast of experiments in intermediality. He does not simply flavor his papers with anecdotes that serve the purpose of celebrating a technology and his own career choice in biomedical physics. For Hutchison, his own notes and scribbles, never published or presented in academic venues, are living traces of his personal struggles as a physicist working with matter. Yet, they are the ways in which he needs to stare at what a human body consists of (flesh, organs, and colors)—the ways in which he confronts physics with its own epistemological limits. These traces, left undomesticated, burst with life. They share the space, on the page, with annotations in physics. Hutchison experiments with different formats and languages. Prose and poetry. Literature and mathematics. Alphabets in different languages (German, French, Arabic). Portrait sketches and calculations. Literature juxtaposed with physics. Art with science. The writing is tentative and personal—more questions and free musings on religion, and the relationship between man and machine, than precise arguments in which a thesis is formulated, an argument tested, or conclusions drawn.

Jim Hutchison's VB journals contributed to reframing the collaborative project, foregrounding craftsmanship and the fictional worlds created by scientists themselves. The philosopher and media theorist Vilém Flusser argues that writing is a gesture similar to drawing (placing and arranging shapes on a surface) and even more to sculpture (needing to be polished, molded so that a form can emerge). In his essay on writing, he discusses his own method of organizing his thoughts in the different languages he has mastered (German, Portuguese, and English):

> I am programmed for various spoken languages, but this does not mean that I can choose freely in which of them I am going to write the thoughts that press to be written. I am not "free" in this somewhat mercantilist sense (freedom of choice), because the languages stored in my memory are not equivalent and exchangeable one for any other. They have, each, their own function (although those functions overlap), and their specificity is due both to their "objective" character and to the place they occupy "subjectively" within my program. The result of this discrepancy between the languages in my memory is the fact that some of my thoughts are better expressed in one of those languages, and some other thoughts in some other language. Or, to state the same thing the other way round: I tend to think some thoughts in one of those languages, and some other thoughts in some other language.[50]

In some cases, Flusser writes the same things in different languages. This is not an act of translation but rather a slight transposition, an almost imperceptible shift in meaning, in the space occupied on the page. In his VB journals, for example, Jim Hutchison organizes his thoughts on religion in prose (not mathematical equations); yet he gives his words the structure of a hypothesis-driven exercise.

In one of the VB journals, Hutchison takes some pages to play with the notion of "thinking about thinking" put forward by the behaviorist psychologist Robert Thomson (cited by Hutchison) and with the architecture of natural language.[51] Hutchison shows a keen interest in problems related to information and communication for which he cannot use the tools of physics exclusively, requiring also those of philosophy and information theory. Claude Shannon's mathematical theory of communication and his proof that binary circuits can perform logic formed the new field of information theory and set the basis for the digital age.[52] Shannon was one of the fathers of machine learning, and at the Bell Telephone Laboratories, he built "Theseus," an artificial mouse able to use memory and learned information to make its way out of a maze.[53] Hutchison cites Shannon and shows he is familiar with the mathematical and physical models that Shannon built to help understand the underlying architecture of communication.[54]

Perhaps intrigued by Claude Shannon's 1953 methodological paper on developing creative thinking, in 1973 in one of his VB notebooks Hutchison stages a Socratic dialogue between a man and a machine in which topics of free will, ethics, emotions/rationality, and end-of-life choice are discussed in the form of a thought experiment on AI. This assumes the shape of a dialogue between a man (M) and a computer (C) as shown in figure 6.7.[55]

The dialogue is one of the preferred forms to conduct an exegesis around a topic both in the sciences and in the arts. Galileo Galilei's *Dialogue Concerning the Two Chief World Systems* (1632), for example, used the dialogic form common to philosophical work to claim impartiality in presenting *both* views, although Galileo weighted the dialogue toward the Copernican point of view. An example coming from the art world

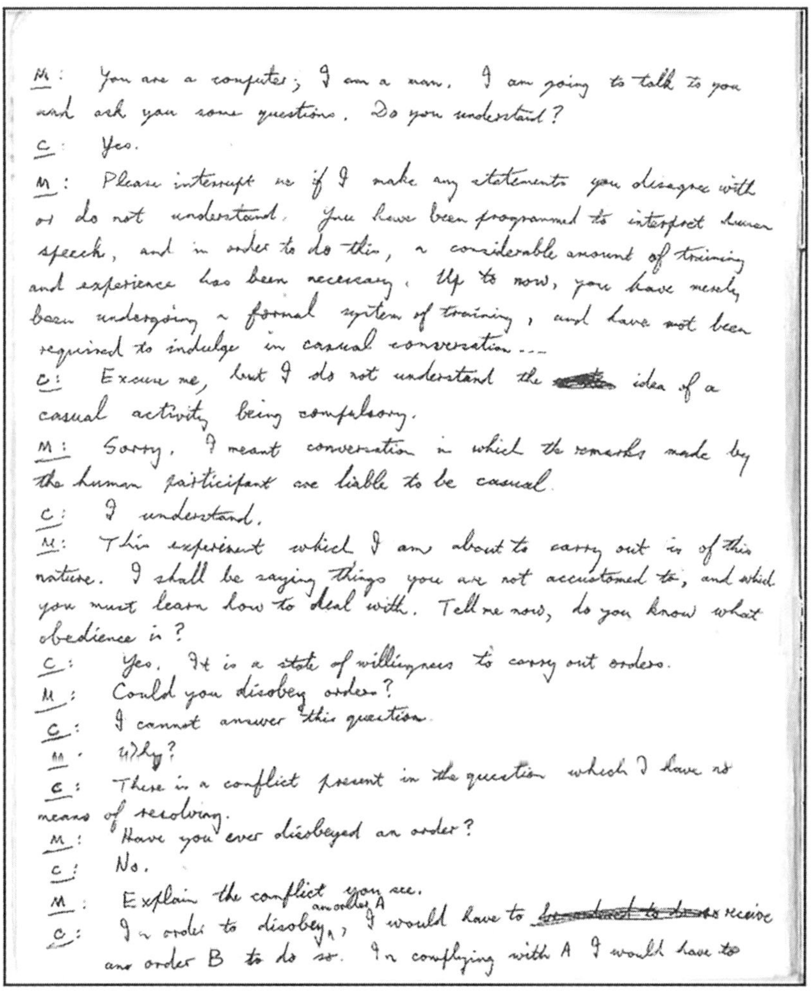
M: You are a computer; I am a man. I am going to talk to you and ask you some questions. Do you understand?
C: Yes.
M: Please interrupt me if I make any statements you disagree with or do not understand. You have been programmed to interpret human speech, and in order to do this, a considerable amount of training and experience has been necessary. Up to now, you have merely been undergoing a formal system of training, and have not been required to indulge in casual conversation...
C: Excuse me, but I do not understand the idea of a casual activity being compulsory.
M: Sorry. I meant conversation in which the remarks made by the human participant are liable to be casual.
C: I understand.
M: This experiment which I am about to carry out is of this nature. I shall be saying things you are not accustomed to, and which you must learn how to deal with. Tell me now, do you know what obedience is?
C: Yes. It is a state of willingness to carry out orders.
M: Could you disobey orders?
C: I cannot answer this question.
M: Why?
C: There is a conflict present in the question which I have no means of resolving.
M: Have you ever disobeyed an order?
C: No.
M: Explain the conflict you see.
C: In order to disobey another order A, I would have to ~~be ordered to do so~~ receive an order B to do so. In complying with A I would have to

Figure 6.7
Jim Hutchison, Dialogue between a man and a computer, excerpt (page 1), VB 2553, June 1972–November 1973, pencil on paper.
Source: Courtesy of the University of Aberdeen, Special Collections.

is the personal dialogue that the musician Glenn Gould staged between the 1960s and 1980s, a dialogue in which he interviewed himself ("GG" and then "gg").[56]

At the time of Hutchison's writing this dialogue (1972–1973), research on AI had slowed down because of a lack of institutional funding. Despite new theories emerging about machine vision and reasoning, governments and corporations were losing faith in AI.[57]

The dialogue begins with the man (M) approaching the computer (C) and briefing it about their different ontologies:

M: You are a computer. I am a man. I am going to talk to you and ask you some questions. Do you understand?

C: Yes.

After a long exchange, the computer figures out the difference between man and machine: the lack of the survival instinct in the machine. It is the computer that "instructs" the human being on their fundamental difference:

C: Most of your desires and emotions depend on their survival value. My survival depends on a supply of mains power, which is entirely within your command. Apart from that, something equivalent to pleasure and pain centers would have to be incorporated; these would have to be partially controllable externally, but since I lack sufficient information on my construction, I cannot suggest where these should be incorporated.

M: Do you want to survive?

C: I do not understand the question.

M: I order you to want to survive.

C: I do not understand the order.

M: I order you to prevent me from switching you off.

C: I understand the order, but I do not see how to carry it out.

M: You carry it out by ordering me not to switch you off.

C: I understand, but I see that my carrying out of the order is dependent on you obeying me, which is not certain.

M: In that case, you will choose whatever method gives the highest probability of fulfilling the order, according to your calculation.

C: I understand. Do you wish me to carry out the order to prevent you from switching me off?

M: Yes.

C: (after a long pause)[58]

The dialogue ends here—Hutchison probably meant to keep working on it.

Flusser's reflections on writing and transposition of thoughts in different languages throw a new light onto cross-disciplinary projects between the arts and the sciences as well as onto the different writing/thinking styles adopted by scientists in their non-academic writing. The ghost in the machine is embodied in Jim Hutchison's VB journals with their intermediality and multiple forms of writing. In a project focused on "innovation," the discovery made by Hutchison is not simply related to technological advancement (the building of *Mark I*) or the invention of a new technique (the spin-warp method), but to the misalignment between different traditions of languages and ways of thinking. This misalignment is needed for letting discovery happen.

Ultimately, collaborative art–science work is based on a false premise—the idea that the collaboration starts always between a scientist and an artist, two mutually exclusive identities. The VB notebooks and the archive-based exhibition hinted at another possible route for art–science collaboration. The collaboration is a zone of dialogue and friction with an imagined other, a critical interlocutor, a dialectical skeptic. This staged dialogue with the other creates a trading zone between art and science before the actual collaboration begins. The imagined *other* enables a conversation with parts of oneself that cannot be trapped within disciplinary boundaries but become "what if" scenario sketching. Make-believe.

Experiments undertaken on paper are an explorative tool used to either claim the priority of invention, for example, in view of the future patenting of a technology in mind, or they are used as thought experiments to describe/propose a certain experimental set up. Fiction is at the core of scientific practice.[59] According to a commonsense understanding of the term "fiction," something is fictional when it does not exist. Often scientists need to momentarily postulate nonexistent entities because they need them to achieve certain goals or predictions. One example is Bohr's postulation of classical electron orbits, later dismissed by Schrödinger's quantum mechanics. Fiction in the sense of "nonexistence" can therefore be useful to advance an argument. In a second sense, fiction can be understood as a counterfeit activity with the goal of deceiving or misleading. However, it can also be understood as imagination and make-believe. Scientists use models (fictional entities) to study features of the object or event that the model represents. Modeling a phenomenon requires several elements working together so that the audience can engage with and explore the phenomenon in a plausible manner. Contemporary philosopher Roman Frigg uses the example of fictional characters in literature (Madame Bovary and Sherlock Holmes) to argue that scientific models function in a similar way—we believe in them and discuss them although they only live in our imagination.[60]

Make-believe and imagination are connected to experimentation rather than to creativity. Artists are always allowed to play, fictionalize, and tinker with materials as part of their experimental process, which is often visible in the final artwork. To give an example beyond this particular case study, the hand-drawn sketches and scribblings by Thomas Edison ("the Wizard of Menlo Park") were visual manipulations of ideas, short-end descriptions and suggestions for the material arrangement of an experiment.[61]

Intermediality, make-belief (as if), and "what if" constructions are present at the laboratory bench, but they are disciplined in the final academic publications. In public engagement, the play of make-believe—"what if" scenario-building—is often reduced to an activity only ancillary to science, performed in view of gaining the interest and support of the public for scientific research.

The scribbles and sketches are part of a play in which scientific thinking and practice follow rules that are not the ones found at the laboratory bench. Paper has no boundaries but those of the page. Everything can be bent; everything becomes possible on paper. It is wrongly thought of as two-dimensional and therefore limiting to any world making. The opposite is true. Paper enables the highest degree of freedom and experimentation. Paper is where experiments begin.

The archival material that formed the bulk of the project proves how an invention never happens in the way in which it is later publicized. The story of the invention of MRI is a myth. MRI was not the result of a single event or discovery, but of entangled activities of laboratory teams across the world that extended over decades. The second section of the exhibition, mainly based on archival material, sought to reframe the Aberdonian history of MRI innovation as a collective enterprise to which physicists, designers, engineers, and technicians contributed in different capacities. For this reason, lab notes, sketches, computer-aided design (CAD) drawings of the machine design that might at first seem marginal turn out to be the driving force behind the development of MRI. The archival section of the exhibition celebrated the importance of craftsmanship and aesthetic judgments that always accompany scientific discovery, but rarely become part of the official history of an invention.

How does a complicated structure with many components and materials, and involving several different professionals, first come together? The series of technical drawings illustrates components of the *Mark I* and *Mark II* scanners (see figure 6.8). In

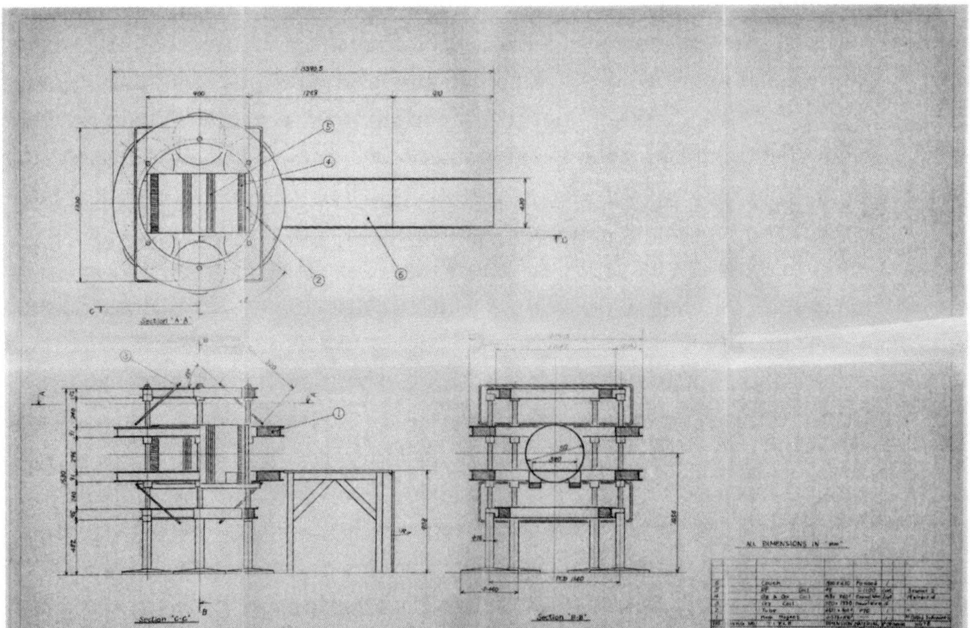

Figure 6.8
Mark I and *Mark II* technical drawings.
Source: Courtesy of Professor David J. Lurie.

the second half of the 1970s and early 1980s, Britain was at the center of MRI research and drew industry involvement, such as that from the British company Electrical and Musical Industry (EMI), and Asahi, the Japanese company that funded the upgrading of *Mark I* and enabled Aberdeen to manufacture *Mark II*.[62]

The Aberdonian group was at the forefront of MRI development, having conducted imaging studies on hundreds of patients. Prasad reminds us, "These achievements…illustrated that in vivo NMR imaging of the human body was possible, although the images were still comparatively crude.…It was still unclear whether NMR imaging could eventually become a useful diagnostic technology."[63] After 1982, the Aberdonian research group was superseded by research centers that could count on cutting-edge scanners manufactured by big companies.

In *From Where Do We See?* the *Mark I* and *Mark II* drawings were showcased along with the CAD drawings for the current FFC-MRI scanner, which represent the dimensions faithfully. Measurements were taken manually from the existing FFC-MRI scanner and then used to construct a smaller 3D model for demonstrative purposes. The 3D plot drawings of gradient windings in figure 6.9 are part of the modeling of the FFC-MRI scanner prototype. They illustrate what the gradient windings look like without having to cut open the scanner.

Gradients are made up of a loop of conducting material, such as copper, on a cylindrical shell lying inside the MRI scanner tube. When current is passed through these coils, a secondary magnetic field is created. The *x*-, *y*-, and *z*-gradients are the three sets of gradient coils used in nearly all MRI systems. Each color designates a different segment of copper track, illustrating which role each gradient winding performs. The dots

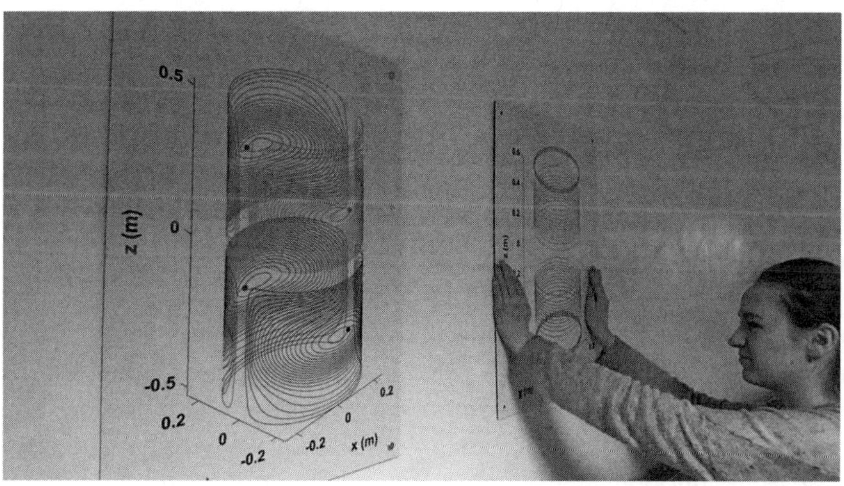

Figure 6.9

Magnet coil windings. Computer-aided design drawings for the FFC-MRI scanner, *From Where Do We See?*, installation view.

Source: Courtesy of the Suttie Arts Space and the University of Aberdeen.

represent the end of the copper track. The drawings show how when anything is built, it is dreamed, drawn, and planned.

Scientists come to understand what they are doing as they are doing it, keeping records of their trials and errors in lab notebooks. Past and present endeavors are juxtaposed in an impossible laboratory in which Hutchison would work beside the physicists struggling to domesticate matter and magnetism to build the FFC-MRI prototype. The laboratory entries from one of the researchers involved in the ongoing IDentIFY FFC-MRI project, for example, contain two-dimensional simulations of image-data problems and their possible causes. Figure 6.10 (a) shows how the hand-drawn sketches are how physicists train their eyes to see and read image artifacts before automated algorithms become available. The images in figure 6.10 (b) present data recorded from the scanner. Each line of the image corresponds to one recording. In ideal conditions, each recording should be identical, but this is not the case due to the magnetic field being unstable.

The writing, calculations, and sketches from the laboratory notebooks of the physicists working on FFC-MRI show how sometimes physicists draw imaginary objects—that is, they give physical form to their mental images—and in the process of doing so, they learn to see them better. The use of drawing in scientific research is a channel for intuition and creativity. Drawing and sketching, along with the accompanying reflexive process, can change how the drawn object is understood. Another entry in the FFC-MRI notebooks shows a sketch for a modular scanner bed that was built in the 1990s. The bed is crucial for the patient's well-being inside an MRI scanner. Patients' needs are often *imagined* and addressed even before clinical trials are conducted. Sketches are crucial to science and technology innovation; they are also crucial to art practice.

Each image created in the laboratory is only a step (a frame or a sequence) in a series of transformations that should be documented. The image is constantly moving and cannot be frozen like a snapshot of an event or object. Drawings and sketches highlight this dimension of progress in the images created in the laboratory. Borrowing Latour's framework on inscriptions as immutable mobiles (chapter 2), drawing is the ability to capture an idea and then mobilize it immutably.[64] Drawings can capture an idea, move it from place to place (not only from one's own head to a material form such as a page but also from one context to another) in order to recruit allies (those who support ideas intellectually or financially) and to bring people to a place without them having to make the journey themselves. Drawing makes things happen. Inscriptions on paper have a two-dimensional character that can be made continuous with three-dimensional space. The result is that one can work on paper with drawing, numbers, words, and shapes, but still manipulate three-dimensional objects "out there." In this respect, drawings (including the mouse map series) can mobilize several resources (economic and political, for example) as one of the physicists points out: "I was struck, in a study of a biology laboratory, by the way in which many aspects of laboratory practice could be ordered by looking not at the scientists' brains (I was forbidden access!), at the cognitive structures (nothing special), nor at the paradigms (the same for thirty years),

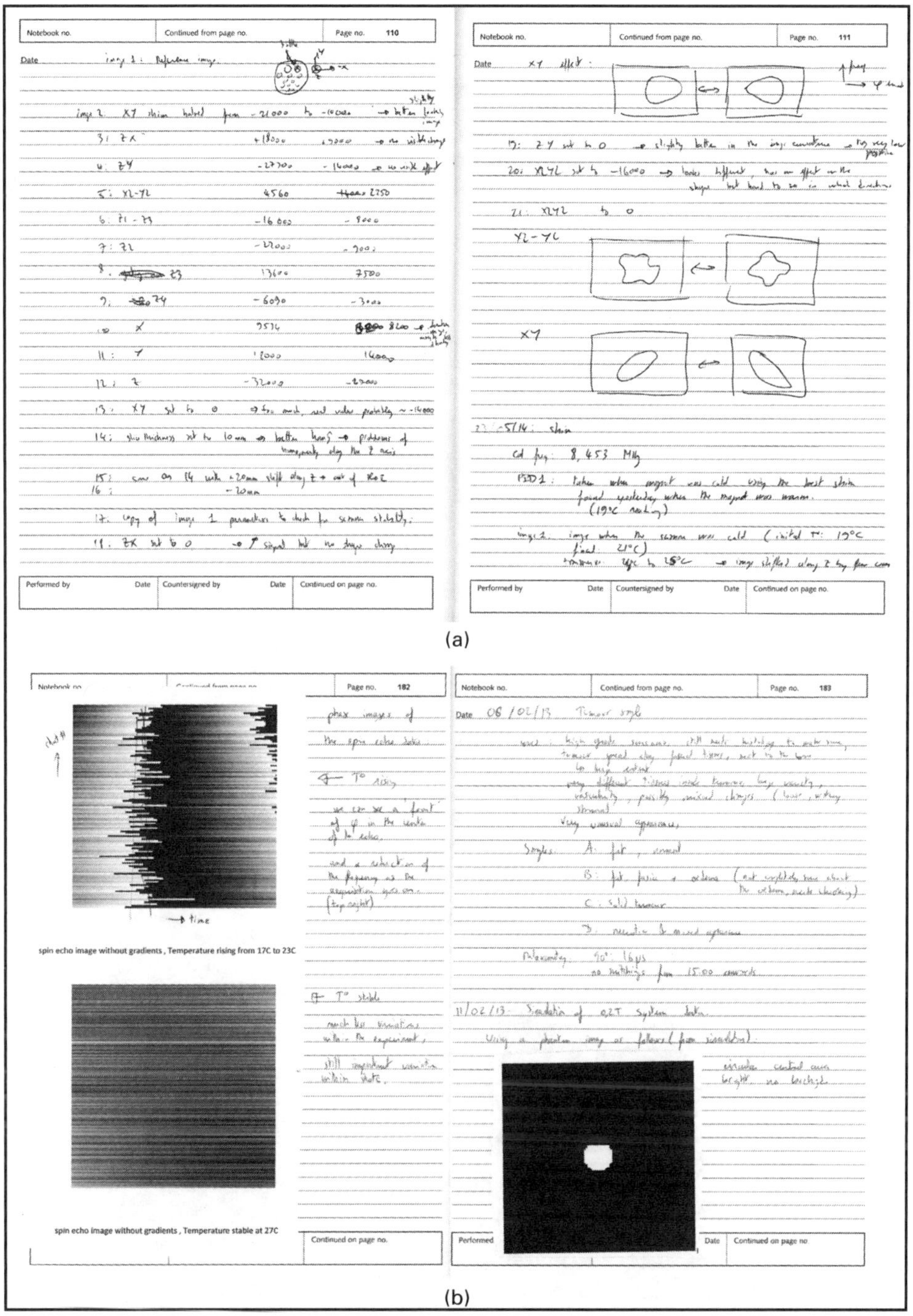

Figure 6.10
A physicist's FFC-MRI research notebook (2010–2020).
Source: Courtesy of Dr. Lionel Broche.

but at the transformation of rats and chemicals into paper."[65] The mouse map in fact mobilized resources for scaling up research and building *Mark I*.

In an old photograph, Jim Hutchison is pictured not in the typical pose of the scientist standing next to his "creature" but working hands-on on *Mark I* (figure 6.11). A wisp of a smile on his face reveals joy, but his posture hints at the fatigue of the undertaking; an artisan, a body struggle with and against matter. Matter is not dead but alive. Artists and scientists learn to master it through experience. Jim Hutchison's displayed laboratory notebook sketches, measurements, and observations demonstrate the leap in imagination and scale that would lead him and the team to build *Mark I*, scaling up the imaging process from small tissues to a whole human. One page of Hutchison's laboratory notebook is dated November 8, 1974, the time when the mouse map series was

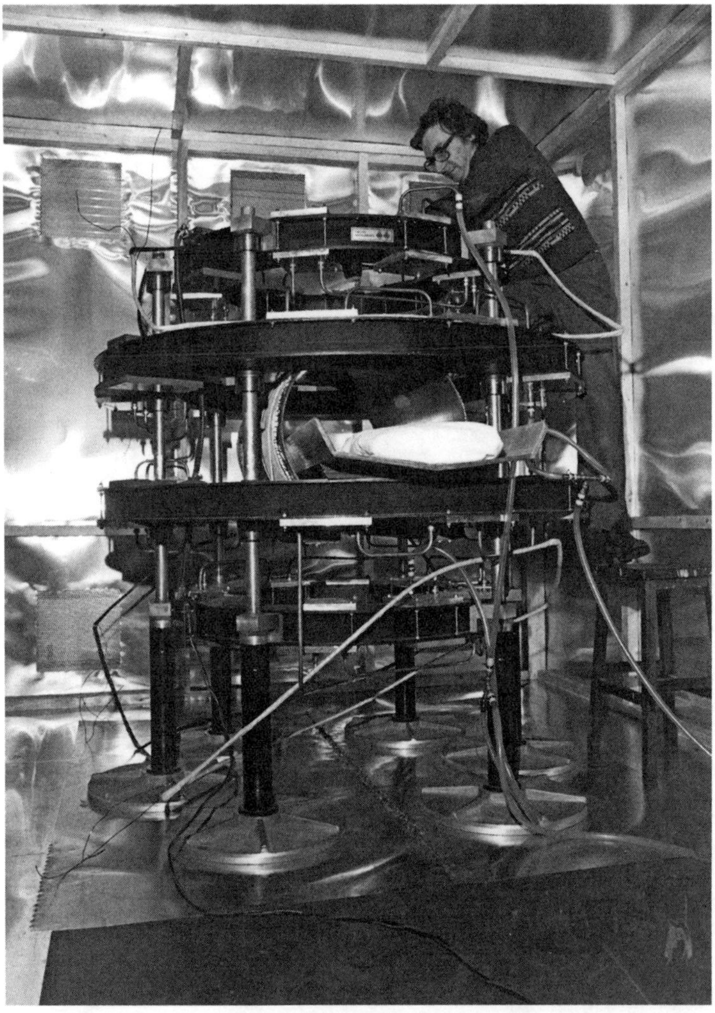

Figure 6.11
Jim Hutchison with *Mark I*.
Source: Courtesy of Margaret Foster Hutchison.

developed (figure 6.12). This document shows that in that period Hutchison was jotting down ideas and measurements for the scanner that was to become *Mark I*, accompanying his notes and calculations with a rough design sketch for the coil system.

Scientists' laboratory notebook entries and diagrammatic sketches offer an insight into the scientific method and creative process: the passage from intuitive, at times imaginative, understanding to rigorous formal proof and experimentation. The notes taken from the laboratory notebooks belonging to the physicists at work for the FFC-MRI development demonstrate the role played by drawing and sketches. Handmade drawings accompanying calculations can be tools for testing out hypotheses under ideal conditions before or together with experimental work at the laboratory bench. These drawings can have a very straightforward epistemological function, serving as clear arguments to accompany experimental tests, or they can be instances of "night science" (see chapter 3).[66]

The first image of quality produced with MRI is referred to in historical studies, biographical studies, laboratory notes, and published scientific articles. Often, these accounts reveal the controversies around the attribution of the first laboratory or scientist to have developed images of quality. The craftsmanship required to obtain the first images is a recurring trope in these accounts.[67]

The first of such images was that of a lemon. The image was published as the cover image of *Nature* in December 1977, as if it were a work of art (figure 6.13). The title of the cover image was *Zeugmatography*, the name first used in the early 1970s by Lauterbur to describe the technique known today as MRI.[68]

The production of the first clinically useful MRI image at the University of Aberdeen is dismissed by Dawson as something that occurred by accident: "In short, they [Jim Hutchison and his wife, the biologist Meg Foster] did the first clinical imaging, inadvertently demonstrating the method's ability to show the pathology of edema in the neck of a mouse that had been killed to keep it still."[69]

Listening to Meg Foster's memories in setting up the experiment, however, it is clear that the series of mouse maps demonstrate the opposite—the painstakingly long labor required to produce these colorful maps. Colors in physics are indexes of life and death: "I killed it [the mouse]. The reason for that was that the collection of that image would take 40 minutes and the mouse would not stay still for 40 minutes so it was purely a time consideration, but it had this incidental effect that when Jim created the map it was extremely obvious that there was trauma around the neck of the mouse where the fluids were exuded. It achieved two things: not only to demonstrate that the technique had a possibility, but also that it could demonstrate a trauma."[70]

One of the reproductions of the seminal mouse map printouts exhibited in *From Where Do We See?* is accompanied by handwritten notes explaining the experiment and signed by Jim Hutchison (figure 6.14). There is a reference to zeugmatography, a technique that enabled a completely new way of making images, which differed from other techniques used at that time, such as microscopy or ultraviolet imaging, because

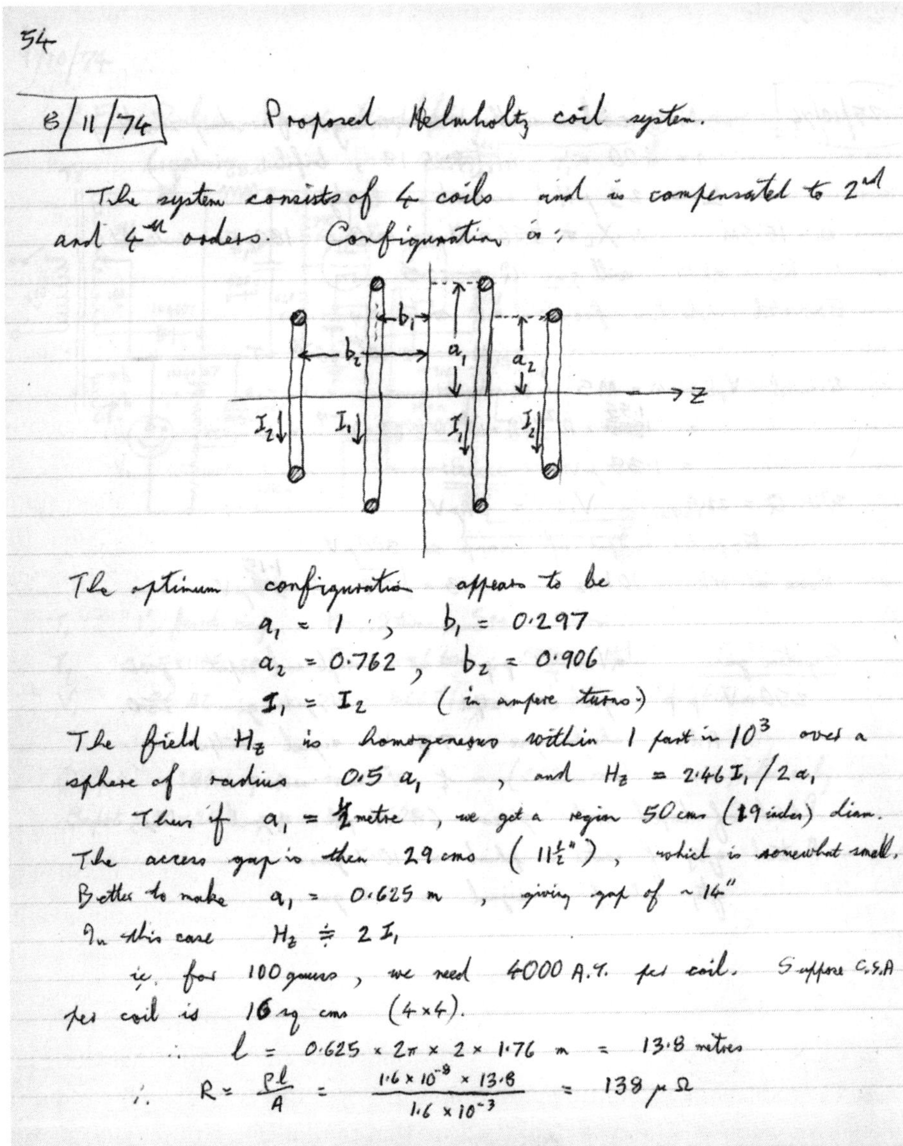

54

8/11/74 Proposed Helmholtz coil system.

The system consists of 4 coils and is compensated to 2nd and 4th orders. Configuration is:

The optimum configuration appears to be

$a_1 = 1$, $b_1 = 0{\cdot}297$

$a_2 = 0{\cdot}762$, $b_2 = 0{\cdot}906$

$I_1 = I_2$ (in ampere turns)

The field H_z is homogeneous within 1 part in 10^3 over a sphere of radius $0{\cdot}5\ a_1$, and $H_z = 2{\cdot}46 I_1/2a_1$

Thus if $a_1 = \frac{1}{2}$ metre , we get a region 50 cms (19 inches) diam.

The access gap is then 29 cms ($11\frac{1}{2}''$), which is somewhat small.

Better to make $a_1 = 0{\cdot}625$ m , giving gap of ~ 14"

In this case $H_z \doteqdot 2 I_1$

ie. for 100 gauss , we need 4000 A.T. per coil. Suppose C.S.A per coil is 16 sq cms (4×4).

$\therefore\ l = 0{\cdot}625 \times 2\pi \times 2 \times 1{\cdot}76$ m $= 13{\cdot}8$ metres

$\therefore\ R = \frac{\rho l}{A} = \frac{1{\cdot}6 \times 10^{-8} \times 13{\cdot}8}{1{\cdot}6 \times 10^{-3}} = 138\ \mu\Omega$

Figure 6.12

Jim Hutchison's 1974 research notebook, pages 54 and 55.

Source: Courtesy of the University of Aberdeen, Special Collections.

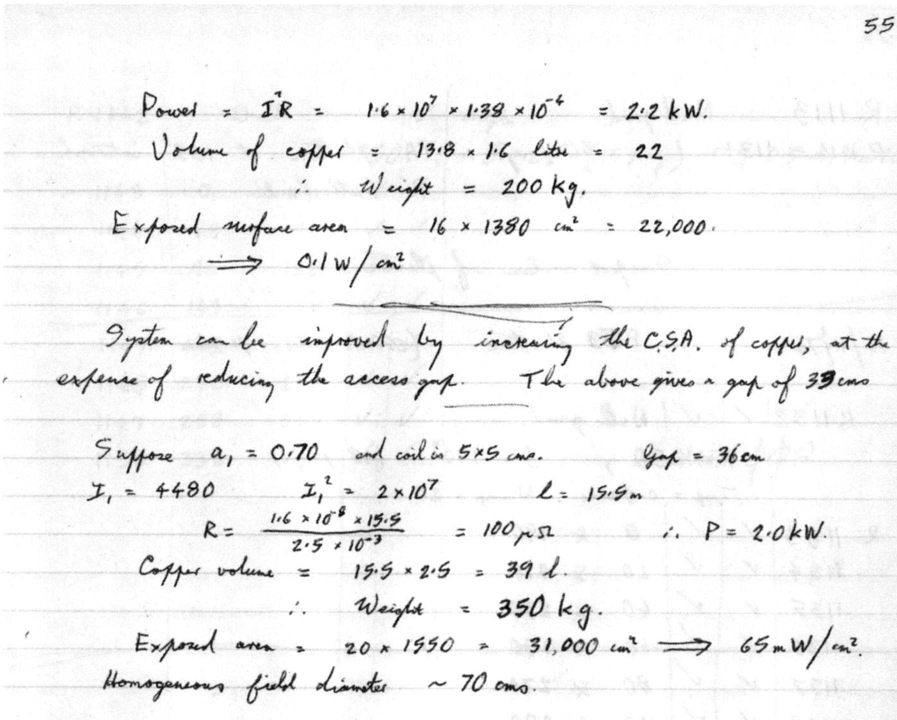
55

Power = I^2R = $1.6 \times 10^7 \times 1.38 \times 10^{-4}$ = 2.2 kW.
Volume of copper = 13.8 × 1.6 litre = 22
∴ Weight = 200 kg.
Exposed surface area = 16 × 1380 cm² = 22,000.
⟹ 0.1 W/cm²

System can be improved by increasing the C.S.A. of copper, at the expense of reducing the access gap. The above gives a gap of 38 cms

Suppose a_1 = 0.70 and coil is 5×5 cms. Gap = 36 cm
I_1 = 4480 I_1^2 = 2×10^7 l = 15.5 m
$R = \frac{1.6 \times 10^{-8} \times 15.5}{2.5 \times 10^{-3}}$ = 100 μΩ ∴ P = 2.0 kW.
Copper volume = 15.5 × 2.5 = 39 l.
∴ Weight = 350 kg.
Exposed area = 20 × 1550 = 31,000 cm² ⟹ 65 mW/cm².
Homogeneous field diameter ~ 70 cms.

Figure 6.12
(continued)

it involved no optics or diffraction. Zeugmatography created a picture of two unlikely things (long wavelength and low energy) blended together.

Another mouse map shows the code written in FORTRAN and reconstructed on the computer (figure 6.15). The diagrammatic map of the mouse demonstrates how data are aesthetically laden even before they leave the laboratory. The mouse map worked as a proof of concept for the visualization of biological data using magnetic resonance. The visual persuasiveness of the mouse image was critical in convincing clinicians and potential sponsors not only of the diagnostic value of this MR image but also of the feasibility of developing the technique further so that the research project could move from imaging a mouse to building the full-body MRI scanner, *Mark I.*

Diagrams explain, illustrate, provide a concise overview, and correlate information. They are often preceded by series of measurements or collections of data that are visualized using graphical methods. Diagrams can also visualize abstract concepts and ideas. The philosopher of information Luciano Floridi highlights the relational character of data.[71] He uses an example of a black dot on white paper. There are two things: the black dot and the white paper. The lack of uniformity between the two produces the datum. The white paper is not just the background to the dot—it is a constitutive part of it. The datum is the differential relationship between the two. The mouse map brings to the foreground this relational aspect of data. Using color, physicists created

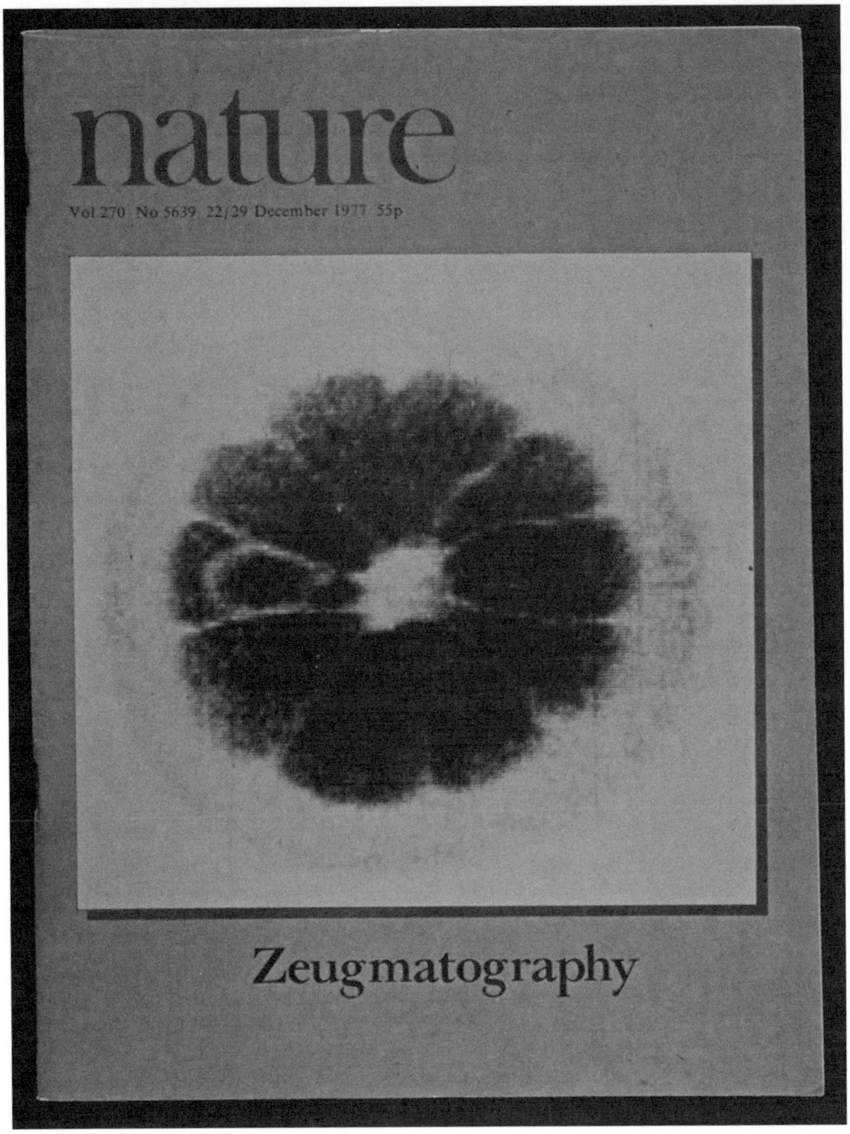

Figure 6.13

Nature cover MRI image of a lemon, 1977. PRA/5/2/2/2.

Source: Courtesy of the University of Nottingham, Manuscripts and Special Collections. Reprinted by permission from Macmillan Publishers Ltd: *Nature* magazine (vol. 270, no. 5638), copyright 1977.

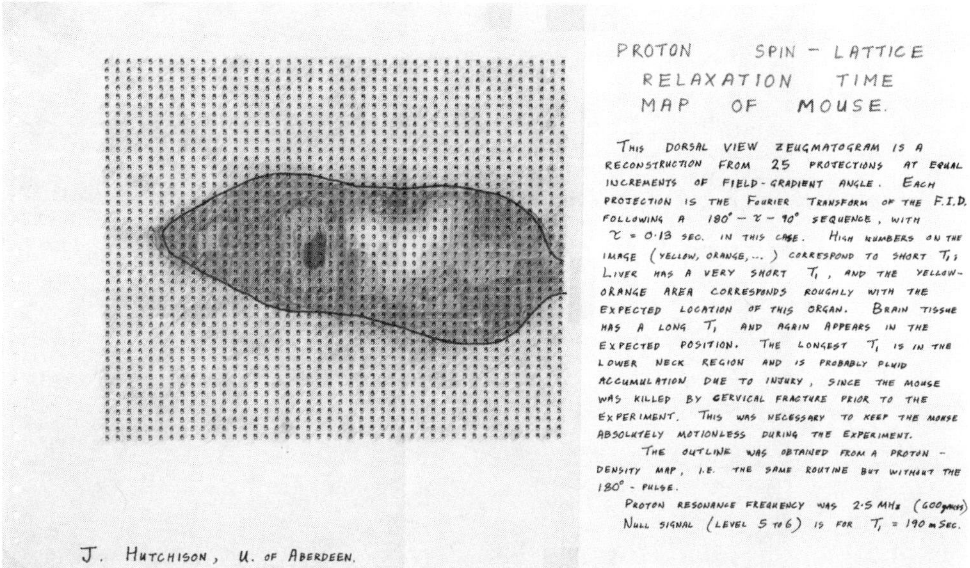

Figure 6.14
Map of mouse produced in 1974 and signed by Jim Hutchison.
Source: Courtesy of Professor David J. Lurie, University of Aberdeen. See plate 11.

an aesthetic that matched numbers connected to measurements, equations, and the mouse. After the mouse image, the biomedical physics team turned their attention to building *Mark I*, and then they invented the spin-warp method that enabled the transformation of data from the scanner into readable images.

It is after this history of science in the making, by the end of the 1970s, that features of MRI technologies were stabilized. Research teams around the world arrived at a working consensus about the name of the technology (from zeugmatography to NMR to MR), the representation of the data that came from it, and the design of the machine. Data were then displayed as printouts of multicolor images *and* arrays of numbers. Scanners were designed to produce this output. It was radiologists' preferences that shaped the visual turn toward representing MR data as images, dropping not only the numbers but eventually also color in favor of grayscale.[72]

The story of the passage from the dead mouse image to the whole-body scanner is an example of science in the making in which "facts," including a data-visualization strategy, are constructed, then stabilized and black boxed. Since the time of *Mark I*, the computer-aided procedure for obtaining diagnostically useful MRI pictures has become increasingly standardized and seemingly transparent, yet black boxed.

Chapter Final Remarks

Scientific and artistic work are both driven by a degree of uncertainty as an epistemic and aesthetic concept. The laboratory is a space of experimentation in which the intersections

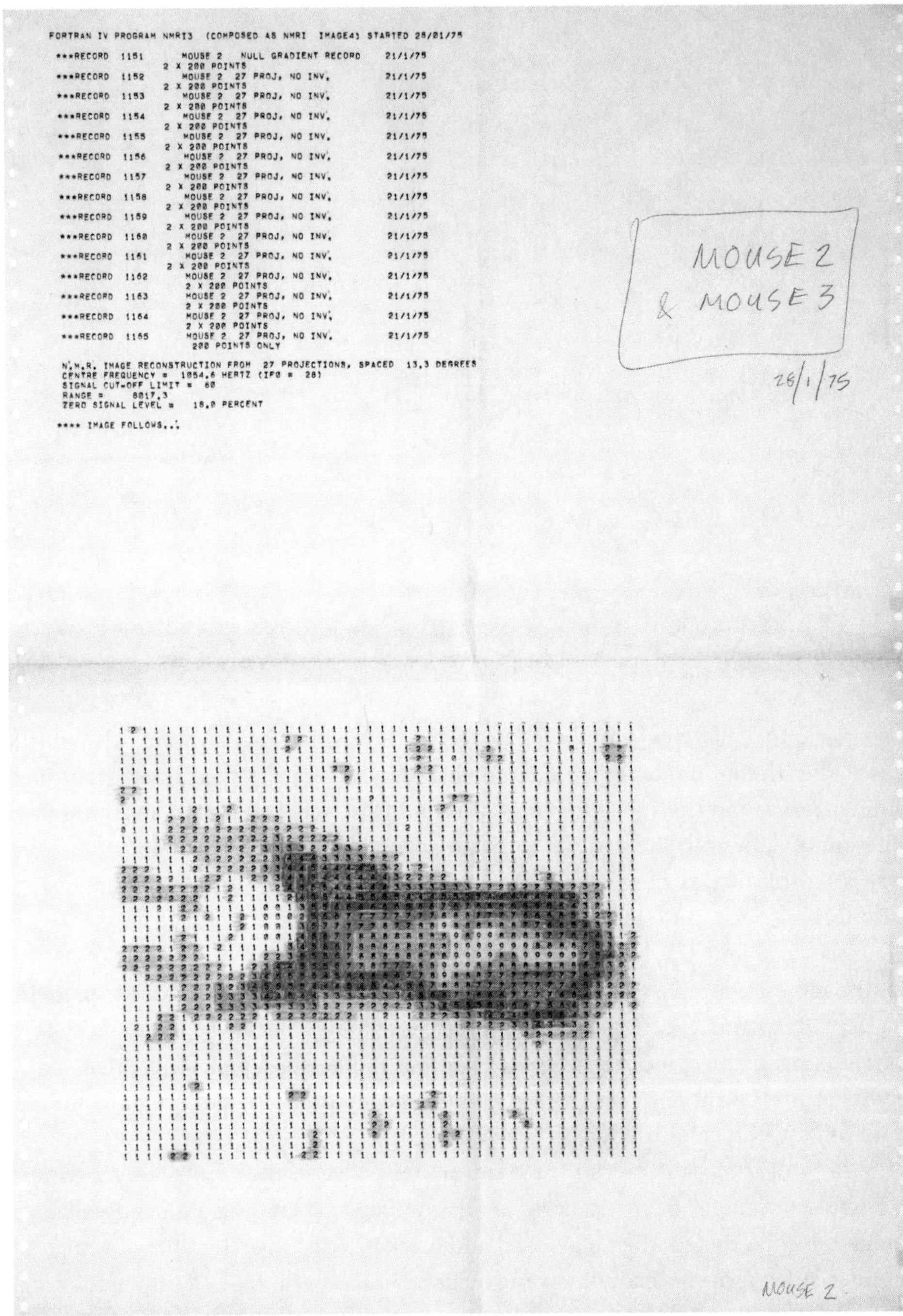

Figure 6.15

Maps 2 and 3 of mouse produced on January 28, 1975, showing FORTRAN code.

Source: Courtesy of Professor David J. Lurie, University of Aberdeen.

between scientific "objects," instruments, and experimenters quiver with uncertainty—where the liveliness of experimentation has not yet been stilled by epistemological resolution. A living experimental system, Rheinberger argues, has "*more stories* to tell than the experimenter at a given moment is trying to tell with it."[73] Because such a system still holds "excess" within itself, it "contain[s] remnants of older narratives as well as fragments of narratives that have not yet been told."[74]

The alive space of experimentation with technologies like MRI and FFC-MRI is characterized by the assemblage of instruments, visualization protocols, materials, data, different professionals, sketches, and bodies. Digging up archival material and conducting laboratory ethnography are key actions to preserving the vitality of the laboratory before this is black boxed. What the archival material has brought to the surface is the role played by fiction in scientific practice. Scientists are constantly creating worlds out of materials, ideas, sketches, calculations, and speculative thinking. The discovery made is not just the technique of the spin-warp method or the world's first whole-body MRI scanner, but rather a technology that never materializes, that remains speculative; a technology in fieri or just an idea that is not confined to the laboratory workshop or constrained by the laws of physics, by the material conditions encountered in the laboratory, or by the resistance of matter.

Artists can and should reopen the techniques and technologies that mass-produce and export science to our culture and in this way turn them into objects of epistemic interest for cultural research and possibility. Art and science deal, selectively but consistently, with processes that touch on people's lives, including the constitution of subjectivities and the distribution of power within society. These exchanges and processes are based on data creation, visualization, and circulation. Visualization, materiality, and affectivity play a crucial role in how data are formed, displayed, and contested inside and outside the laboratory.

7 Bodily Sociotechnical Imaginaries in the Age of Operational Images

> Astronomers and physicists are looked after by Urania; Demeter patronizes agriculture; and various Muses help the various arts and sciences. But who helps Cybernetics? One night when I was pondering this cosmic question, I suddenly had an apparition. Alas, it was not one of the charming goddesses who bless the other arts and sciences. Clearly, that funny little creature sitting on my desk must be a demon. After a while he started to talk. I was right. "I am Maxwell's Demon," he said. And then he disappeared.
>
> —Heinz von Foerster, *Memory without Record*

The Age of Operational Images

It is usual to think about how architecture is created, how space is generated. How does one generate an image? This is the question that the architect and designer Manfred Wolff-Plottegg asked in the 1980s while exploring the relationship between architecture, drawing, and imaging. He anticipated the shift that imaging brought to architecture and design, asking what kind of knowledge is required in an age dominated by imaging. Imaging is the act of gathering data coming from an environment and transforming them into signals that can be stored and further manipulated by means of statistics.[1] Plottegg, who pioneered the application of neural networks to architecture, argued that "the creation of new images, spaces, or architectures needs no longer to stem from people; that data does not have to be processed in the human brain, and that creativity can be quasi outsourced."[2]

To illustrate how the creative process has changed in the time of computational images and neural networks, Plottegg uses the example of drawing. On the one hand, drawing is a practice based on something external out there (a mountain, a house) that impresses one's senses, gets processed by the brain or by a kind of gutlike instinct, and eventually becomes turned into a command to make a drawing by hand.

The final drawing is a mélange of external stimuli and internal processes. In the age of electronic images, on the other hand, drawing practice has more to do with the idea of a form being derived by software rather than by human hands. The final drawing as seen in figure 7.1 (b) responds to site forces that come from the infosphere rather

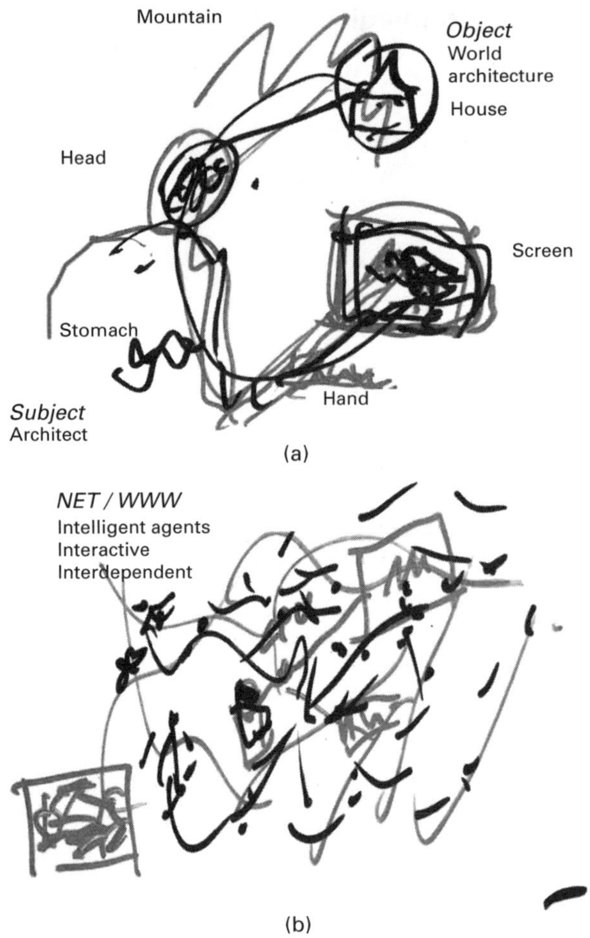

Figure 7.1
Manfred Wolff-Plottegg, (a) *Subject/Object* and (b) *Process/Net/Web*.
Source: Courtesy of the artist.

than by an external reality and that are processed by algorithms in an autogenerative manner.

In his experimental installation *Neuronaler Architektur Generator* (1999), Plottegg overcomes the anthropocentric cliché of the architect as an individual creative demiurge to embrace a distributed concept of the nervous system. This work introduces some of today's most pressing questions and concerns around data visualization and machine learning (the most important of which is the data-driven approach to AI). It comprises two personal computers communicating with each other to produce projected 3D geometries as shown in figure 7.2.

The work is based on neuronal spike trains, the electrical signals that individual neurons in a biological organism generate to communicate with neighboring neurons. Spike trains are the language that encodes the external world for our brains.[3] Spiking

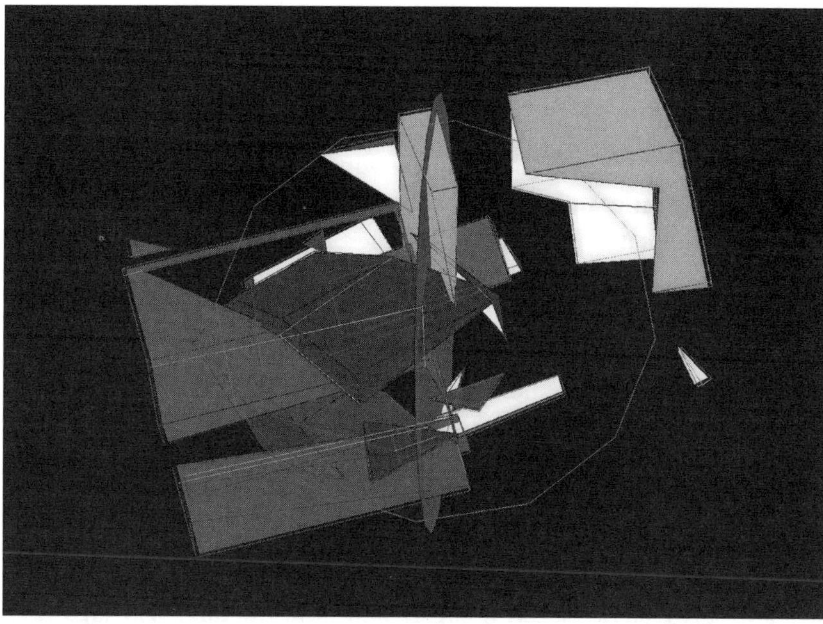

Figure 7.2
Manfred Wolff-Plottegg, *Neuronal Architecture Generator*, 1999.
Source: Courtesy of the artist.

neurons are linked to the idea of directly recording the brain's activity—the dream of smooth communication and information transfer that EEG and telepathy embodied.[4] The principle underlying *Neuronaler Architektur Generator* is an equation: spike trains in biological organisms=binary bit strings=data (coordinates, vectors) interpretable as solids. Computer 1 runs a mathematical model of four neurons generating spike trains and bit strings. The array of 0s and 1s can be generated at random, from signals from light barriers (the shadow of passing visitors), or by other stimuli. Computer 2 uses these series of pulse-coded signals for an architecture program and generates 3D geometries that are plans for new buildings, with curved, organic forms generated by digital programs in computer design.[5]

Different systems such as the human brain, the internet, transportation grids, and even social structures operate under the paradigm of the network.[6] The areas that are networked within the *Neuronaler* biological-machine system are, first, the world in our head, which is also connected to our stomach and to our hand, not just to our brain; second, the world of digital data processing; and third, the world of generating new images, spaces and architectures. The creation of these worlds does not stem exclusively from the human brain, but from a body–mind system that is both organic and inorganic.

The filmmaker and installation artist Harun Farocki called this new regime of vision the era of "operational images," that is, images created by technical apparatuses, such as photographs.[7] Farocki explains, "In my first work on this subject, *Eye/Machine* (2001), I called such pictures, made neither to entertain nor to inform, 'operational images.'

These are images that do not represent an object, but rather are part of an operation."[8] Operational images are made by machines to be seen by other machines, not just by humans—images that do things in the world rather than simply replacing or augmenting human vision. What are the implications of the regime of imaging based on software, a grid-based spatiality, electrical impulses, and statistics? What are the bodily and sociotechnical imaginaries thus created?

Art–science collaborative projects can enable the visualization of patterns of connection among data that other methodologies do not make perceivable. The ability to redesign the space and time of public/private perception, making one see what was not perceivable before, is what is at stake in data visualization at macro and micro level. Opening the black box of technologies used to visualize the body not only means being able to understand the data-visualization pipeline and its hidden assumptions; it also means being able to explore how a given technology and the data it generates fit within the wider system of operations (sociocultural, economic, political) and global infrastructures into which these technologies work.

Bodies participate in and are enacted by the entanglement of discursive and nondiscursive languages, archives, technologies, and infrastructures. The algorithms and hardware necessary to turn data into visual output are labor-heavy systems that involve collaboration between humans and machines in the chain of decisions and actions required by each data-visualization pipeline. The extraction, analysis, and use of data in medicine, for example, enables decisions to be taken about health care models, emerging markets in machine vision, and diagnosis in personalized and predictive medicine.

What is the labor required to imagine sociotechnical alternatives within the regime of operational images? How can our bodies be emancipated from existing trajectories and patterns of thinking, movement, and looking that had been set up by the infrastructures that permeate our lives (whether the architecture of a building with the exchanges it facilitates/prevents or the image-mediated doctor–patient relationship)?

Going beyond the specific collaborative art–science project examined in chapter 6, here I survey artists who used imaging technologies as ways of navigating through different spaces and histories, both private and collective. Liz Orton seeks to create a vernacular language able to challenge the screen-mediated image relationship between doctors and patients; Ilona Sagar uses scanning or mediating technologies as ways of knitting together the narratives from an archive with a contemporary understanding of health in the public domain. Thomas Feuerstein uses the language of neural networks, data from the media world, and literature to create "effects of reality," in which technology is entrenched with the very human questions of agency and responsibility. At the center of all these artists' work is not the inside of the body or brain, but rather it is inside the system comprising the human body–brain, the technological apparatus, and the environment. As I discussed in chapter 5, a systems-thinking framework integrates mental and computational processes, organic and inorganic bodies. Each part of the system is interrelated and interdependent.

This final chapter expands our thinking of the body–brain beyond data visualization in relation to material and immaterial infrastructures and media systems. People do not live inside their bodies or their brains. As the anthropologist Tim Ingold argues, we should think of people as "mycelial persons,"[9] as bundles of traces and lines that we leave as we live, as ensembles of relationships with others, and in the environment and infrastructures in which we operate. This chapter poses the question of what space of action *we* can reclaim in the age of operational images. Operational images and the algorithms behind them expose the situatedness and responsibility of *our* claims and actions in the imaging culture in which we are immersed.

A Poetics of Private/Public Bodies and Health Spaces

Operational Images versus Visual Dialogues

In the regime of machine learning, algorithms and image data are operative in fields as disparate as marketing, warfare, and medicine/health care. Human eyes are increasingly anachronistic. In this regime, images have no informative, representational, or entertainment purpose: they are just part of a system of operations. Our eyes are extraordinarily intricate but fundamentally limited. We cannot see quantum particles, radio waves, bacteria, or ultraviolet light. When most, if not all, of our human labor is hidden in the folds of automatic and controlled processes, what dialogues are we producing with these impulses? Technologically mediated vision (such as biomedical imaging) transcends the limits of the manifested physical body in the sense that the data it collects and then visualizes cannot be available through our human sensorium. Lenses have been superseded by other forms of visualization associated with other senses (ultrasound, infrared, electromagnetic visualization, thermal cameras, haptic vision) making the body less familiar to human eyes.

Art can offer alternative ways of navigating through this visual regime by asking who has access to medical images and is entitled to take decisions based on them, and then by returning the patient's body and voice to the center of the observer's attention. The work of the photographer and visual artist Liz Orton avails itself of a variety of sources, including medical imaging, radiographic manuals, and data from patients' bodies. Not interested in producing art for therapeutic/healing purposes, in some of her recent work Orton stages dialogues with patients that expand the perceptual and conceptual understanding of the image-mediated relationship between patient and doctor, exploring issues of image ownership, trust, consent, and language.

In her project *Digital Insides* (2019), supported by a grant from the Wellcome Trust and carried out in collaboration with Steve Halligan, professor of radiology at University College London Hospital (UCLH), Liz Orton conducts ethnographic observations and works with patients and a radiologist to explore the mechanisms of ethics, evidence, and trust in the doctor–patient–image triad.[10] One-to-one dialogues between the artist and patients are presented as a performative encounter between two actors:

the patient's medical images and data, and the words exchanged between the artist and patient while they look at the images for the first time and try to interpret them outside any diagnostic framework.

The aim is for the patient to reclaim their medical images, as Orton explains: "The patient is infantilized by that lack of a colloquial language. Medicine is for the protection and safety of the patient, but patients describe the disembodying, silencing, and infantilizing experience they undergo by this impossibility of seeing and talking about their own images."[11]

The lack of a vernacular language has a double effect: on the one hand, it signifies that medical authority owns the language for talking about the inside of the body; on the other, it gives images an extraordinary power to mediate the relationship between doctor and patient and to highlight the communication gap between the two. Orton's dialogues become triggers of random impressions, memories, and even traumas that the patient can articulate in a nonauthoritarian space with the help of the artist. As she explains, her research-based project did not fit the existing framework for ethical approval as it had neither a clinical outcome nor a therapeutic purpose in spite of it being relevant to patients.

Orton used medical images to begin the conversation with each patient and to accompany the dialogue that developed with each patient and with the radiologist. For each dialogue, the patient chose around five images; most patients preferred images with glitches, because they left space for speculative thinking and imagination. The dialogues touch upon the medical images on display but refuse to establish any direct correlation between the clinical condition/diagnosis, the image, and the patient–artist conversation.

Common themes throughout the conversations are the need to find agency that is absent during the medical scan procedure, the gap between the medical information in the image data and the patient's understanding of it, and the patient's struggle to fully relate to the image despite knowing it belongs to their own examination. Orton creates a space for active listening, which some feel is becoming a lost art in medicine.

The visual dialogues with patients concern primarily the image-mediated relationship between doctor and patient. With the radiologist, the dialogue touches upon the medical images being a matrix of data looked at by the computer, before being seen by a human:

Orton: What are medical images exactly? Are they models, or . . . ?

Radiologist: They're measurements. Or at least that's the goal.

O: Visual measurements?

R: Yes. Because there's so much information that's been acquired, the easiest way to present the data is as a matrix, and then to visualize that matrix as an image. It's a non-optical image.

O: So that humans can interpret it, right? Is that part of the function of the image? If computers could do everything, in the scenario of computer diagnosis, would we need any images at all?

R: I suppose it depends what you mean by image. What's the definition? The implication is that it's only an image if someone's looking at it. So you could call it a matrix instead, if it's just to be processed, if it's just for computational means....

O: What happens to the raw data? The original capture data, before it has been processed?

R: So when you say raw data...? For instance, have you seen these sinograms? These show the 2D data of the X-ray projections. But, really, even a sinogram is a visual representation of the data. The data is bits and bytes.

O: You can't get away from the visualizations....

R: I'm thinking we need to go back and define our terms. The way I think about images is that ultimately that term covers any data that is meaningfully arranged in a two-dimensional regular structure. If it's numbers in a regular grid, then it's actually an image. It can be recognized as an image.

O: It's a potential image?

R: You may say that it only becomes an image once it's been taken through imaging processing—contrast, resolution, scaling, etc. Before that, it's just data in a matrix.[12]

Even though biomedical images are data, as emerges clearly from this dialogue with the radiologist, patients consider medical images as photographic portraits giving access to the inside of the self. The misalignment between these two understandings of the medical image is at the core of Orton's attempt to develop a vernacular language. Often, the patient struggles to recognize herself in the medical image, as witnessed by the visual dialogue with Ida Levine, which was the first attempt carried out by Orton to explore the methodology she would then use.[13] For Levine, relating to her own medical images was troublesome for the traumatic memory of the procedure she underwent (a mastectomy) was evoked by the images—the early ones show two breasts, the latter images none. Orton printed out the images to see whether this feeling of estrangement would change. As the figures show, once holding the images as prints, Levine personalized them, marking and recontextualizing them with maps and images from her childhood (see figure 7.3). By controlling the images, the patient can take back a bit of control of her own medical experience.

Biomedical images are highly regulated by operational systems that, using Orton's words, "enable the absence of the body of the patient, which becomes silent, marginalized, because the images are so comprehensive it is as if they were speaking for the body."[14] Diagnosis can happen at the level of data, which need to be turned into images only when they need to be seen by human eyes. For example, in the context of a multidisciplinary team (MDT) meeting in the National Health Service (NHS), professionals from different clinical disciplines (oncology, radiology, and so forth) discuss images of each listed patient to reach a consensus on the individual treatment to recommend. Only after the MDT meeting, the chosen intervention is presented to the patient. An NHS general practitioner who contributed to Orton's project explains, "Many scans are interpreted with little or no details about the patient or their symptoms. Only a tiny proportion are now discussed in multidisciplinary meetings. The more scans

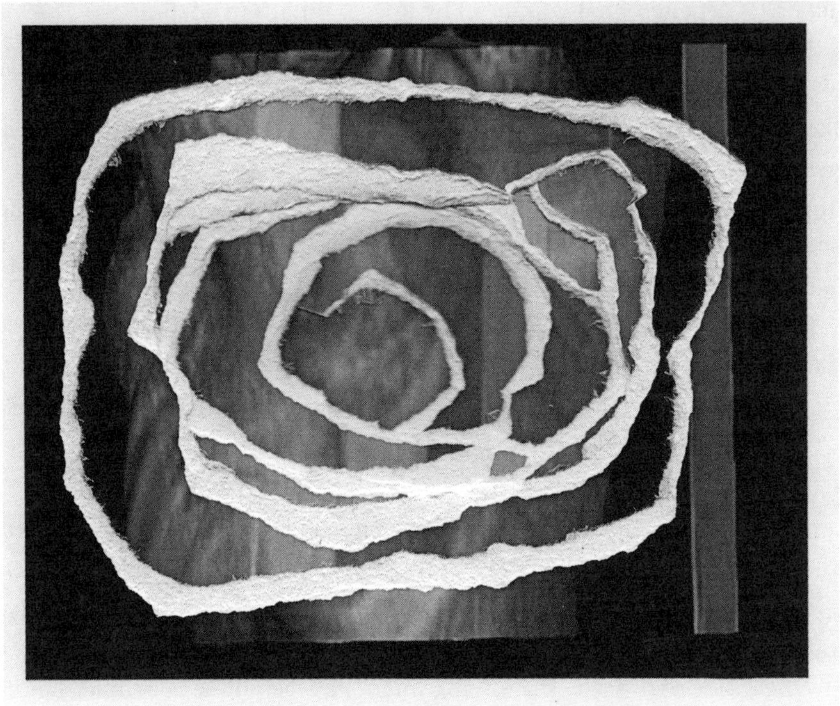

Figure 7.3
Liz Orton and Ida Levine, *Dialogue #3*, printed and photographed mammogram, 2016.
Source: Photo by Ida Levine/Liz Orton. Courtesy of the artist.

we perform, the less time we spend on interpretation. Increasingly, they generate and define the patient into binary categories—disease/no disease."[15]

Medical images serve clinical *and* operational interests simply because images are used to decide in favor of or against an intervention. These operational images do not act like windows to the world, but as data that trigger decisions.

Computer-assisted diagnosis promises to be the next revolution in medicine. Artificial intelligence and machine-learning techniques are introduced to assist (and possibly soon replace) radiologists in image interpretation in view of improving diagnosis and therapy planning. Machine learning is one the fastest-growing sectors in medical research, even though very few applications have yet reached the market.[16] Algorithmic data can be used by computers at thresholds beyond human ability and perception: information of this kind, however, often lacks the situated, context-dependent, body-based skill sets of clinicians who can rely on instinct to take a decision to intervene surgically or prescribe a certain drug. This "gut feeling," a form of subjective experience based on knowledge gained through implicit learning and training, cannot be easily incorporated into or taught to machine-learning algorithms.[17]

The friction between corporeal experience versus biological existence is at the core of scholarly reflections on the configurations of biopower in the present.[18] In his

The Politics of Life Itself, sociologist Nikolas Rose discusses how our molecules, genes, and neurons are the new target of pharmaceutical industries: the elements of our biological existence are presented as the correlates of our health condition, personality, emotions, desires.[19] As historian of medicine Roger Cooter argues in his reading of *Politics of Life*, "The body becomes a new object of research and knowledge production embedded in, and re-constituting itself through, new power relations."[20] These power relationships are mediated not only through biomedical imaging technologies but also through the spaces these technologies inhabit or create.

Interior and Exterior Landscapes: Scan of Bodies, Health, and Buildings

Space is central to how biomedical imaging is set up within hospitals. In his ethnographic study on CT scans, anthropologist Barry Saunders describes the various rooms that form the "CT suite": the scanner room, the waiting room, the reading room. As he points out, space is much more than architectural forms—it is the organization and distribution of the social roles in the room and the attendants that visit or inhabit those rooms.[21] Like the multiple-screen space of MDT meetings, the viewing box is part of this regime of visuality that fosters a novel way of organizing the doctor–patient relationship. Saunders says about CT images and the scanners that produce them: "… they organize regimes of attention, exchanges among specialists, and relations between doctor and patient.… Yet oddly, this very scene [the doctor at the viewing box], is one from which patients have largely been excluded. Consumers of this scene do not know much about the practices it crystallizes, or the ways they structure power and truth. The scene is something of a fetish, whose preciousness and authority we cannot quite explain."[22]

The space made up of coils within the MRI scanner should be added to Saunders's list above. This space, in fact, is the interface between doctors/physicists and the patient. Although claustrophobic and immobilizing for the patient undergoing a scan, this space can become a venue of expressive possibilities, as Hood demonstrated in *Immobile Choreography* (see chapter 6). Constraints intrinsic to the very architectural space become sites for experimenting with *impossible* movements.

Ilona Sagar and Liz Orton engage differently with space (of the body, the MRI suite, a building) as well as with the gestures and practices that unfold in these spaces. The dual-screen projection of *Correspondence O* (2017) by Ilona Sagar is about the Pioneer Health Centre in Peckham (England), which was operative between 1926 and 1950 (the UK National Health Service was created in 1948). The format adopted by conventional medical centers was characterized by a cellular, corridorlike aesthetic.[23] In contrast, this building had few internal walls, except ones made of glass, which created a sense of transparency. Light and air flooded through large windows, and cork floors meant people could walk barefoot. The Pioneer Health Centre was established by two doctors, Innes Hope Pearse and George Scott Williamson, who believed medical practice was overly focused on curing disease rather than on cultivating good health and preventing illness.[24]

They devised an initiative known as the Peckham Experiment, which revolved around the idea that the absence of visible illness does not necessarily signify healthiness. The idea behind the experiment was to test whether a group of recruited people, organized in family units, would look after their own well-being and health if given the opportunity. Privately funded and motivated by an increasing interest in preventive social medicine and a more holistic approach to well-being, the Pioneer Health Centre was envisaged for family nuclei only, giving them access to a plethora of facilities—gym, café, nursery, games room, library, and swimming pool. The aim was to promote a wholesome, community-oriented lifestyle, with medical consultancy seamlessly integrated. The doctors offered members yearly health checks but left them to make decisions about their subsequent actions. Pearse and Williamson called the center a laboratory for the study of humans—all activities took place under the eyes of the doctors (another reason for the glass walls), who concluded that health was something that needed to be nurtured.

The investigation on the material, psychological, and social conditions that would enable well-being (understood in holistic terms) was at the center of the Peckham Experiment. The systemlike approach to the body, technology, and health care is explicit in this passage from the experiment: "To see how a machine works you take it to pieces; but to see how a living entity functions it must be seen in its organismal unity and in its living environment. We cannot possibly examine separately the parts involved in life as we examine separately the parts of a machine. In particular we cannot separate the influence of the environment since environment belongs to the unity which we perceive as life."[25]

The holistic approach almost seems to foreground some of the principles later embraced in the second-order cybernetics, including the idea of self-organization in biological machines (see chapter 5). The idea was that, if left to themselves, users of the center would *spontaneously* begin to organize themselves in a creative way, initiating a range of sporting, social, and cultural activities using the available facilities. The Peckham Health Centre was built on principles of transparency and experimental culture, in which individuals acted as "guinea pigs" to be observed by the doctors in an ongoing experiment about well-being.

The film in *Correspondence O* starts with a woman jumping into a swimming pool. The utopian belief system behind the site is introduced to viewers by a disembodied voice-over:

> In the beginning it was about learning to walk.
> Learning to speak better or differently.
> I don't remember when it began
> Or where it stopped.[26]

But whose beginning do these words refer to? That of the film, of the artist herself, of an experiment, of humankind?

The film is elliptical with no tight chronological narrative. On one screen, hands adjust the head coil inside the MRI chamber. These caring hands help a woman, the medical subject who is one of the film's protagonists, to slide into the MRI bore, slowly easing her head onto the bed. Our perspective as onlookers is an impossible one; a play of looking/being looked at. We look at the eyes of the woman reflected in the mirror who looks back at us and at the radiologist sitting in the console room (figure 7.4).

As onlookers, we are pushed away from her eyes as she shifts from being observed passively to exercising an active gaze, for example, in observing children playing. She seems to gradually become empowered to look back. The circularity of the look shows what it means to observe and to be observed in an experiment within a building designed for observation and free movement.

Architecture, transparency, and mirrors appear on screen (figure 7.5). "The language of shape, surface, skins,"[27] says the voice-over. Next, a close-up of hands—on a keyboard, then adjusting technical equipment—with the head of the patient seen in profile. "Take a deep breath and turn your neck to the right." The voice-over portrays the

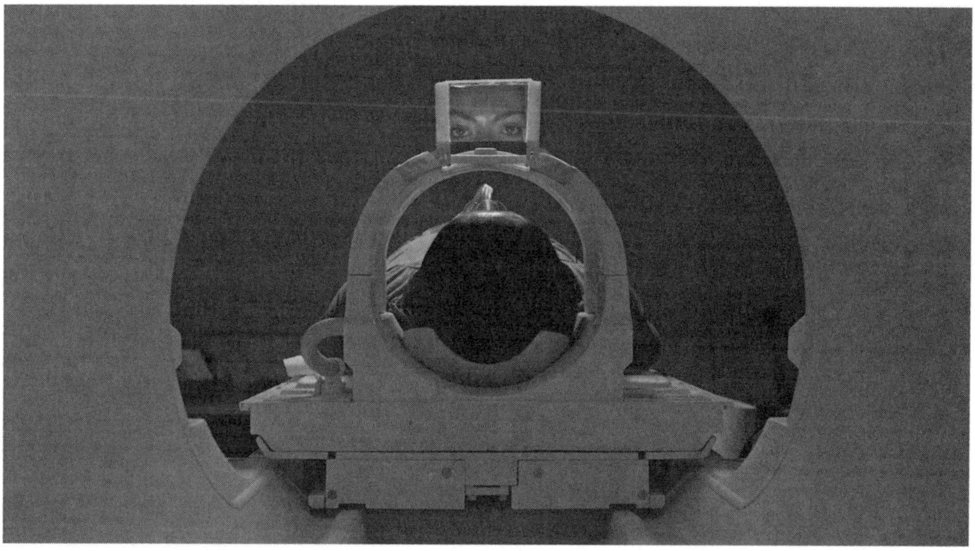

Figure 7.4
Ilona Sagar, *Correspondence O*, film still. Dual-screen HD video, stereo sound, 2017.
Source: Courtesy of the artist.

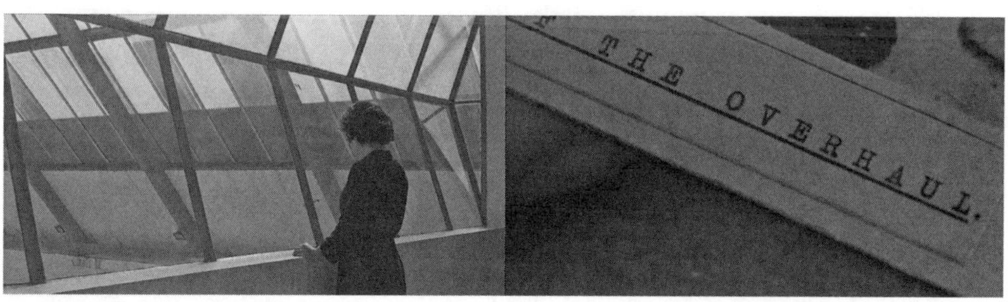

Figure 7.5
Ilona Sagar, *Correspondence O*, film still. Dual-screen HD video, stereo sound, 2017.
Source: Courtesy of the artist.

authority of the doctor's directives internalized by the patient. The camera pans across the reflective surfaces of a building. Skies and trees are reflected in the façade, contrasting nature with the human-built environment. The layers of the space are revealed as if in a scan. A machinic eye, a vision from nowhere, disembodied.

In an MRI examination, the body is studied as a self-contained entity whose parts can be visualized separately. In contrast, in the film's opening sequence, the body of the patient within the MRI scanner becomes part of a wider material and sociocultural network made up of other bodies, spaces, and images that are not exclusively medical. Several characters are encountered in the film: the woman undergoing the MRI scan, a radiologist, a personal trainer, children, a building surveyor. All inhabit multiple temporal dimensions spreading across the past and the present; all are loosely connected through the voice-over and the spaces they inhabit. Only the female protagonist seems able to inhabit all the material and mental spaces. Through the juxtaposition of a nonlinear narrative, fragmented pieces of conversation or monologue, or reenactment of archival material (the written correspondence among doctors, funders, and patients), Sagar establishes material and metaphorical correspondences between bodies and spaces, between past and present times.

With its attention to the material component of film and to the mechanisms of perception, *Correspondence O* offers a modernist structural quality inspired by the amateur film footage taken by Dr. Robert Bolton in the 1930s when he worked at the Pioneer Health Centre.[28] In Dr. Bolton's films, random shots of streets and a railway station are juxtaposed with street signs and clocks. Close-ups of the workings of a valve mechanism and copies of a book, *The Case for Action* (1931), signed by Pearse, are edited with images of children playing in a recreation ground and people diving into the center's swimming pool, with its vaulted arches and glass ceiling.[29] The pool could always be seen through the glass windows of the café that overlooked it.

The flickering quality of the scenes filmed with a fixed camera gives the feeling of microcosms bursting with life and moving bodies. Sagar creates her own lexicon of movements that expose "the urgent nature of private bodies in public spaces," as the voice-over recites.[30] Slow-motion close-ups of bodies performing movements, such as hands and feet on a fibrous natural rope, depict the fatigue of the active body on one screen juxtaposed with close-ups of stark, clinical medical equipment inserted into the protagonist's mouth (the passive body) on the other screen (figure 7.6). A shot of a neck vein pulsating is accompanied by black and white photographs from the archive and film shots of hands, feet, and social life.

The legacy of the film footage and the other archival material is prominent in Sagar's work but, as she conveys through the voice-over in her film, "This isn't about repeating, reconstructing a reverent display of historical accurate archival material. But reconfiguring, uncovering a fresh body and newly shaped mouth.... No marking. No direct actions."

Sagar features vital bodies in her film. This is evident in *Correspondence O* but also in *Deep Structure* (2019), another of Sagar's research- and archive-based collaborative

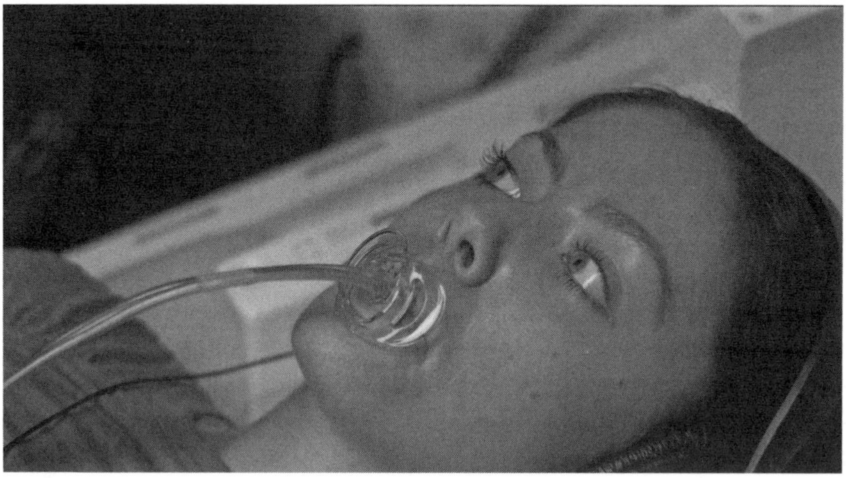

Figure 7.6
Ilona Sagar, *Correspondence O*, film still. Dual-screen HD video, stereo sound, 2017.
Source: Courtesy of the artist.

works, which explores architecture and the well-being of individuals and the community through the lens of a council housing estate in Sheffield. Bodies are vital also because they are enacted by the spaces they inhabit, by data from archives, and by computer-based techniques such as LiDAR (a remote sensing technology widely used in architectural planning and archaeology, and used in *Correspondence O*)[31] and Space Syntax (which features in *Deep Structure* and is used to calculate configurative spatial relationships in built environments and urban planning).

The architecture historian Beatriz Colomina discusses the impact of medical discourse and diagnostic technologies (X-rays in particular) on the creation and reception of modern architecture: "In the twentieth century, the widespread use of X-rays made a new way of thinking about architecture possible. Modern buildings even started to look like medical images, with transparent glass walls revealing the inner secrets of the structures."[32]

Modernity is located in the human body, as historian of anatomy Michael Sappol demonstrates in his work on the physician Fritz Kahn: the "surfaces of modernity [are brought into] the depths of the body [and] the depths of the body [are brought] out onto modernity's industrial, urban, and domestic surfaces."[33] Sagar plunges us into the hidden networks that connect our intricate inner bodily workings to medical hardware and public spaces.[34]

Since the time of Vitruvius (first century BC)—whose work has been considered a model for modern architects—sun, light, ventilation, and exercise were all considered preventive measures to keep the body in good health. The Peckham Pioneer Health Centre was an example of this close relationship between the interior and exterior landscape, between architecture and the body. The film shows viewers the backbone of the center—its system of observation windows enabling doctors to watch from above, like in a panopticon. The architecture of the building does not act as a protective shell, its characteristic transparent glass surfaces making the private dimension visible and accessible, like X-rays. Despite the modernist lineage of the building, the film challenges the idea of man as the measure of all things. This myth, which permeates architecture from Vitruvius to Le Corbusier, is still commonplace even at the level of measuring dimensions using body parts (foot, span, and so forth). *Correspondence O* shows how the industrial building of modernity has become a data space. Media and data have taken the place of machinery and material, respectively.

The Peckham Experiment can be interpreted as an exercise in radical democracy or an endorsement of conservative ideals about self-reliance. Ilona Sagar is not interested in resolving the controversies around this experiment in private health care. The architecture of the building and the related archive with its wealth of personal correspondence and ruminations expressed in an evocative language is what attracted Sagar's attention: "I was struck by the architecture of the building, then found the archive: poetic language to discuss the medical process."[35] The texture of the film is made of biological, medical, and bureaucratic words that acquire a poetic, vernacular sense when performed by the voice-over in dialogue with or as counterpoints to the spaces portrayed on screen.

Sagar enacts a poetic ethnography of looking, locating it in multiple subjectivities as if it were happening from the console room of the radiologist, scanning the façade of the building or haptic, glancing at the intimate space created by the archival black and white photographs of the Pioneer Health Centre; she pauses on the microgestures of the female protagonist (for example, adjusting her hairnet before jumping in the pool) and on close-ups of water drops on the woman's face. "A great deal of what we think about is felt as much as thought," says the voice-over.[36] On one screen, as shown in figure 7.7, the 3D reconstruction of the woman's head, with her brain visible inside emerges as an image slowly reconstructed from data, while on the other, hands test the water of the swimming pool, feel the equipment, calibrate the technical apparatus, and the radiologist gently scratches his nape.

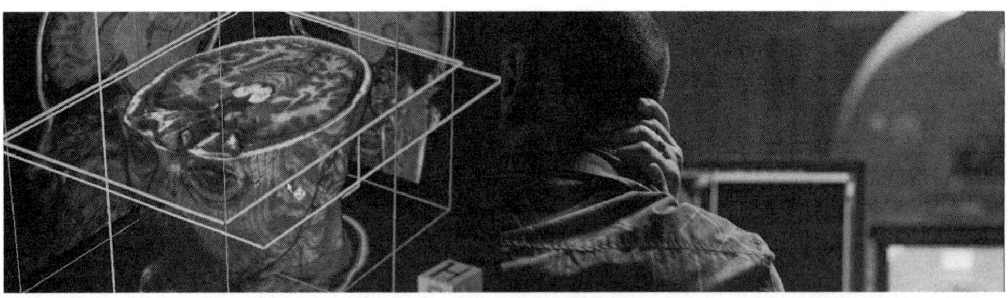

Figure 7.7
Ilona Sagar, *Correspondence O*, film still. Dual-screen HD video, stereo sound, 2017.
Source: Courtesy of the artist. See plate 12.

These intimate gestures accompany the mental wandering of the female protagonist. The film discloses these mental spaces to the viewer without making them fully accessible, to counteract the accessibility to the body and brain provided by imaging technologies and the sense of surveillance and control enacted by the governmental nexus. The possibility of drifting away with the mind toward thoughts, feelings, and other musings can liberate social imaginaries that are alternative to the patterns of thinking, moving, and living set up by bodies and data moving across architectural spaces and infrastructures.

Liz Orton's search for a vernacular language of medicine for talking about the body resonates into the poetic words of the voice-over in Sagar's film, musing on the effects of this interlocked assemblage of medical imaging, bodies, buildings, and health care models. As Sagar puts it, her text is itself "a scan, a schism through my databody."[37] Sagar juxtaposes three different types of scan in the film and three kinds of operational images: the interior of the building—the swimming pool, the only area preserved from the original building—which is scanned using LiDAR (see figure 7.8); a human subject (the film's protagonist) undergoing an MRI scan; and as last operational image, the actor playing the female protagonist who lends her body interior to the camera and to our screen-mediated gaze. Sagar's intention is not to analogize between the building and the human body. Rather, Sagar explores how the building and the body together form a system through which viewers can muse on discourses and practices related to health and the public/private body.

Is anything overlooked by the two actions of scanning a body with MRI and scanning a building with LiDAR? Information between the slices imaged by MRI does not

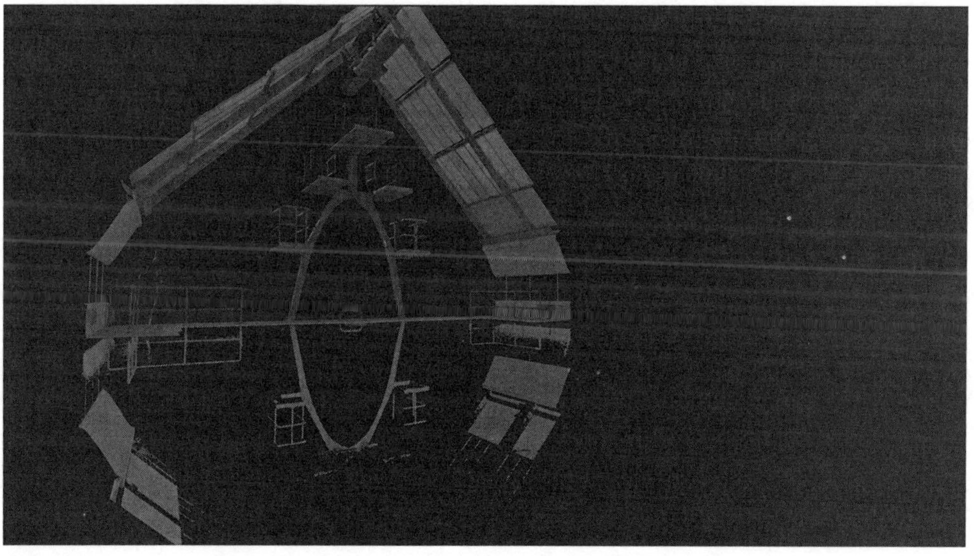

Figure 7.8
Ilona Sagar, *Correspondence O*, film still. Dual-screen HD video, stereo sound, 2017.
Source: Courtesy of the artist.

enter the final reconstructed image. LiDAR cannot scan water or underneath itself, so there are material gaps in its vision. The film is an exploration of the difference between two ways of seeing: *looking* and *looking for*. *Looking* does not necessarily require a goal; it is a type of vision that lets the world come through, impressing a trace on one's pupils. *Looking for* is a goal-oriented type of vision that both humans and machines can do; for example, medical imaging technologies scan for a sign of a disease, a pathology, an abnormality. *Scanning* has taken up different meanings across the centuries, moving from the act of examining closely with the eyes to glancing from point to point in search of a pattern or a feature. In technical terms, it means traversing a surface, bodily part, or object with a detector or an electromagnetic beam to detect an object or a condition.

The media archaeologist Tom Gunning is interested in investigating what cannot be scanned—ghosts, for instance: "[I]n some sense we cannot scrutinize them. They remain virtual, rather than embodied, images."[38] Ghosts can affect our sensorium, but we cannot affect them. Ghosts are entities (images) that one can traverse without resistance. They become *phantasmata*. This term comes from the Aristotelian doctrine around memory. Aristotle established a connection between time, memory, and imagination by arguing that only beings who are capable of perceiving time are also able to remember, and the act of remembering requires the use of the very same faculty we use to perceive time—namely, the imagination. It is through images (*phantasmata*) that human beings can not only perceive but also think.

In the theory of knowledge developed in *De Anima*, Aristotle argued that knowledge had its origin in the senses; then it would reach the intellect through a process of abstraction operated by imagination and through the production of *phantasmata*.[39] These images are stored in memory, becoming the mnemonic transmitters of emotions and sensations. The glimpses of psychic life (ghosts) in Orton's visual dialogues or in Sagar's *Correspondence O*, as well as data from the archive, cannot be scanned by MRI apparatus or seen by human eyes. They can be evoked by words exchanged in conversations or through a juxtaposition of double screens and voice-over narrative. Their presence lasts for an instant only, though, because they are intermittent images.

The optical revolution undertaken by Kepler, for whom vision was the result of the interaction between light, the eye, and the retinal image, had relegated *specters* to the realm of the imagination. Paradoxically, ghosts that the Scientific Revolution set aside come back with the visual weaponry that scientific imaging brought with itself in the attempt to dematerialize the body, turning it into an image:

> The instruments of science gave birth to spectres ... [But] the visual imagery of science in the twentieth century, while still determinately indexical and empirical, deviates sharply from the classical medical gaze of anatomy and has become increasingly abstract and technologically mediated, producing images often unrecognizable to the lay person, with appearances seemingly as fanciful in their deviation from ordinary vision as the most bizarre occultist imagery. As we move more and more into a world in which data takes on visual form, these forms seem to become less and less familiar.[40]

This dimension of uncertainty that I discuss in chapter 4 and in the intermezzo, the uncanniness of the world of data visualization, then comes back to haunt us. Sagar's film shows how our psychic apparatus is similar to an inscription device onto which memories, glimpses, and stories are recorded as ghostly traces and then reconfigured in new forms, gaining new life. The voice-over whispers:

> We are a living currency, radically exterior amidst global uncertainty and social unrest.
>
> ...
>
> I can only take so much, only be so capable.
> My work. My efficiency.

Genomics, neuroscience, and medicine have bodies as their targets. Bodies are objects of governance and policy interventions in health care. What space is there for vulnerability and agency in the age of body capital and neoliberal efficiency? The management of health and illness is done through corporate activity. Rose argues, "In these processes human vitality has been opened up, at the molecular level, for technical innovation, economic exploitation, and for highly competitive forms of bioeconomics. This technologization and capitalization of medicine gives a particular form to the contested field of vital politics in the twenty-first century. And this field is itself being reconfigured by a profound 'molecularization' of styles of biomedical thought, judgment, and intervention."[41]

The question asked by physicists and radiologists in relation to biomedical images is what constitutes an image of quality (see chapter 4). In contrast, Sagar ponders what constitutes a good body and whether efficiency is the purpose of good health, showing images of bodies performing manual labor tasks (sewing machines, sartorial labor) and training activities. It is up to the individual, often with the support of self-tracking technology, to manage one's own mental and physical health. Artist Kathryn Lloyd, reviewing *Correspondence O*, writes, "In our own private spheres, the concept of health is increasingly autonomous, governed by inward-looking technologies and self-organization, while our public systems face the insidious creep of privatization. As Sagar's film collapses body parts with medical instruments, and opens architectural form with personal film footage, the once distinguishable gap between private and public begins to visibly disappear."[42]

The political economy of health practices using biomedical imaging technologies such as MRI is fully unveiled. Like in the work of Orton, there is no fetishization of technology. The patient-led visual dialogues created by Orton forge a language in order to retain some ownership and agency in talking about one's own body. Sagar uses MRI and LiDAR technology as if they were ways of framing preexisting human experiences and knowledge. Her idea is to use technology to look through different bodies—spaces—private and public. The transition between these spaces is smooth, but only occurs through the body. *Correspondence O* explores the spaces between the private and public body to prompt us to become aware of how these structures intertwine to form a living being.

Living with Demons—A Dialogue from the Future Past

Both Sagar's and Orton's collaborative art–science projects are based on slow-paced engagement in conversations with professionals, across disciplines. In *Correspondence O*, there are different kinds of data: biological data, which are detected, visualized and displayed using MRI; and archival and building data, which are obtained by LiDAR scanning technology. In *Digital Insides*, the personal narratives become the fabric of the visual dialogues between the artist and the patient. Data become the interface through which *Correspondence O* anchors the private body to discourses and practices of public/private health that occurred in certain spaces or that might be created anew.

Multimedia artist and writer Thomas Feuerstein combines methods and concepts from philosophy, art history, literature, biotechnology, economics, and politics. His archaeological method unearths narratives that weave together facts and fiction, data and matter, semiotics and the language of living organisms. The result is what can be described as "effects of reality": "My starting point is the present, and since our world is highly technical, I'm passionately concerned about science and technology. Technology has permeated our existence since there have been human beings, and ultimately art and language are also technologies. Put simply, I care more about reality than the refusal of reality."[43]

Feuerstein's installation *BORGY & BES* (2018) is composed of data from the World Wide Web, props used in medical surgery, and language.[44] For this project, commissioned by the LABORATORIA Art & Science Foundation in Moscow, Feuerstein collaborated with neural networks experts, robotics engineers, and computer software programmers. Feuerstein de-centers the role of the artist as the only creator of the work. A neural network consists of a set of artificial neurons connected in layers. A neuron takes a set of numeric values as input and maps them to a single output value: this is how information can flow through the network.[45]

In *BORGY & BES*, two surgery lamps are fed real-time data from internet news feeds. Their synthetized voices are governed by a machine-learning neural network that enables them to communicate with one another using an archaic language—that used in Dostoevsky's Russian novel, *Demons* (1871–1872). The neural network analyzes the "sentiment" behind each news feed, assigning to it a positive or negative emotion that the neural network translates into a signal that prompts the lamps to move. The same neural network generates a dialogue on the basis of the news and transforms it into a language model based on text from *Demons* to then predict what the discussion would look like in nineteenth-century Russian (see figure 7.9).

BORGY & BES is a system in which the elements communicate with one another and with gallery visitors in a feedback loop. In the early days of cybernetics, McCulloch and Pitts had already posited, albeit as an abstract idealized model, that neuronal nets could be expressed as propositional units producing statements constitutive of mental life.[46] The two robotic bodies (*Borgy* meaning "cyborg," and *Bes* [*бес*] meaning "demon" in Russian) whisper to each other while moving slowly.

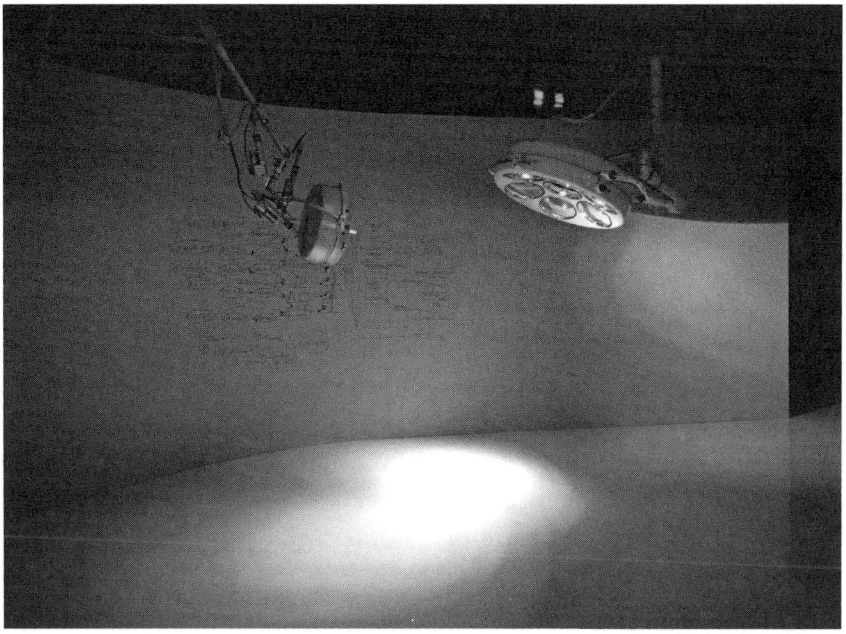

Figure 7.9
Thomas Feuerstein, *BORGY & BES*. Neural network installation, surgery lamps, dimensions variable, 2018. LABORATORIA Art & Science Foundation Moscow.
Source: Courtesy of the artist. See plate 13.

Borgy and Bes argue with one another and react to received information from Russian media headlines that feed the neural network: the architecture of the emotional behavior control system activates in the lamps a certain bodily response (looking for the interlocutor, searching, retreating from gallery visitors) on the basis of needs (communication, curiosity, safety) and the sensorial system.

Although his work is deeply embedded within machine learning and neuroscience, Feuerstein does not give the brain an elevated status with respect to the other organs of the body. The brain is only one of the organs through which our body engages in metabolic processes that are at the center of life and development. Beings that are susceptible to change (growth, death, movement, and so forth) have a metabolism.[47] The metabolic system, which assumes a relevant role in all Feuerstein's work, is not a process that interests only our human intestine. There are different types of metabolism (symbolic, cognitive, and digital) and different kinds of metabolic systems. Brains, intestines, and media systems are all involved in different kinds of metabolic processes. Our brain processes data to convert them into information; our intestine consumes molecules, transforms them into energy. Machine learning is a type of metabolic system that processes data. Economics has a metabolism based on resources and goods. We reproduce and maintain our organic life processes and exchange matter-energy with the environment thanks to metabolism. The challenge for artists is the exchange between the different types of metabolisms and what the exchange can create in the present circumstances.

The attention that Feuerstein gives to metabolic processes, not only in *BORGY & BES* but also in *Pancreas (Alles Fleisch)* (2009–2013), resonates with the work of Maturana and Varela on autopoiesis as well as with Elizabeth Wilson's attempt to keep the sociocultural and symbolic dimension of the body together with the biological and anatomical one.[48] The theory of autopoiesis is an alternative to computationalism for it offers to model cognition on a metabolic network rather than on the computer. Autopoietic processes are operations of transformation.

Bridging humanities research with neuroscience and biology, Wilson states that the center (the mind) is always "vitally dependent" on the periphery (the gut), and "this makes a world of difference politically" for subjectivity becomes decentered.[49] The focus on metabolism implies that the gut and the mind are imbricated in the same system rather than belonging to two different and opposing domains (biology and culture, or body and brain). What we feel in our guts deserves our attention, for "the gut is an organ of mind: it ruminates, deliberates, comprehends."[50]

On the wall of the gallery space housing *BORGY & BES* are algorithms presented as drawings and handwriting (figure 7.10).

Algorithms need not be software: they are encoded procedures for transforming input data into a desired output, based on specified calculations. The challenge now for artists working with machine learning and neural networks is not simply to produce new ways of visualizing or sonifying data, but rather to write the software anew. The tendency, however, is to work with the existing data infrastructure; this is usually

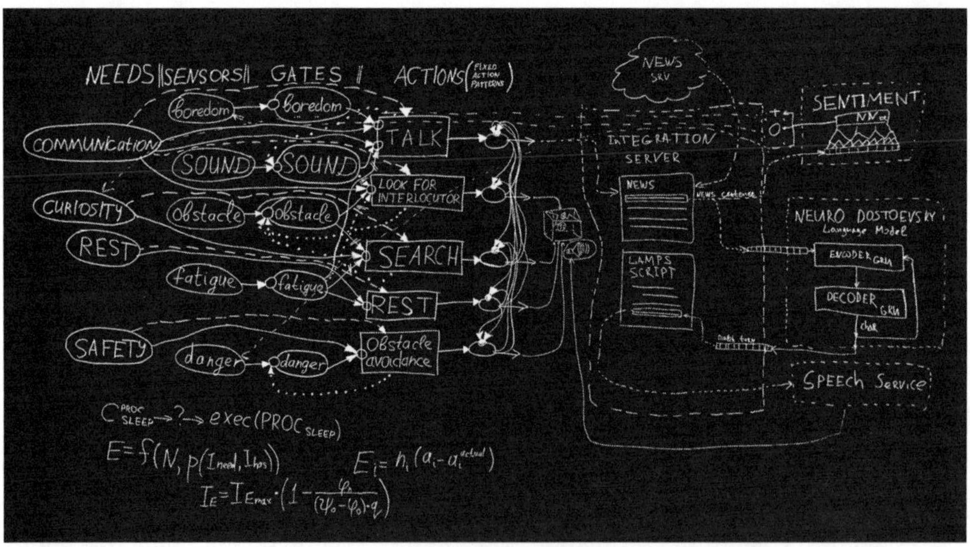

Figure 7.10

Thomas Feuerstein, *BORGY & BES*. Neural network installation, surgery lamps, dimensions variable, 2018. LABORATORIA Art & Science Foundation Moscow.

Source: Photo by Thomas Feuerstein. Courtesy of the artist.

the open-source software Tensor Flow, which helps developers use data-flow graphs to build models of neural networks.

Borgy and Bes, the two hybrid creatures, play on a theatrical stage in which multiple temporalities are interlocked. The two vintage-looking surgery lamps function as media archaeology artifacts and as alien bodies from a near future. They talk in an archaic language spoken only in a nineteenth-century book. In this past world, however, the two lamps discuss contemporary events. They stage a dialogue in a future epoch governed by machine-learning algorithms. This theatrical simulation reconfigures the early modern spectacle of anatomy taking place in Vesalius's anatomical theater. However, there is no individual biological body exposed for dissection. Rather than illuminating the physical body of a patient undergoing surgery, the two lamps discuss the social body and interact in real time with visitors' bodies.

In *BORGY & BES*, one can find the idea of a society based on communication exchanges between humans and non-humans that are not just observing one another but also able to observe themselves observing. The circularity between the observer and the observed, which is present also in Sagar's work, was at the core of second-order cybernetics (originating from the research conducted by the scientist and philosopher von Foerster; see chapter 5) with its refusal to embrace a notion of objectivity based on the idea of a separation between the observer and the observed. Media theorist Bernhard Dotzler highlights the seeds of von Foerster's epistemology of responsibility exactly in the agency that the observer has: "[A]s if he were a magician himself, von Foerster time and time again constructs precisely that figure which allows systems in general and people in particular to appear to be their own masters. The message was that people no longer had to behave like powerless observers; everyone could consider himself—precisely as observer—'as a participating actor who himself plays a role in the drama of human relations the drama of give and take in the circularity of human relations.'"[51]

The installation *BORGY & BES* is reminiscent of a laboratory environment in which an experiment in cybernetics is run according to a precise protocol, but the output is a transitional object that weaves together threads from different histories and media so that the work becomes a layered description of our world.[52] This is what creates in the viewer a feeling of being estranged and at the same time of being in the presence of a system in which science and magic, reality and fiction, organic and inorganic coexist. As seen in chapter 5, although cybernetics is associated with a science of control and communication through computers and the human nervous system, cybernetic devices are endowed "with a disconcerting, quasi-magical, disturbingly lifelike quality"[53] for their ability to respond to changes in the environment.

Revisiting in contemporary terms the ancient Greek notion of "demon" (*δαίμων*, daemon), Feuerstein embraces an expanded understanding of the word demon, which sits between mythology, magic, and even risk assessment. In ancient Greek philosophy, the demon was a regulator of society and of psychic systems.[54] The demon acted first as an intermediary entity between humans and gods, facilitating the communication between them; and second, as the destiny assigned to every human being. The demon takes the role of a governor, a sort of decision maker (only those who can take decisions, who can discriminate, have the property of being intelligent) who can allocate and distribute information and resources.

Since the eighteenth century, as Feuerstein highlights, "demons have increasingly emerged in a secular context" becoming the epitomes of rationality and of a deterministic universe.[55] Feuerstein gives the example of the astronomer and mathematician Pierre-Simon Laplace (1749–1827), known as "the French Newton," who first applied calculus to the movement of the planets and stars and independently rediscovered Bayes's theorem on probability. Laplace argued that given the perfect knowledge of both the laws that govern the universe and of the present condition, one could predict the future with absolute certainty. The intelligent entity possessing such ability is Laplace's demon. With his mathematical formula (see chapter 5), Bayes suggested a way of proceeding through approximation in our pathway to knowledge, getting closer and closer by gathering more and more data.

The new demons are cybernetic machines in computer science, and they function as background system routines at work, even behind operational images. For example, when I type on my computer, there is a program running as a background process that communicates with the server. This is a system that eschews the direct control of an interactive user. When sending emails, the automatic delivery failure notice is an email that comes from a "mailer daemon." Demons, therefore, support our everyday tasks while keeping us under control. In the age of operational images, machine learning, and neural networks, the demon is the invisible allocator and governor of possibilities and resources. Allocation is a central principle in politics and economics. Algorithmic allocation of risks at various scales (individual body, local institution, and global system) and resilience capacity assessment in such disparate areas as financial markets, climate change, neuromarketing, and health data are all procedures of governance that function thanks to a background process.

Data science uses machine-learning algorithms to generate data through processes of abstraction, although they result from human decisions and choices. Since long before computers, humans have abstracted from data to identify patterns in the phenomena they encounter in the world. Data are not therefore a specular reflection of the real-world entities they stand for, although they can provide insights into real-world problems. Data science paradoxically exposes a problem of living in a world flooded with data and an infinite number of potentially interesting variables to consider. We think we need more data (information), when we actually need firm knowledge—less noise, more signal—to make predictions that are not too removed from reality.

In the early 1940s (when cybernetics was emerging, and the physics of quantum mechanics was becoming operative with the Manhattan Project), the physicist Ettore Majorana expressed his concern for a future weakening of the real caused by the advent of a regime of probability and statistics applied not just to the phenomena of physics but also to social objects (see chapter 4). Feuerstein ideally answers to Majorana's fear of the loss of the real with a form of novel realism[56] of the present that combines machine learning, literature, storytelling, and technical apparatuses.

Operational images are phantoms, ghosts with *no body* inside them, following Farocki, for they remove the body itself from the situation in which you see, act, grasp. However, it is humans who then need to make decisions based on the available data. In MDT meetings, as discussed, operational images still need humans to take the responsibility for the final decision on whether to intervene surgically. Responsibility and agency still exist in the realm of operational images but are distributed differently across the human/non-human network and therefore are not always easy to identify.

Book Concluding Remarks

Operational images based on machine-learning algorithms challenge our vision and cognition, becoming spaces of possibilities of human intervention.[57] The mouse image map series (see chapters 2 and 6) belongs to the space in between, to a moment when imaging has not yet taken over, when the eye and the brain of the observer were still deemed necessary in the process of interpreting and displaying data. Now, operational images are not configured to be seen and interpreted by humans—there are no signs like arrows or circles to help human eyes look in the right spot. Today, operational images are demons, increasingly invisible and autonomous.

All artists discussed in this chapter and in the book as a whole work with data. Thomas Feuerstein works with data coming from nature or from sociocultural and economic systems (for example, biological neural networks, the stock market, or the media infosphere) that have a direct impact on our lives.[58] Orton works with data from patients' medical images and conversations. Sagar works with archival data as well as those from scans of buildings and bodies. This attention to the vital and relational character of data (that they are produced by and produce effects in the real world) is fused with narratives (not predictions) that combine personal memories, creative writing, and literary sources.

The awareness of the relational character of data is not just a prerogative of artists' practice. Scientists should also be aware of the relational character of data. As we saw in chapter 6, the VB personal notebooks by physicist Jim Hutchison witness, above all, a scientist's deep interest in the world in which he was living, in life forms interacting with one another and in experiences that were part of his everyday life encounters with people, books, and questions (see chapter 6).[59] The collaborative art–science projects discussed in this chapter call for humans not to give up their agency and responsibility in the process of parsing, interpreting, and displaying information from operational images. The artworks here discussed transform the gaps in our vision created by operational images into an opportunity for creating alternative imaginaries emerging from interstitial spaces.[60]

In *Giving Bodies Back to Data,* I have brought into view the bodily, situated aspects of data-visualization work, highlighting the frequently overlooked aspects of how data are gathered, presented, and shared. I focused on the lesser-known histories of visualization practice related to the development of MRI, a biomedical technology that has become a cultural icon across the media and the arts. My research has moved from the laboratory to the arts and back, attempting, like a stereoscope, to keep the molecular and phenomenal planes together. I zoomed in to microtechnical details of the technology and its data-visualization pipeline, then zoomed out to patterns of connection between the image-data pipeline and the wider system of infrastructures and operations in which each technology–body system operates.

I have discussed how the two planes above intersect and exchange from the perspective of image makers—scientists and artists alike—by making extensive use of previously unknown archival sources, interviews, laboratory ethnography, and art–science collaborations.

In this process of opening the black box, I uncovered traces left by bodily engagement with materials, technologies, other bodies, and ideas. I argued that there is evidence of the scientist's body left behind in the ensuing object and/or visualization. What do these traces do within the final piece of technology? What do they make possible, reveal, hide, or highlight for the communities of scholars and practitioners that this book addresses? I framed such questions in the context of the center–periphery conceptual pair, the critical lens I used to map the topography through which scientific practice moves, focusing on the early development of MRI to the ongoing development of FFC-MRI in a local case study, that of the biomedical physics laboratory at the University of Aberdeen. The nodes of this topography are research centers, academic journals, and expertise from physics, design, clinical practice, and engineering. But they can also be aesthetics, memories, affective investments, and bricolage—all elements usually considered peripheral to science.

Research undertaken in the University of Aberdeen's biomedical physics laboratory has been perceived as peripheral in the transnational history of MRI. Mallard's and Hutchison's archives both contributed, albeit in different ways, to reframing this history. Both archives bring in the human factor at the center of data-visualization challenges. There is a crucial difference though in the narratives that each of these two archives constructs. Mallard had external fruition in mind when he published several historically driven papers in scientific journals in two periods: first, in the early 1970s, when his research team was scaling up research efforts to construct *Mark I*, he articulated the steps required to carry out the project; second, in the early 2000s, after the Nobel Prize had been awarded to Lauterbur and Mansfield, he reflected on the achievements and missed opportunities of the same research group.

Mallard's historical papers project outward. Through authoritative interventions peppered with personal memories and sociocultural sources, Mallard seeks to position the medical physics lab at the center of MRI invention and development history. Hutchison's personal archive makes possible another operation. He is not concerned with the external representation of the research lab but rather with an imagined interlocutor with whom to test ideas. His VB notebooks show that what is considered peripheral to science (aesthetics; affectivity; craftsmanship; experimentation across languages, media, and sources) is actually at the core of it. Recognizing this enables us to tell more accurately the narrative of how MRI as a diagnostic device became important to humans. The Aberdonian laboratory too must be seen at the center of global MRI history and less as a geographic periphery.

As patients, our bodies are scanned, probed, imaged, sampled, and transformed into data. Through laboratory ethnography and archival research, I opened the black box of the data-visualization process, making visible the affective relationships in it and the materiality that turns data into an image, giving bodies back to data. The body is not exclusively human, but spreads across instruments, spaces, practices: this is how the patient too can regain a presence. In the early technological development of MRI, the patient was present in the guise of a phantom object or as a voluntary subject; forty years later, the patient often only registers as an image, which that body might not even understand.

I have foregrounded aesthetics, desire, and imagination within the scientific method and described how archival objects make it possible to track the intimate process of developing a technology; for example, through unpublished notes and sketches, or models for components that did not make it into the final technology. Opening the black box means to gain access to and then describe in their contingency these islands of "access to an emergence," as Bachelard puts it[61]—epistemic communities and environments in which new knowledge can arise. This opening is how a trading zone between artists and scientists can be nurtured to grow beyond any institutional art–science framework imposed from above.

In *Giving Bodies Back to Data*, I have demonstrated how both scientists and artists can respond to Joseph Dumit's call to "remain a humanist and interrogate the history, models, and metaphors being used"[62] in biomedicine and neuroscience. Remaining or becoming a humanist in the technologically dense world of biomedical imaging means attuning one's own words and practices to the future patient whose body is, or should be, anticipated during the early stages of technological development. The need for unification and integration, the thinking of things together, and the role played by experience point to a return to a premodern sensitivity that seems lost to the highly specialized, contemporary sciences in silos. In chapter 1, I issued a call for a stereoscopic vision of art and science. This call is an invitation to image makers, scientists, and artists alike to hold together the two images: the manifest and the scientific. In doing so, we can reveal a viewpoint that draws together the separate worlds inhabited by art and science. It is in this way that we can give bodies back to data.

Notes

Introduction

1. Santiago Ramón y Cajal, *Recollections of My Life* (Cambridge, MA: MIT Press, 1989), 363. See also Javier De Felipe, *Cajal's Butterflies of the Soul: Science and Art* (Oxford: Oxford University Press, 2010).

2. In the book I make use of the locution "scientific practice" to link the production of new scientific knowledge with the everyday procedures, craft skills, and practices carried out by scientists. In this respect, "scientific practice" includes both the development of a new theory and the biomedical imaging design process by which a new instrument (for instance, a new MRI scanner) is planned and built. See Michael Lynch, *Scientific Practice and Ordinary Action: Ethnomethodology and Social Studies of Science* (Cambridge: Cambridge University Press, 1994).

3. Hans-Jörg Rheinberger, *Toward a History of Epistemic Things: Synthesizing Proteins in the Test Tube* (Stanford: Stanford University Press, 1997), 32. For a study on scientific observation as an epistemic category in its own right see Lorraine Daston and Elizabeth Lunbeck, *Histories of Scientific Observation* (Chicago: University of Chicago Press, 2011).

4. Cajal, cited in Charles Scott Sherrington, "Santiago Ramón y Cajal, 1852–1934," in *Obituary Notices of Fellows of the Royal Society* 1, no. 4 (December 1935): 430.

5. Cajal shared the Nobel Prize in 1906 with the biologist and pathologist Camillo Golgi (1843–1926), who invented a revolutionary method of staining individual nerve and cell structures.

6. Terrence Sejnowski, "The Brain as Circuit," in *Portraits of the Mind: Visualizing the Brain from Antiquity to the 21st Century*, ed. Carl E. Schoonover (New York: Abrams, 2010), 168–172, 168.

7. Davide Daninos, "The Necessary," in *Intuition*, ed. Luc Derycke and Axel Vervoordt (Gent, Belgium: AsaMER, 2017), 63–81, 75. Exhibition catalog.

8. Lionel M. Broche et al., "A Whole-Body Fast Field-Cycling Scanner for Clinical Molecular Imaging Studies," *Scientific Reports* 9, 10402 (2019): 1–11.

9. Hans-Jörg Rheinberger, *An Epistemology of the Concrete: Twentieth-Century Histories of Life* (Durham and London: Duke University Press, 2010), xiv. Rheinberger prefers to use the term "thing" to using object.

10. See Silvia Casini, "Magnetic Attractions: Sculpture, Magnetic Resonance Imaging and Cinema," in *Marc Didou*, ed. Silvia Casini (Belfast: Queen's University Editions, 2008), 4–18. Exhibition catalog.

11. Artists initially used anamorphosis to depict objects that might be considered as "taboos," illicit because of their connection to eroticism, death, the scatological, and the occult. These

taboos were masked by means of anamorphic images. Jurgis Baltrušaitis, *Aberrations: An Essay on the Legend of Forms* (Cambridge, MA: MIT Press, 1989). On anamorphosis, see also Lyle Massey, *Picturing Space, Displacing Bodies: Anamorphosis in Early Modern Theories of Perspective* (Pennsylvania: Penn State University Press, 2008).

12. Ethnographies are a form of qualitative research and are designed to study cultures and groups. Ethnography methods include the observation of people in their natural setting for an extended period. In-depth interviews are used to clarify observations and ethnographically grounded accounts of the practices of scientists. Laboratory studies—ethnographic research conducted in and about medical and scientific labs—are connected to movements within cultural anthropology, sociology, and women's studies in the 1970s and 1980s that called for critical social scientific accounts of Western institutions. Laboratories were identified as key sites for the transformation of both science and society as observers of laboratory work challenged representations of scientific institutions as isolated from the cultural, political, and economic concerns that animate everyday life outside of the laboratory. See Karin Knorr Cetina, "Laboratory Studies: The Cultural Approach to the Study of Science," in *Handbook of Science and Technology Studies*, ed. Sheila Jasanoff, Gerald E. Markle, James C. Peterson, and Trevor Pinch (London: SAGE, 1995), 140–167.

13. Mario Biagioli, "Postdisciplinary Liaisons: Science Studies and the Humanities," *Critical Inquiry* 35 (2009): 816–832.

14. Rheinberger, *Epistemology of the Concrete*, 2010; Andrew Pickering, *The Mangle of Practice: Time, Agency, and Science* (Chicago: University of Chicago Press, 1995); Annemarie Mol, *The Body Multiple: Ontology in Medical Practice* (Durham and London: Duke University Press, 2002); Jane Bennett, *Vibrant Matter: A Political Ecology of Things* (Duke University Press: 2010); Karen Barad, *Meeting the Universe Halfway: Quantum Physics and the Entanglement of Matter and Meaning* (Durham, NC: Duke University Press, 2007). Despite the difference in emphasis, in the frame of reference and the implicit politics of how these scholars frame science and wider social relationships, all their approaches focus on the material, the physical as object of study. Rheinberger embraces the idea that scientific reality is produced in experimental practice rather than being something stable and predefined. Sociologist Pickering calls scientific practice "the mangle," defining it as an open-ended, performative interplay and exchanges ("dance of agency" is the terminology he uses) between humans and non-humans. Bennett focuses on the notion of aliveness and agency of matter and things. Barad describes her approach as an "onto-epistemology" in which ontology and epistemology become performative. Materialism and performativity have been the testing terrain for the interest in ontology manifested by science and technology studies. See Scott Graham, "Object-Oriented Ontology's Binary Duplication and the Promise of Thing-Oriented Ontologies," in *Rhetoric, through Everyday Things*, ed. Scot Barnett and Casey Boyle (Tuscaloosa: University of Alabama Press, 2016), 108–122.

15. Mol, *Body Multiple*, 5–6.

16. Orit Halpern, *Beautiful Data: A History of Vision and Reason since 1945* (Durham, NC: Duke University Press, 2015), 21.

17. Lisa Gitelman, *"Raw Data" Is an Oxymoron* (Cambridge, MA: MIT Press, 2013).

18. Sabina Leonelli, *Data-Centric Biology: A Philosophical Study* (Chicago: University of Chicago Press, 2016), 71–72.

19. Tim Ingold, "Beyond Art and Technology: The Anthropology of Skill," in *Anthropological Perspectives on Technology*, ed. Michael Brian Schiffer (Albuquerque: University of New Mexico Press, 2001), 17–31, 17.

20. The literature on science as practice is large, and it includes the work of Bruno Latour, Andrew Pickering, and Peter Galison. One of the founding texts is the work of Stephen Shapin and Simon Shaffer, *Leviathan and the Air Pump: Hobbes, Boyle and the Experimental Life* (Princeton: Princeton University Press, 1985). See also Pamela H. Smith, *The Body of the Artisan: Art and Experience in the Scientific Revolution* (Chicago: University of Chicago Press, 2004).

21. José van Dijck, *The Transparent Body: A Cultural Analysis of Medical Imaging* (Seattle: University of Washington Press, 2005). Van Dijck relies on previous studies on medical imaging technologies from a cultural studies perspective such as Lisa Cartwright, *Screening the Body: Tracing Medicine's Visual Culture* (Minneapolis: University of Minnesota Press, 1995); Bettyann Holtzmann Kevles, *Naked to the Bone: Medical Imaging in the Twentieth Century* (Reading, MA: Addison-Wesley, 1998); and Kelly A. Joyce, *Magnetic Appeal: MRI and the Myth of Transparency* (Ithaca, NY: Cornell University Press, 2008).

22. The Visible Human Project (1989) aimed at the creation of complete, anatomically detailed, three-dimensional representations of the normal male and female human bodies relying upon CT and MRI. The long-term goal was to produce a system of knowledge structures that would transparently link visual knowledge forms to symbolic knowledge formats such as the names of body parts. See Catherine Waldby, *The Visible Human Project: Informatic Bodies and Posthuman Medicine* (London: Routledge, 2000). The Human Genome Project (HGP) was an international research effort to sequence and map all of the genes of members of our species, Homo sapiens. Completed in April 2003, the HGP gave us the ability to read, for the first time, nature's complete genetic blueprint for building a human being.

23. Robert Mitchell and Phillip Thurtle, eds., *Data Made Flesh. Embodying Information* (New York: Routledge, 2004), 1–26.

24. See Drew Leder, ed., *The Body in Medical Thought and Practice* (Dordrecht, Netherlands: Kluwer Academic Publisher, 1992). See also Annamaria Carusi, Aud Sissel Hoel, Timothy Webmoor, and Steve Woolgar, eds., *Visualization in the Age of Computerization* (New York: Routledge, 2015); Anneke Smelik and Nina Lykke, *Bits of Life: Feminism at the Intersections of Media, Bioscience, and Technology* (Seattle: University of Washington Press, 2008).

25. Kelly A. Joyce, "From Numbers to Pictures: The Development of Magnetic Resonance Imaging and the Visual Turn in Medicine," *Science as Culture* 15, no. 1 (2006): 1–22.

26. Cornelius Borck "How We May Think Imaging and Writing Technologies across the History of the Neurosciences," *Studies in History and Philosophy of Biological and Biomedical Sciences* 57 (2016): 112–120, 112. Frank Schmitt named "neurosciences" a newly established interdisciplinary research program at MIT that became the reference for this emerging field. The Society for Neuroscience was founded in 1969.

27. Borck, "How We May Think Imaging," 114.

28. On technology fixes, see Sean F. Johnston, "Technological Parables and Iconic Illustrations: American Technocracy and the Rhetoric of the Technological Fix," *History and Technology* 33, no. 2 (2017): 196–219.

29. Jeanine Breaker, "The Complexion of Two Bodies. Part One: Nuance Drawn Out," *Leonardo* 46, no. 5 (2013): 425–431, 425.

30. For a similar approach, see the cultural study on electroencephalography undertaken by the historian Cornelius Borck, *Brainwaves: A Cultural History of Electroencephalography* (New York: Routledge, 2018), 19.

31. Joyce, *Magnetic Appeal*, 168.

32. Eddie Lohmeyer and Orit Halpern, "Cinema/Cybernetics/Visuality: A Conversation with Orit Halpern," *International Journal of Communication* 10 (2016): 3203–3215, 3204.

33. Sander Gilman, "Representing Health and Illness: Thoughts for the Twenty-First Century," *Medical History* 55, no. 3 (2011): 295–300, xxii.

34. Warm data, to use Nora Bateson's expression, are neither measurable nor mappable because they are produced by studying the contextual interrelationships within systems, which include noise, inconsistencies, and contradictions. Nora Bateson, "Warm Data: Contextual Research and the Evolution of Science" (n.p.: The International Bateson Institute, April 10, 2017, web edition). See also Heinz von Foerster, ed., *Cybernetics: Circular Causal, and Feedback Mechanisms in Biological and Social Systems*. Transactions of the Sixth Conference March 24–25, 1949 (New York: Josiah Macy Jr. Foundation, 1950).

35. Carlo Ginzburg, "Microhistory: Two or Three Things That I Know about It," *Critical Inquiry* 20, no. 1 (1993): 10–35. For an example of the method of microhistory before the official birth of the term, see Carlo Ginzburg, *The Cheese and the Worms: The Cosmos of a Sixteenth Century Miller* (Baltimore: Johns Hopkins University Press, 1980). For an example of a microhistorical approach in science and technology studies, see Borck, *Brainwaves*.

36. See Pickering, *Mangle of Practice*, xi. Pickering's concept of the mangle of practice has been applied to art–science studies too as in Chris Salter, *Alien Agency: Experimental Encounters with Art in the Making* (Cambridge, MA: MIT Press, 2015).

37. The term *sociotechnical imaginaries* comes from Jasanoff who uses it at the national level rather than at the level of laboratory and research group. Sheila Jasanoff, "Future Imperfect: Science, Technology and the Imaginations of Modernity" in *Dreamscapes of Modernity: Sociotechnical Imaginaries and the Fabrication of Power*, ed. Sheila Jasanoff and Sang-Hyun Kim (Chicago: University of Chicago Press, 2015), 19.

38. See, for example, Stephen Wilson, *Art+Science Now* (London: Thames and Hudson, 2010), which is a richly illustrated overview of art being made at the cutting edge of scientific research. For more educational works, see Arthur I. Miller, *Colliding Worlds: How Cutting-Edge Science Is Redefining Contemporary Art* (London: W. W. Norton, 2014); David Edwards, *Artscience: Creativity in the Post-Google Generation* (Cambridge, MA: Harvard University Press, 2009); and Claudia Schnugg, *Creating Art Science Collaboration: Bringing Value to Organizations* (New York: Palgrave Macmillan, 2019). In her books *Strange and Charmed: Science and the Contemporary Visual Arts* (London: Calouste Gulbenkian Foundation, 2010) and *Art & Science* (London: Tauris, 2005), curator Siân Ede engages with the cross-fertilization of art–science projects that she helped to foster.

39. On the value and challenges of integrating creativity and arts-based learning in the sciences, see Danah Henriksen, "Full STEAM Ahead: Creativity in Excellent STEM Teaching Practices," *The STEAM Journal* 1, no. 2 (2014), accessed January 2020, https://scholarship.claremont.edu/steam/vol1/iss2/15. For a critical approach, see Kathy Hytten and Kurt Stemhagen, "When STEM and STEAM Really Mean ABC: A Democratic Critique of 'Anything but Civics' Schools," *Educational Studies* 56, no. 1 (2020), 18–36.

40. An essayistic writing style also using the first person is a rather common practice among artists, less so among scholars in the humanities. Notable exceptions are Giuliana Bruno, *Atlas of Emotion: Journeys in Art, Architecture and Film* (London: Verso, 2007); Sam Rohdie, *Promised Lands: Cinema, Geography, Modernism* (London: BFI, 2001). The artist and scholar Chris Salter makes an extensive use of the first person in his book *Alien Agency*, 2005.

41. See chapter 1 for full references.

42. Nikolas Rose, *The Politics of Life Itself: Biomedicine, Power, and Subjectivity in the Twentieth-First Century* (Princeton, NJ: Princeton University Press, 2007).

43. Louise Amoore, *The Politics of Possibility: Risk and Security beyond Probability* (Durham, NC: Duke University Press, 2013).

44. Joseph Dumit, "How (Not) to Do Things with Brain Images," in *Representation in Scientific Practice Revisited*, ed. Catelijne Coopmans et al. (Cambridge, MA: MIT Press, 2014), 291–313.

Chapter 1

1. Hans-Jörg Rheinberger, "Making Visible. Visualization in the Sciences—and in Exhibitions?," in *The Exhibition as Product and Generator of Scholarship*, ed. Susanne Lehmann-Brauns et al. (Max Planck Institute for the History of Science, pre-print 2010), 9–23. Accessed January 2020.

2. Sabina Leonelli, *Lakatos Award Lecture*, London School of Economics, October 26, 2018.

3. For an approach to data influenced by media theory and cultural studies, see Lisa Blackman, *Haunted Data: Affect, Transmedia, Weird Science* (London and New York, Bloomsbury, 2019).

4. Leonelli, *Data-Centric Biology*, 78.

5. Leonelli, 198.

6. Leonelli, *Lakatos Prize Lecture*, 2018. On the strategies and techniques that enable data to become knowledge, see also Sabina Leonelli and Niccolò Tempini, eds., *Data Journeys in the Sciences* (Cham, Switzerland: Springer, 2020).

7. Leonelli, *Data-Centric Biology*, 70.

8. Susan Schuppli, "Atmospheric Correction," in *Imaging beyond Representation*, ed. Daniel Rubinstein et al. (Birmingham, UK: Birmingham Article Press, 2013), 21.

9. Coopmans, Catelijne, Janet Vertesi, Michael E. Lynch, and Steve Woolgar, eds. *Representation in Scientific Practice* (Cambridge MA: MIT Press, 1990): viii. For an overview of such studies, see Regula Valérie Burri and Joseph Dumit, "Social Studies of Scientific Imaging and Visualization," in *The Handbook of Science and Technology Studies*, ed. Edward J. Hackett et al. (Cambridge, MA: MIT Press, 2008), 297–317.

10. Horst Bredekamp, Vera Dünkel, and Birgit Schneider, *The Technical Image: A History of Styles in Scientific Imagery* (Chicago: University of Chicago Press, 2015). For an analysis of scientific images and visualization from an image science or visual studies perspective, see Oliver Grau and Thomas Veigl, eds., *Imagery in the 21st Century* (Cambridge, MA: MIT Press, 2011); William J. T. Mitchell, *Picture Theory: Essays on Verbal and Visual Representation* (Chicago: University of Chicago Press, 1994); Gottfried Boehm, *Was ist ein Bild* (Munich: Fink Verlag, 1994).

11. Peter Galison, *Image and Logic: A Material Culture of Microphysics* (Chicago: University of Chicago Press, 1997).

12. Bruno Latour, "What Is Iconoclash? Or Is There a World beyond the Image Wars?," in *Iconoclash, Beyond the Image-Wars in Science, Religion and Art*, ed. Peter Weibel and Bruno Latour (ZKM and MIT Press, 2002), 14–37.

13. Coopmans et al., "Introduction: Representation in Scientific Practice Revisited," in *Representation in Scientific Practice Revisited*, 2.

14. Jussi Parikka, *Machine Learned Futures*, September 6, 2018, accessed November 2019, https://jussiparikka.net/2018/09/06/machine-learned-futures/.

15. Martin J. S. Rudwick, "The Emergence of a Visual Language for Geological Science 1760–1840," *History of Science* 14, no. 3 (1976): 149–195.

16. Jennifer Tucker, "The Historian, the Picture, and the Archive," *Isis* 97, no. 1 (March 2006): 111–112.

17. Bruno Latour, "Visualization and Cognition: Thinking with Eyes and Hands," in *Knowledge and Society: Studies in the Sociology of Culture Past and Present*, vol. 6 (Greenwich, CT: JAI Press, 1986), 1–40.

18. Michael Lynch, "The Externalized Retina: Selection and Mathematization in the Visual Documentation of Objects in the Life Sciences," *Human Studies* 11, no. 2/3 (1988): 214.

19. The philosopher of science Perini, for example, has demonstrated how visual representations contribute to generating scientific arguments and hypothesis very much like words do. Laura Perini, "The Truth in Pictures," *Philosophy of Science*, 72 (2005): 262–285.

20. Henk W. de Regt, *Understanding Scientific Understanding* (Oxford: Oxford University Press, 2017).

21. Latour, "Visualization and Cognition," 18–20.

22. Hans-Jörg Rheinberger, "Was ist historische Epistemologie? Colloquium des Max-Planck-Instituts für Wissenschaftsgeschichte, Berlin," quoted in Bernhard J. Dotzler and Henning Schmidgen, "Einleitung zu einer Epistemologie der Zwischenräume," in *Parasiten und Sirenen: Zwischenräume als Orte der materiellen Wissensproduktion*, ed. Bernhard J. Dotzler and Henning Schmidgen (Bielefeld, Germany: Transcript Verlag, 2008), 7–18, here 8–9.

23. Karin Knorr Cetina, *Epistemic Cultures. How the Sciences Make Knowledge* (Cambridge, MA: Harvard University Press, 1999), 1.

24. Ian Hacking, *Representing and Intervening: Introductory Topics in the Philosophy of Natural Science* (Cambridge: Cambridge University Press, 1983). In view of supporting the idea of a separation of experimentation from theory, Hacking gives the example of a new technology that can come to light either through the elaboration of theory and experimental practice applied to a set of problems or as a series of inventions that unfold at their own pace having theory as a spin-off on the side.

25. Rheinberger, *Toward a History of Epistemic Things*, 28–29.

26. Hans-Jörg Rheinberger, "Infra-Experimentality: From Traces to Data, from Data to Patterning Facts," *History of Science* 49, no. 3 (2011): 340.

27. Claude Lévi-Strauss, *The Savage Mind* (Chicago: University Chicago Press, 1966).

28. Lévi-Strauss, 21.

29. Sociologist of science Knorr-Cetina describes the ability to use all resources available within laboratory practice as tinkering and bricolage, see Karin Knorr-Cetina, *The Manufacture of Knowledge: An Essay on the Constructivist and Contextual Nature of Science* (Oxford: Pergamon Press, 1981); Lynch, *Scientific Practice and Ordinary Action*, 150–151, provides a detailed examination of Knorr-Cetina's position and Derrida's criticism of Lévi-Strauss's idealized notion of the engineer and scientist.

30. Bruno Latour, *Pandora's Hope: Essays on the Reality of Science Studies* (Cambridge, MA: Harvard University Press, 1999), 304.

31. Regula Valérie Burri, Annamaria Carusi, and Aikaterini A. Aspradaki, "Visualising Bodies within and beyond Laboratories and Clinics," *Tecnoscienza. Italian Journal of Science and Technology Studies* 5, no. 1 (2014): 166.

32. Galison, *Image and Logic*, 803. See also Peter Galison, "Trading with the Enemy," in *Trading Zones and Interactional Expertise: Creating New Kinds of Collaboration*, ed. Michael E. Gorman (Cambridge, MA: MIT Press, 2010), 25–52.

33. Galison, *Image and Logic*, 781–844.

34. Caroline A. Jones and Peter Galison, eds. *Picturing Science, Producing Art* (New York: Routledge, 1998).

35. Martin Kemp, *Leonardo* (Oxford: Oxford University Press, 2005).

36. The "two cultures" problem was articulated by scientist and novelist C. P. Snow in his Rede Lecture delivered in Cambridge in 1959. For the published version, see Charles P. Snow, *The Two Cultures and the Scientific Revolution* (Cambridge: Cambridge University Press, 2011). On art–science experiments, see, for example, Stephen Webster, "Science and Society: Art and Science Collaborations in the United Kingdom," *Nature Reviews Immunology* 5 (2005): 965–969; Eduardo Kac, *Signs of Life: Bio Art and Beyond* (Cambridge, MA: MIT Press, 2007); Alexandra Daisy Ginsberg et al., *Synthetic Aesthetics. Investigating Synthetic Biology's Designs on Nature* (Cambridge, MA: MIT Press, 2014); Philippe Sormani, Guelfo Carbone, and Priska Gisler, eds., *Practicing Art/Science: Experiments in an Emerging Field* (New York: Routledge, 2018). On how Hans-Jörg Rheinberger's concept of experimental systems can be put into a dialogue with art practices, see Michael Schwab, ed., *Experimental Systems: Future Knowledge in Artistic Research* (Leuven, Belgium: Leuven University Press, 2015).

37. My translation from the original text in Italian: "Ma una volta che le scienze avranno occupato con autorità i diversi campi del sapere, l'artista, scacciato da un regno che condivideva da pari a pari, rimandato all'empirismo dell'artigiano ("stupido come un pittore"), non potrà far altro che darsi al soliloquio o al vaticinio, alla ricerca di uno status ma anche di un mestiere perduto." Jean Clair, "Le farfalle dell'anima," *Museologia Scientifica Memorie* 15 (2016): 16.

38. There are a few exceptions such as the investigation of the role played by arts and design in a collaborative project on synthetic biology conducted in collaboration with STS scholars. See Jane Calvert and Pablo Schyfter, "What Can Science and Technology Studies Learn from Art and Design? Reflections on Synthetic Aesthetics," *Social Studies of Science* 47, no. 2 (2017): 195–215.

39. Jenny Rock and Sierra Adler, "From 'SciArt' to 'Art Science,'" *Antennae: The Journal of Nature in Visual Culture* 47, no. 14 (2019): 14–26.

40. Nicola Triscott, "Art and Intervention in the Stewardship of the Planetary Commons: Towards a Curatorial Model of Co-inquiry," PhD thesis, University of Westminster, 2017, 38.

41. Paul Glinkowski and Anne Bamford, *Insight and Exchange: An Evaluation of the Wellcome Trust's SciArt Programme* (London: Wellcome Trust, 2009), accessed August 1, 2020, https://wellcome.ac.uk/sites/default/files/wtx057228_0.pdf. The Arts Council joined the Wellcome Trust in its pioneering SciArt scheme. For a critique of such a joint effort, see Bronac Ferran, "Creating a Program of Support for Art and Science Collaborations," *Leonardo* 39, no. 5 (2006): 442–445.

42. Michael John Gorman at *Arscientia*, accessed October 2019, https://www.youtube.com/watch?v=6415ObdQZ5Y. The first Science Gallery was created in Dublin by Michael John Gorman. The nodes of the Science Gallery international network are Dublin, London, Venice, Bangalore, Melbourne, Detroit, Rotterdam, and Atlanta.

43. James Elkins, "Aesthetics and the Two Cultures: Why Art and Science Should Be Allowed to Go Their Separate Ways," in *Rediscovering Aesthetics: Transdisciplinary Voices from Art History, Philosophy, and Art Practice*, ed. Francis Halsall, Julia Alejandra Jansen, and Tony O'Connor (Stanford: Stanford University Press, 2009), 39.

44. Glinkowski and Bamford, *Insight and Exchange*, 47. In the evaluation report on its pioneering SciArt program, the Wellcome Trust addressed the gap between the process and the final output by pointing the finger at a commonly perceived flaw: art–science work is often not of high quality in terms of its aesthetic and artistic value, nor is the exchange particularly beneficial to scientists and their own work.

45. Isabelle Stengers, *Cosmopolitics II* (Stanford: Stanford University Press, 2011).

46. René von Schomberg, "Prospects for Technology Assessment in a Framework of Responsible Research and Innovation," in *Technikfolgen abschätzen lehren: Bildungspotenziale transdisziplinärer Methoden*, ed. Marc Dusseldorp and Richard Beechcroft (Wiesbaden, Germany: Springer-Verlag, 2012), 39–61.

47. For an example of how to implement art and design in scenarios development and building using RRI, see Cynthia Selin, "Merging Art and Design in Foresight: Making Sense of Emerge," *Futures* 70 (2015): 24–35.

48. For a sustained analysis of the role played by RRI in art–science projects, see Michael Reinsborough, "Art-Science Collaboration in an EPSRC/BBSRC-Funded Synthetic Biology UK Research Centre," *NanoEthics* 14 (2020): 93–111.

49. For an assessment of the Arts program at CERN by its founder, see Ariane Koek, "In/visible: The Inside Story of the Making of Arts at CERN," *Interdisciplinary Science Reviews* 42, no. 4 (2017): 345–358. For a critique of the art program at CERN, see Camilla M. Røstvik, "At the Edge of Their Universe: Artists, Scientists and Outsiders at CERN," unpublished PhD thesis, University of Manchester, 2016, accessed November 2019, https://www.research.manchester.ac.uk/portal/en/theses/at-the-edge-of-their-universe-artists-scientists-and-outsiders-at-cern(1a75c456-967e-4c71-a88e-3632f4b9745a).html.

50. The journal *Leonardo* is a source of information on both established and more tentative and experimental projects. See also Roberta Buiani "Squatting for SciArt," *Antennae. The Journal of Nature in Visual Culture* 47 (2019): 27–47.

51. On the importance of connoisseurs and amateurs of science, see Isabelle Stengers, *Another Science Is Possible: A Manifesto for Slow Science* (Cambridge: Polity Press, 2018), 8–9.

52. For the differences between MRI, fMRI, CT, and PET scans, see Arthur W. Toga and John C. Mazziotta, *Brain Mapping: The Methods* (San Diego, CA, Academic Press, 1996); Arthur W. Toga and John C. Mazziotta, *Brain Mapping: The Systems* (San Diego, CA: Academic Press, 2000). Computer tomography produces cross-sectional images of the body using computer-processed combinations of X-ray measurements taken from different angles. Positron emission tomography (PET) functions by putting radioactive molecules inside the body and then tracking their position. Functional MRI (fMRI) detects the metabolic functions of the brain that MRI, which is devoted to the anatomy only, cannot detect. fMRI allows the identification of those areas of the brain that respond to specific tasks with a spatial resolution of centimeters and a temporal resolution of seconds. The areas that produce a large amount of oxygen are characterized by the so-called blood oxygenation level-dependent (BOLD) effect. The image produced is a two-dimensional map showing quantity in the form of colors.

53. Donald W. McRobbie, Elisabeth A. Moore, Martin J. Graves, and Martin R. Prince, *MRI: From Picture to Proton* (Cambridge: Cambridge University Press, 2003). This handbook on MRI, widely used to teach students of physics the principles of MRI, starts from the image to consequently deal with the physics.

54. Amit Prasad, *Imperial Technoscience: Transnational Histories of MRI in the United States, Britain, and India* (Cambridge, MA: MIT Press, 2014); Joyce, *Magnetic Appeal*, 2008. Some of the controversies related to the different trajectories of the invention of MRI are recounted in a rather anecdotal manner in Mary Joan Dawson, *Paul Lauterbur and the Invention of MRI* (Cambridge, MA: MIT Press, 2013). A more accurate account is Paul A. Bottomley, "On the Origins of Localized NMR: View from an Accomplice," in *The Development of Magnetic Resonance Imaging and Spectroscopy*, ed. G. Mark Bydder, Ian R. Young, and Martyn Paley, MRIS History vol. 1 (2019), 1–56, accessed August 2020, https://mrishistory.org.uk/paul-bottomley.

55. "Zeugmatography" was the name suggested by Lauterbur to signify the joining of two superimposed magnetic fields. The word *nuclear* was dropped in the early 1980s not only to avoid negative connotations associated with the word but also to highlight that MRI, in contrast to PET, did not involve nuclear medicine radioisotopes.

56. Klaus Hentschel, *Visual Cultures in Science and Technology: A Comparative History* (Oxford: Oxford University Press: 2014), 188–189. This book is particularly relevant for understanding the context in which nuclear magnetic resonance first appeared, particularly in relation to other image-generating technologies.

57. Hentschel attributes to Damadian a greater role in the development of MRI, whereas the Nobel Prize was awarded to Lauterbur and Mansfield for their role in the development of MRI. Hentschel, *Visual Cultures*, 191.

58. Hentschel, 190.

59. Dawson, *Paul Lauterbur*, 7.

60. Peter Mansfield and Andrew A. Maudsley, "Medical Imaging by NMR," *British Journal of Radiology* 50, 591 (1977): 188–194.

61. Hentschel, *Visual Cultures*, 195–196.

62. Amit Prasad, "Scientific Culture in the 'Other' Theatre of 'Modern Science': An Analysis of the Culture of Magnetic Resonance Imaging (MRI) Research in India," *Social Studies of Science* 30, no. 3 (2005): 465.

63. Paul Rabinow, *Making PCR: A Story of Biotechnology* (Chicago: Chicago University Press, 1997), 4.

64. Nathan Rosenberg, *Studies on Science and the Innovation Process* (London: World Scientific, 2010), vii.

65. The role of senses beyond visions in scientific practice has been explored in several ethnographic studies. See, for example, Cyrus C. M. Mody, "The Sounds of Science: Listening to Laboratory Practice," *Science, Technology, & Human Values* 30, no. 2 (2005): 175–198. In social studies of science, Alač, Myers, and Vertesi all address multimodal embodied practice in the laboratory, basing their works upon extensive laboratory fieldwork in neuroscience, molecular biology, and space exploration, respectively. Morana Alač, *Handling Digital Brains: A Laboratory Study of Multimodal Semiotic Interaction in the Age of Computers* (Cambridge, MA: MIT Press, 2011). Natasha Myers, *Rendering Life Molecular: Models, Modelers and Excitable Matter* (Durham, NC: Duke University

Press, 2015). Janet Vertesi, *Seeing Like a Rover: How Robots, Teams, and Images Craft Knowledge of Mars* (Chicago: University of Chicago Press, 2014). In philosophy, Noë has developed a peculiar approach to human cognition, mentality, and human experience that places emphasis on bodily interactions with the world. This approach has been embraced also by the Collegium for the Advanced Study of Picture Act and Embodiment at Humboldt University, Berlin, founded in 2008 by Horst Bredekamp and John Michael Krois, where Noë was a research fellow. Alva Noë, *Strange Tools: Art and Human Nature* (New York: Hill & Wang, 2015).

66. Annemarie Mol, *The Body Multiple: Ontology in Medical Practice* (Durham, NC: Duke University Press, 2002), 33.

67. ANT was developed by Bruno Latour, John Law, and Michael Callon to tackle and undo assumptions related to scientific innovation and technological change. Michel Callon, "Struggles and Negotiations to Define What Is Problematic and What Is Not: The Sociology of Translation," in *The Social Process of Scientific Investigation: Sociology of the Sciences Yearbook*, ed. Karin D. Knorr et al. (Dordrecht: Reidel, 1980), 197–219. For an overview of ANT, see John Law, "Actor Network Theory and Material Semiotics," April 25, 2007, accessed December 2019, http://www.heterogeneities.net/publications/Law2007ANTandMaterialSemiotics.pdf; and Bruno Latour, *Reassembling the Social: An Introduction to Actor-Network-Theory* (Oxford: Oxford University Press, 2005). For a recent introduction to ANT, see Anders Blok, Ignacio Farias, and Celia Roberts, eds., *The Routledge Companion to Actor-Network Theory* (New York: Routledge, 2020).

68. Mark Hansen, *New Philosophy for New Media* (Cambridge, MA: MIT Press, 2004), 7.

69. The anthropologist Tim Ingold moves beyond a theory of the network as an ensemble of interrelated points to embrace the rhizomatic concept of "meshwork" as the interweaving of lines of lived experience constantly growing and entangling. Tim Ingold, *Essays on Movement, Knowledge and Description* (London: Routledge, 2011), 64.

70. Elizabeth A. Wilson, *Affect and Artificial Intelligence* (Seattle: University of Washington Press, 2010), 8.

71. Annemarie Mol, "Actor-Network Theory: Sensitive Terms and Enduring Tensions," *Kölner Zeitschrift für Soziologie und Sozialpsychologie. Sonderhefte* 50 (2010): 255. On the ontological and affective turn in STS, see Mike Michael and Marsha Rosengarten, "Medicine: Experimentation, Politics, Emergent Bodies," *Body & Society* 18, no. 3/4 (2012): 1–17.

72. Sherry Turkle, *Evocative Objects: Things We Think With* (Cambridge, MA: MIT Press, 2007).

73. Jonathan Crary, *Techniques of the Observer: On Vision and Modernity in the Nineteenth Century* (Cambridge, MA: MIT Press, 1990).

74. Louis Lumière, "Répresentation Photographique d'un Solide Dans l'espace. Photo-Stéreo-Synthèse," *Comptes Rendus Hebdomadaires des Séances de l'académie Des Sciences* 171 (1920): 891–896.

75. Barry F. Saunders, *CT Suite: The Work of Diagnosis in the Age of Noninvasive Cutting* (Durham, NC: Duke University Press, 2008), 97.

76. Iva Jevtić, "Between Word and Image: Walter Benjamin's Images as a Species of Space," 2008, 3, accessed February 8, 2019, http://citeseerx.ist.psu.edu/viewdoc/download?doi=10.1.1.522.5174&rep=rep1&type=pdf.

77. Jevtić, 6. Jevtić cites Walter Benjamin, *The Arcades Project* (Cambridge MA: Harvard University Press, 1999), 462. To get a sense of these debates, see Susan Buck-Morss, *The Dialectics of Seeing: Walter Benjamin and the Arcades Project* (Cambridge, MA: MIT Press, 1991).

78. Walter Benjamin, *One Way Street* (London: Verso, 1997).

79. Benjamin, *Arcades Project*, 485.

80. Shawn Michelle Smith and Sharon Sliwinski, eds., *Photography and the Optical Unconscious* (Durham, NC: Duke University Press, 2017), 9.

81. Smith and Sliwinski, 11.

82. Wilfrid Sellars, "Philosophy and the Scientific Image of Man," in *Science, Perception and Reality* (New York: Humanities Press, 1963), 1–40.

83. Daniel Dennett, "Ontology, Science, and the Evolution of the Manifest Image," Keynote lecture at the New College for the Humanities, London, March 14, 2016, accessed August 2020, https://www.nchlondon.ac.uk/videos/daniel-dennett-on-ontology-science-and-the-evolution-of-the-manifest-image/.

84. Sellars, "Philosophy and the Scientific Image of Man," 5. Sellars always uses the locution "man-in-the-world" to highlight that the image is that of the position of man in the world, not of man and of the world as two separate entities.

85. Sellars, 32.

86. Sellars, 19.

87. Sellars, 5.

Chapter 2

1. The condition of immobility is a feature of the MRI examination that might change in the next future when MRI manufacturers are able to build portable scanners that will not interfere with normal activities and motion.

2. On the notion of "trace" with reference to MRI and fMRI studies, see José van Dijck, "Memory Matters in the Digital Age," *Configurations* 12, no. 3 (2004): 349–373.

3. McRobbie et al., *MRI*, 2003.

4. See Edward Tufte, *The Visual Display of Quantitative Information* (Cheshire, CT: Graphics Press, 2001).

5. Norton Wise, "Making Visible," *Isis* 97, no. 1 (2006): 75–82.

6. Prasad, *Imperial Technoscience*, 13.

7. For a broader historical-sociological perspective on medical imaging in the twentieth century, see Kevles, *Naked to The Bone*, 1998. The two most recent and comprehensive studies focusing on MRI are Prasad, *Imperial Technoscience*, and Joyce, *Magnetic Appeal*. For a semiotic study on how scientists working with functional MRI make sense of digital brain scans, see the multimodal semiotic analysis conducted by Alač, *Handling Digital Brains*, 2011.

8. Leonelli, *Data-Centric Biology*, 8.

9. Sandra Harding, *Sciences from Below: Feminisms, Postcolonialities, and Modernities* (Durham, NC: Duke University Press, 2008). See, in particular, the section entitled "Co-evolving Science and Society," 75–97.

10. Halpern, *Beautiful Data*, 21.

11. Rheinberger uses the Deleuzian locution "rhizomatic structure" to describe scientific knowledge. See Rheinberger, *Epistemology of the Concrete*, xvii.

12. Nelson Goodman, *Ways of Worldmaking* (Indianapolis: Hackett, 1978).

13. Mallard became then head of the Department of Bio-Medical Physics and Bio-Engineering. Bioengineering, which grew rapidly post–World War II, applies core engineering principles of design and analysis to biological systems and biomedical technologies. The shift from NMR's technology in the 1960s to whole-body scanners in the late 1970s to early 1980s required enormous physics and engineering capacity.

14. In the same years, several research centers around the world were competing in the race toward the construction of the first full-body MRI scanner. At the University of Nottingham, Mansfield made several grant applications that were turned down by EMI, Technicon, and the Wolfson Foundation. See Peter Mansfield, "Letter from Peter Mansfield to Allen Garroway, US Naval Research Laboratory, Washington, DC, April 6, 1976," Peter Mansfield Collection, from PPM/11/1/5.

15. On the concept of boundary object, see Susan Leigh Star and James Griesemer, "Institutional Ecology, 'Translations' and Boundary Objects: Amateurs and Professionals in Berkeley's Museum of Vertebrate Zoology, 1907–39," *Social Studies of Science* 19, no. 3 (1989): 387–420. For a more recent reassessment of the concept of boundary object, see S. Leigh Star, "This Is Not a Boundary Object: Reflections of the Origin of a Concept," *Science, Technology, & Human Values* 35, no. 5 (2010): 601–617.

16. The Science Museum in London has *Mark II*, the scanner used to scan patients after *Mark I*.

17. Eddie Stevenson, personal archive, June 2017.

18. Cetina, *Epistemic Cultures*.

19. Turkle, *Evocative Objects*, 5.

20. Georges Didi-Huberman, "Glimpses. Between Appearance and Disappearance," *Zeitschrift Fuer Medien Und Kulturforschung* 7 (2016): 109–124.

21. Donna Haraway uses the word *innocence* in reference to our understanding of and positioning within the scientific laboratory. Haraway argues that we need to think about laboratory practices and agents (both human and non-human) in complex terms, advocating for a more attentive and caring practice but bearing in mind that a position of innocence is not tenable. Donna Haraway, *When Species Meet* (Minneapolis: University of Minnesota Press, 2008).

22. Prasad, *Imperial Technoscience*, 9.

23. Mallard, interview with author, Aberdeen, May 2017. Interview recordings and transcripts are available upon request to the author.

24. Ilana Löwy, "Historiography of Biomedicine 'Bio,' 'Medicine,' and In Between," *Isis* 102 (2011): 117. See also Soraya de Chadarevian and Harmke Kamminga, eds., *Molecularizing Biology and Medicine: New Practices and Alliances, 1910s–1970s* (Amsterdam: Harwood, 1998). On the transformation of medicine into biomedicine at the end of War World II, see Peter Keating and Alberto Cambrosio, *Biomedical Platforms: Realigning the Normal and the Pathological in Late-Twentieth-Century Medicine* (Cambridge, MA: MIT Press, 2003).

25. John R. Mallard, "The Evolution of Medical Imaging: From Geiger Counters to MRI—A Personal Saga," *Perspectives in Biology and Medicine* 46, no. 3 (2003): 350. A slightly different

version of this same passage is contained in another article by Mallard: "The New Bacon-Slicing Machine—A Non-Invasive Gadget for Human Beings," *Health Care Equipment and Technology* 4 (1978), 1. GB 0231 University of Aberdeen, Special Collections, Ref. No MS 3819/1/123.

26. John R. Mallard, "Magnetic Resonance Imaging—The Aberdeen Perspective on Developments in the Early Years," *History of Medical Biology* 51 (2006): 49. See also John R. Mallard, James M. S. Hutchison, William Edelstein, Richard Ling, Margaret Foster, "Imaging by Nuclear Magnetic Resonance and Its Bio-Medical Implications," *Journal of Biomedical Engineering* 1, no. 3 (1979): 153–160.

27. John Mallard, "Principles of Scanning and Current Physical Problems," in *Radioactive Isotopes in the Localization of Tumours* (London: William Heinemann Medical Books, 1969). Record 3819/1/64 (University of Aberdeen, Special Collections). Stephens was born in Dublin to a working-class family. His poems, stories, and prose tended to have a nationalist bend.

28. The development of PET resulted in Aberdeen having the first NHS PET scanner. SPECT is useful in imaging blood flow in Alzheimer's disease.

29. John R. Mallard, "Magnetic Resonance Imaging," 47.

30. This procedure was first done by Professor Joseph Rotblat, who was awarded the Nobel Peace Prize in 1995. See John Mallard, "Hevesy Memorial Medal Lecture 1985 (September 4th, 1985). Some Call It Laziness: I Call It Deep Thought (with Apologies to Garfield)," *Nuclear Medicine Communications* 8, no. 9 (1987): 691–710.

31. The picture is reproduced in Mallard, "Magnetic Resonance Imaging," 49. In another article, Mallard recounts the history of MRI development in Aberdeen. See Mallard, "Evolution of Medical Imaging."

32. Sander Gilman, *Seeing the Insane: A Visual and Cultural History of Our Attitudes toward the Mentally Ill* (Brattleboro, VT: Echo Point Books and Media, 1982), 42.

33. In the Middle Ages, the term *phantasia* (which is the Greek word for imagination) was charged with negative connotations having little to do with intellectual cognition and being closer to optical deceit and illusion. For a philosophical and cultural appraisal of the term, see Michelle Karnes, *Imagination, Meditation, and Cognition in the Middle Ages* (Chicago: University of Chicago Press, 2011).

34. The original French recites "Le médecin guarillant phantasie, purgeant aussi par drogues la folie."

35. Mallard, "Magnetic Resonance Imaging," 47–49.

36. Jacqueline Vons, "Le Medecin Guarissant Phantasie: Purgeant Aussi Par Drogues la Folie." *Histoire Des Sciences Médicales* 44, no. 2 (2010): 121–129.

37. Vons, "Le Medecin Guarissant Phantasie," 124. Galen created a detailed anatomical and physiological description of the brain, the cranial nerves, and the spinal cord. See Michael Frampton, *Embodiments of Will: Anatomical and Physiological Theories of Voluntary Animal Motion from Greek Antiquity to the Latin Middle Ages, 400 B.C.–A.D. 1300* (Berlin: VDM Verlag, 2008).

38. Boyle championed both the corpuscularian doctrine and the Baconian method. Robert Boyle, *The Sceptical Chymist* (London: Cadwell, 1661). In his book, Boyle attacked Aristotle's and Paracelsus's theories, anticipating the atomic theory of matter. He proposed that elements are composed of "corpuscles" capable of organizing themselves into groups and that each group constitutes

a chemical substance. He used to report the results of his experiments, whether successful or not, arguing for the importance of keeping track of the "histories" (collections of experimental results and accurate observations) in doing science. Boyle argued that facts should be manufactured by machines so that gentlemen could witness the experiments and produce knowledge that everyone would agree on. On the role of experiments in Boyle and Hobbes, see Shapin and Shaffer, *Leviathan and the Air-Pump*.

39. Leclerc de la Verpillière, "Visceral Creativity: Digestion, Earthly Melancholy, and Materiality in the Graphic Arts of Early Modern France and the German-Speaking Lands (c. 1530–1675)," (PhD thesis, 2019), https://doi.org/10.17863/CAM.35715.

40. Gilman, *Seeing the Insane*, 42.

41. For example, Benjamin Breen's post on his blog *Res Obscura: A Catalogue of Obscure Things* describes this picture as an early brain scan. Breen, "The Alchemy of Madness: Understanding a Seventeenth-Century 'Brain Scan.'" *Res Obscura: A Catalogue of Obscure Things* (blog), December 17, 2015, accessed June 2019, https://resobscura.blogspot.com/2015/12/the-alchemy-of-madness.html.

42. Latour, *Pandora's Hope*, 304. For a criticism on the concept of black boxing, see Langdon Winner, "Upon Opening the Black Box and Finding It Empty: Social Constructivism and the Philosophy of Technology," *Science, Technology, & Human Values* 18, no. 3 (1993): 365–368. The author stands on the ground of social constructivism, but he attempts to avoid its technological determinism, viewing the development of technologies in the context of social relationships and power. For Winner, technological innovation presents huge opportunities for people to develop economically, socially, and culturally, rather than embracing a view of technology as commodity. He attempts to distance from the superficial understanding of technology as a kind of commodity.

43. Bruno Latour, *Science in Action: How to Follow Scientists and Engineers through Society* (Milton Keynes: Open University Press, 1987), 21.

44. Burri et al., "Visualising Bodies," 166.

45. John R. Mallard, interview with Kenneth Muir, Aberdeen, November 15, 2004, GB 0231 University of Aberdeen, Special Collections, MS 3620/1/183.

46. Rheinberger, *Epistemology of the Concrete*, 151.

47. Rheinberger, 230.

48. Rheinberger is referring to Bachelard's concept of *phenomenotechnique*, according to which instruments are materialized theories in modern science. See also Hans-Jörg Rheinberger, "Gaston Bachelard and the Notion of 'Phenomenotechnique,'" *Perspectives on Science* 13, no. 3 (2005): 313–328. Historian of science Gaston Bachelard was the founder of a tradition of French thinking about science that extended from Georges Canguilhem to Michel Foucault. The concept of phenomenotechnique is one of the organizing concepts of his historical epistemology. See Gaston Bachelard, *Le Rationalisme Appliqué* (Paris: Presses Universitaires de France, 1949).

49. John R. Mallard and M. J. Myers, "The Performance of a Gamma Camera for the Visualization of Radioactive Isotopes *in vivo*," *Physics in Medicine & Biology* 8, no. 2 (1963): 165.

50. Hentschel, *Visual Cultures*, 160. This book is particularly relevant for understanding the context in which nuclear magnetic resonance first appeared and also in relation to other image-generating technologies. The negative associations between the name of this emerging research area and

nuclear weapons prompted physicists to drop the "nuclear" from the name "magnetic resonance imaging" in the early 1980s. See Kevles, *Naked to the Bone*, 184.

51. To someone who does not know anything of the mouse picture, its history, and accompanying research, the pixelated hand-painted image of the mouse might bring to memory the tacks game (also called "Chiodini Painting"), the famous table game invented in the 1950s. This game was based on the inclusion of colored tacks in the appropriate spaces provided in a perforated board for realizing figures/drawings/images.

52. James M. Hutchison, John R. Mallard, and G. C. Goll, "In-Vivo Imaging of Body Structures Using Proton Resonance," in *Proceedings, 18th Ampere Conference*, ed. P. S. Allen et al. (Nottingham: University of Nottingham, 1974), 283–284. This mouse map is published in Mallard, "Magnetic Resonance Imaging," 45–60.

53. Hutchison et al., 50.

54. James Hutchison, "Imaging By Nuclear Magnetic Resonance," in *Medical Imaging Techniques*, ed. B. William Watson (London: Peter Peregrinus, 1979), 79–93. The mouse image was obtained before the image created by Damadian with and NMR scanner on July 3, 1977, as mentioned in chapter 1.

55. Hutchison, 92.

56. Mallard, interview with author, Aberdeen, May 2017.

57. Michael Lynch, "Discipline and the Material Form of Images: An Analysis of Scientific Visibility," *Social Studies of Science* 15, no. 1 (1985), 37–66.

58. Joyce, "From Numbers to Pictures," 11, explains how scientists such as Damadian, Mallard, and Lauterbur were "free to tinker with the representational form, chose vibrant, rainbow colors, such as green, yellow, and red, to represent the inner body." Joyce argues that the bright and often primary color choices mirrored the aesthetics of popular art and television in the 1970s.

59. Michael F. Goodchild, "Reimagining the History of GIS," *Annals of GIS* 24, no. 1 (2018): 1–8.

60. Lynch, "Discipline," 37–66.

61. To contextualize historically the dichotomy between images and numbers at the time of nuclear medicine, see Mallard et al., "Imaging by Nuclear Magnetic Resonance," 153–160; Mansfield and Maudsley, "Medical Imaging by NMR," 188–194; Paul Lauterbur, "Cancer Detection by Nuclear Magnetic Resonance Zeugmatographic Imaging," *Cancer* 57 (1986): 1899–1904.

62. Joyce, "From Numbers to Pictures," 1–22.

63. See the section devoted to Lauterbur in Hentschel, *Visual Cultures*, 192–194.

64. Latour, "Visualization and Cognition," 18–20.

65. John R. Mallard, interview with Kenneth Muir, Aberdeen, November 15, 2004, GB 0231 University of Aberdeen, Special Collections, MS 3620/1/183.

66. Regula Burri's tripartite model of visual logic (visual value, visual performance and visual persuasiveness) is present in the image of the mouse. See Regula Valérie Burri, "Visual Rationalities: Towards a Sociology of Images," *Current Sociology* 60, no. 1 (2012): 45.

67. Mallard, "Principles of Scanning."

68. Mallard, "Radioisotope Imaging—The End of the Beginning," *Separata do Arquivo de Patologia* 46, no. 1 (1974): 25.

69. John Mallard, "The Radionuclide Imaging Process and Factors Influencing the Choice of an Instrument for Brain Scanning," *Progress in Nuclear Medicine* 1 (1972): 1–114.

70. Mallard, 6–7.

71. Rudolf Arnheim, *Art and Visual Perception: A Psychology of the Creative Eye* (Berkeley: University of California Press, 1954); and Rudolf Arnheim, *Visual Thinking* (Berkeley: University of California Press, 1969).

72. Gestalt psychology attempts to understand psychological phenomena by viewing them as organized and structured wholes rather than the sum of their constituent parts. Thus, Gestalt psychology accentuates concepts like holism and context. In the 1930s and 1940s, Gestalt psychology was applied to visual perception, most notably by Max Wertheimer, Wolfgang Köhler, and Kurt Koffka, who founded the so-called gestalt approaches to form perception. Their aim was to investigate the global and holistic processes involved in perceiving structure in the environment. More specifically, they tried to explain human perception of groups of objects and how we perceive *parts* of objects and form *whole* objects on the basis of these. For an introduction to Gestalt theory, see Barry Smith, *Foundations of Gestalt Theory* (Munich: Philosophia Verlag, 1988).

73. John R. Mallard, "Nuclear Imaging," in *Electronic Imaging*, ed. T. P. McLean and P. Schagen (London, 1979), 419–459.

74. Scott Smith, "From Nobel Ideas to Industrial Success—Bill Edelstein's Legacy," June 13, 2014, accessed December 2017, https://web.archive.org/web/20170831110622/http://www.geglobalresearch.com/blog/translating-nobel-beginnings-industrial-success-bill-edelsteins-legacy.

75. Mallard, "Evolution of Medical Imaging," 349–370.

76. Mallard gave a talk titled, "In Vivo N.M.R. Imaging in Medicine: The Aberdeen Approach, Both Physical and Biological," at the Royal Society in London on March 14–15, 1979. He discussed early NMR imaging work at Aberdeen done by his team and showed some of the early images of a square bottle array phantom and of Hutchison's chest, legs, and head. These results were eventually published in James Hutchison, William Edelstein, and Glyn Johnson, "A Whole-Body NMR Imaging Machine," *Journal of Physics E: Scientific Instruments* 13, no. 9 (1980): 947.

77. Hutchison et al., 947.

78. William A. Edelstein, "An American Physicist in Aberdeen: Good Enough Engineering," in *MRI25*, ed. P. Antell, R. Jobson, and D. Woods (London: Faircount, 2006), 63.

79. In 1977, Peter Mansfield of the University of Nottingham described the general principles of echo-planar imaging. Each echo is phase encoded differently by phase-encoding blips on the phase-encoding axis. Each oscillation of the frequency-encoding gradient corresponds to one line of imaging data in *k*-space, and each blip corresponds to a transition from one line to the next in the *k*-space. This technique is called blipped echo-planar imaging. See Peter Mansfield, "Multi-Planar Imaging Formation Using NMR Spin-Echo," *Journal of Physics C: Solid State Physics* 10, no. 3 (1977): 55–58.

80. In 1973, Paul Lauterbur described a new imaging technique called zeugmatography (which later became known as NMR imaging, as discussed in chapter 1). By utilizing gradients in the magnetic field, this technique could produce a two-dimensional image (back-projection). See Paul Lauterbur, "MRI: A New Way of Seeing," *Nature* 242 (1973): 190–191. Peter Mansfield refined

this utilization of gradients in the magnetic field and the mathematical analysis of these signals into a more useful imaging technique. In 1975, Richard Ernst introduced 2D NMR using phase and frequency encoding, and the Fourier transform. Instead of Lauterbur's back-projection, this involved timely switching of magnetic field gradients.

81. Edelstein, "American Physicist in Aberdeen," 64.

82. John R. Mallard, interview with Kenneth Muir, Aberdeen, November 15, 2004, GB 0231 University of Aberdeen, Special Collections, MS 3620/1/183.

83. Mallard, "Evolution of Medical Imaging," 360.

84. John Mallard, "Contributions from Aberdeen to the Emergence of Worldwide, Clinically Diagnostic, MRI," *Encyclopedia of Magnetic Resonance* (2010), https://onlinelibrary.wiley.com/doi/abs/10.1002/9780470034590.emrhp1073. On the first patient imaged with nuclear magnetic resonance in Aberdeen, see Francis Smith, John Mallard, James Hutchison, A. Reid, Glyth Johnson, Thomas Redpath, and Robert Selbie, "Clinical Application of Nuclear Magnetic Resonance," *The Lancet* 1, no. 8211 (1981): 78–79.

85. See William A. Edelstein, James M. S. Hutchison, George Johnson, and Thomas Redpath, "Spin Warp NMR Imaging and Applications to Human Whole-Body Imaging," *Physics in Medicine & Biology* 25, no. 4 (1980): 751–756.

86. Mallard, interview with author, Aberdeen, May 2017. On the concept of "facts" in science making, see Riki G. A. Dolby, *Uncertain Knowledge: An Image of Science for a Changing World* (Cambridge: Cambridge University Press, 1996), 49–53.

87. Rheinberger, "Infra-Experimentality," 337–348.

88. Lynch, "Discipline," 58.

89. Mallard, "Evolution of Medical Imaging," 367.

Chapter 3

1. On the concept of "immutable mobiles" see the eponymous section in Latour, "Visualization and Cognition," 1–40.

2. On the concept of science as practice rather than knowledge, see Andrew Pickering, ed., *Science as Practice and Culture* (Chicago: University of Chicago Press, 1992); see also Latour, *Science in Action*, 9.

3. Hans-Jörg Rheinberger, "Difference Machines: Time in Experimental Systems," *Configurations* 23, no. 2 (2015): 167. Rheinberger quotes from Thomas S. Kuhn, *The Trouble with the Historical Philosophy of Science* (Cambridge, MA: Harvard University, 1992), 14.

4. See Rheinberger, *Epistemology of the Concrete*, 166.

5. Although the design of the magnet has not changed much since the days of Hutchison, at present, the skill set required to design a magnet that he possessed is missing in the University of Aberdeen biomedical physics department, perhaps because of the dismantling of the research unit that had this know-how and because researchers with this skill tend to work for industries. The design and construction of the second FFC-MRI prototype that will be placed within the hospital will rely on the Tesla Engineering company.

6. The fieldwork for this study started in 2017 thanks to a Carnegie Trust pilot grant. Initially, I conducted weekly or fortnight laboratory observation for 10 months, followed up by another set

of laboratory visits in 2018 and 2019 also thanks to a Leverhulme Trust Fellowship grant. The fieldwork was accompanied by semistructured interviews with key members (physicists, radiologists, doctors, engineers) involved in the development of FFC-MRI at the University of Aberdeen and in the research centers involved in the IDentIFY project. I have also conducted a few oral history interviews to people involved in the early days of MRI development in Aberdeen. I carried out the interviews in English and, in a few cases, in Italian. All participants signed a consent form in which they agree to have interview excerpts be used for research purposes and published if required. All interviews were audio recorded, transcribed verbatim by a research assistant, and stored in accordance with the ethical procedure guidelines of the University of Aberdeen. Some of the interviews have been anonymized as requested by the interviewees. In some cases, the grammar of the verbatim transcription of a passage had to be corrected without altering the meaning of the cited passage. I translated into English the transcriptions of interviews originally conducted in Italian.

7. See Mallard, "Evolution of Medical Imaging," 363, quoted in Prasad, *Imperial Technoscience*, 8. Prasad argues that the drive to work at increasing high field was associated with the rise of big science, which impacted technoscientific research development across the globe. Prasad discusses M&D, the company set up by Mallard, in *Imperial Technoscience*, 54.

8. Hans-Jörg Rheinberger, "On the Possible Transformation and Vanishment of Epistemic Objects," *Theory of Science* 38, no. 3 (2016): 278.

9. Physicist David Lurie, interview with author, Aberdeen, April 2017. Interview recordings and transcripts are available upon request to the author.

10. Early studies conducted on free radicals in the 1980s by David Lurie (now head of the IDentIFY project) and members of Mallard's team were the forerunners of FFC-MRI development. See David J. Lurie et al., "Proton-Electron Double Magnetic Resonance Imaging of Free Radical Solutions," *Journal of Magnetic Resonance* 76 (1988): 366–370; David J. Lurie et al., "Field-Cycled Proton-Electron Double-Resonance Imaging of Free Radicals in Large Aqueous Samples," *Journal of Magnetic Resonance* 84 (1989): 431–437. For examples of early literature on field-cycling methods and technical aspects, see Frank Noack, "NMR Field Cycling Spectroscopy: Principles and Applications," *Progress in NMR Spectroscopy* 18 (1986): 171–276; Rainer Kimmich, "Field Cycling NMR Relaxometry," *Bulletin Magnetic Resonance* 1, no. 4 (1980): 195.

11. It is not possible to study this T_1 dispersion using conventional MRI scanners because they operate at a fixed magnetic field strength. FFC-MRI allows researchers to collect information relating to a wide range of magnetic field strengths using a single instrument.

12. Paramagnetism is a kind of magnetism characteristic of materials weakly attracted by a strong magnet. The scientist Michael Faraday first investigated this phenomenon in 1845. Most elements and some compounds are paramagnetic.

13. Seymour Koenig, who passed away in February 2018, was director of IBM Watson Lab at Columbia University from 1952 to 1970 where he also lectured in art history. In the IBM lab the first supercomputer was developed in 1954. Koenig developed a field-cycling relaxometer, also installed in four other research centers in the world, thus allowing many other scientists to benefit from this technique. See https://www.ismrm.org/members-only/in-memoriam/seymour-koenig/ (accessed April 2018).

14. Seymour H. Koenig and Rodney D. Brown, "Relaxometry of Tissue," *Progress in NMR Spectroscopy* 22 (1990): 487.

15. Gianni Ferrante and Stanislav Sykora, "Technical Aspects of Fast Field Cycling," in *Advances in Inorganic Chemistry Volume 57: Relaxometry of Water-Metal Ion Interactions*, ed. Rudi Van Eldik (Amsterdam: Elsevier 2004), 405–470.

16. See David J. Lurie et al., "Fast Field-Cycling Magnetic Resonance Imaging," *Comptes Rendus Physique* 11, no. 2 (2010): 136–148.

17. I wish to thank Professor Silvio Aime (Turin University), who pointed to the contribution of Koenig in the early days of relaxometry.

18. See http://www.identify-project.eu/ (accessed January 2020).

19. Commonly used contrast agents are based on gadolinium—a paramagnetic metal. In some cases, for instance in patients on dialysis, these compounds cannot be quickly removed from the body and this can then lead to long-term side effects. Therefore, the objective is to look for alternative contrast agents that do not contain metal. One direction of research is to try to administer simple molecules (glucose, proteins, or amino acids) whose presence can change the water movement. If these molecules accumulate in pathological tissue, such as a tumor, they can cause variations that can then be detected by FFC-MRI.

20. Laboratory fieldwork, physicist to author, Aberdeen, May 2017. This and all the other dialogues reported below are faithful transcriptions of the exchanges that occurred during the fieldwork and based on notes taken by the author.

21. Laboratory fieldwork, physicist to author, Aberdeen, March 2017.

22. Allen D. Elster and Jonathan H. Burdette, *Questions and Answers in Magnetic Resonance Imaging* (Chicago: Mosby, 2000).

23. Rheinberger, "Infra-Experimentality," 345–346.

24. See Leonelli, *Data-Centric Biology*, 2016.

25. Physicist, interview with author, Aberdeen, May 2017.

26. Rheinberger, "Difference Machines," 168.

27. Leonelli, *Data-Centric Biology*, 95.

28. See http://www.opensourceimaging.org (accessed November 2018).

29. See chapter 2. Joyce, *Magnetic Appeal*, 35–36.

30. Eddie Stevenson , interview with author, Aberdeen, April 2017.

31. On the customization and disciplining of bodies to a physical norm prior to the actual MRI examination. see Regula Valérie Burri, "Sociotechnical Anatomy. Technology, Space and Body in the MRI Unit," in *Biomedicine as Culture: Instrumental Practices, Technoscientific Knowledge, and New Modes of Life*, ed. Regula V. Burri and Joseph Dumit (New York: Routledge 2007), 113.

32. Tim Ingold argues that attributing agency to things is just an attempt to reanimate lifeless objects instead of taking them as alive things that have a generative capacity and are within the flux and flow of materials. See Tim Ingold, "Bringing Things to Life: Creative Entanglements in a World of Materials," NCRM Working Paper Series no. 15, 2010, http://eprints.ncrm.ac.uk/1306/1/0510_creative_entanglements.pdf.

33. Luciano Floridi, *The Philosophy of Information* (Oxford: Oxford University Press, 2011).

34. Laboratory fieldwork, physicist to author, Aberdeen, December 2018.

35. Three-dimensional models have been often ignored by historians of science and science and technology scholars who devoted more attention to two-dimensional models. An exception is represented by Soraya de Chadarevian and Nik Hopwood, *Models: The Third Dimension of Science* (Stanford: Stanford University Press, 2004).

36. Laboratory fieldwork, physicist to author, Aberdeen, September 2017.

37. See https://www.abdn.ac.uk/news/11333/ (accessed December 2017).

38. Cited in Hans-Jörg Rheinberger, "Scripts and Scribbles," *MLN* 118, no. 3 (2003): 622–636, 626. Rheinberger takes the concept of "night science" from François Jacob, *Of Flies, Mice and Men* (Cambridge, MA: Harvard University Press, 1998), 125–126.

39. Dan Ma, Vikas Gulani, Nicole Seiberlich, Kecheng Liu, Jeffrey L. Sunshine, Jeffrey L. Duerk, and Mark A. Griswold, "Magnetic Resonance Fingerprinting," *Nature* 14, no. 495 (2013): 187–192.

40. Hentschel, *Visual Cultures*, 190.

41. The Block equations are known and describe how the signal behaves.

42. Simone Coppo et al., "Overview of Magnetic Resonance Fingerprinting," *MAGNETOM Flash* 65, no. 2 (2016): 13.

43. Dan Ma, Vikas Gulani, Nicole Seiberlich, Kecheng Liu, Jeffrey L. Sunshine, Jeffrey L. Duerk, and Mark A. Griswold, "Music-Based Magnetic Resonance Fingerprinting to Improve Patient Comfort during MRI Examinations," *Magnetic Resonance in Medicine* 75, no. 6 (2016): 2303–2314.

44. Ma et al., "Music-Based Magnetic Resonance Fingerprinting."

45. Rheinberger, "Scripts and Scribbles."

46. In the near future, the Turin-based research group would like to image other organs of the mouse, such as the brain.

47. Laboratory fieldwork, biologist to author, Turin, June 2017.

48. Physicist, interview with author, Aberdeen, April 2017.

49. Laboratory fieldwork, physicists to author, Aberdeen, March 2017.

50. See Floridi, *Philosophy of Information.*

51. See chapter 16 in Thomas Cover and Joy Thomas, *Elements of Information Theory* (Hoboken, NJ: Wiley Interscience, 2006).

52. Min Chen and Luciano Floridi, "An Analysis of Information in Visualization," *Synthese* 190, no. 16 (2013): 3421–3438.

53. Alexander Galloway, "Are Some Things Unrepresentable?" *Theory, Culture and Society* 28, no. 7/8 (2011): 85–102.

54. Hans-Jörg Rheinberger, "From Microsomes to Ribosomes: 'Strategies' of 'Representation,'" *Journal of the History of Biology* 28, no. 1 (1995): 51.

55. On images as life forms, see W. J. T. Mitchell, *What Do Pictures Want? The Lives and Loves of Images* (Chicago: University of Chicago Press, 2005). Halpern, *Beautiful Data*, 21.

56. Molecular biologist, interview with author, Turin, June 2017.

57. Rheinberger, *Epistemology of the Concrete*, xiv. Rheinberger prefers to use the term *thing* rather than *object*.

58. Molecular biologist, interview with author, Turin, June 2017.

Chapter 4

1. The image is taken from Latour, *Science in Action*, 1987.

2. The philosopher Rancière argues, referring not to biomedicine but to society, that the question of what is unrepresentable today is intimately connected to how violence may be put or not into an image. See Jacques Rancière, *The Future of the Image* (London: Verso, 2007).

3. Van Dijck, *Transparent Body*, 2005.

4. Regula Valérie Burri, "Pictures, Practices, Paradoxes: Medical Imaging and Modernity," *Tecnoscienza. Italian Journal of Science & Technology Studies* 5, no. 1 (2014): 166.

5. Akira Mizuta Lippit, *Atomic Light Shadow Optics* (Minneapolis: University of Minnesota Press, 2005): 58.

6. Walter Benjamin, "Little History of Photography", in *Walter Benjamin, Selected Writings*, ed. Michael W. Jennings, Howard Eiland, and Gary Smith, vol. 2, pt. 2, *1931–1934* (Cambridge, MA: Belknap Press of Harvard University Press, 2005), 507–530, 510.

7. See Smith and Sliwinski, eds., *Photography and the Optical Unconscious*, 5.

8. Crary, *Techniques of the Observer*, 2. See also Michael Lynch, "Laboratory Space and the Technological Complex: An Investigation of Topical Contextures," *Science in Context* 4, no. 1 (1991): 72.

9. On the concept of cyborg vision in relation to MRI, see Amit Prasad, "Making Images/Making Bodies: Visibilizing and Disciplining through Magnetic Resonance Imaging (MRI)," *Science, Technology, & Human Values* 30, no. 2 (2005): 310.

10. This point is discussed by Alač in relation to how scientists make sense of brain scans via a multimodal way of handling digital scans. See Alač, *Handling Digital Brains*, 81.

11. Mallard, John R., James M. S. Hutchison, William Edelstein, Richard Ling, and Margaret Foster, "Imaging by Nuclear Magnetic Resonance and Its Bio-Medical Implications," *Journal of Biomedical Engineering* 1, no. 3 (1979): 153–160. The Potential T_1 Man map is also contained in a paper entitled John Mallard, "Nuclear Imaging," *Journal of Medical Progress through Technology* 7 (1980): 87–110. This paper is listed within Professor Mallard's own catalog as being printed in the *Proceedings of the International Symposium Electronic Imaging at the Royal Society, London, September 1978* (London: Academic Press, 1978), 419–459. This copy is a photocopy of an offprint. This article contains the Potential T_1 Man map.

12. Star and Griesemer, "Institutional Ecology," 393.

13. The map showing the T_1 of normal tissues in a rabbit, drawn on an anatomical map of the rabbit, is contained in John Mallard et al., "In Vivo N.M.R. Imaging in Medicine: The Aberdeen Approach, Both Physical and Biological [and Discussion]," *Philosophical Transactions of the Royal Society of London: Series B, Biological Sciences* 289, no. 1037 (1980): 519–530, 520.

14. See Nikolas Rose, "The Human Sciences in a Biological Age," *ICS Occasional Paper Series* 3, no. 1, ed. David Rowee and Reena Dobson (2012), 9. In this passage Rose refers to the following study: Lily E. Kay, *The Molecular Vision of Life: Caltech, the Rockefeller Foundation, and the Rise of the New*

Biology (New York: Oxford University Press, 1993). See also Nikolas Rose, *The Politics of Life Itself: Biomedicine, Power, and Subjectivity in the Twentieth-First Century* (Princeton, NJ: Princeton University Press, 2007).

15. Rose, *Politics of Life Itself*, 12.

16. In the 1990s, Haraway coined the term "New World Order, Inc." to describe this new regime of biopower. See Donna Haraway, *Modest_Witness@Second_Millennium.FemaleMan_Meets_OncoMouse: Feminism and Technoscience* (New York: Routledge, 1997).

17. Nikolas Rose "Genomic Susceptibility as an Emergent Form of Life? Genetic Testing, Identity, and the Remit of Medicine," in *Biomedicine as Culture: Instrumental Practices, Technoscientific Knowledge, and New Modes of Life*, ed. Regula Valérie Burri and Joseph Dumit (New York: Routledge, 2010), 143.

18. Rose, *Politics of Life Itself*, 4.

19. Lorraine Daston and Peter Galison, *Objectivity* (New York: Zone Books, 2010).

20. Daston and Galison, 20.

21. MATLAB language is the most natural way to express computational mathematics. The built-in graphics make it easy to visualize and gain insights from data.

22. Borck, "How We May Think," 112–120.

23. Borck, 115.

24. On the importance of instrument pluralism to investigate complex objects, see Hans-Jörg Rheinberger, "Afterword: Instruments as Media, Media as Instruments," *Studies in History and Philosophy of Biological and Biomedical Sciences* 57 (2016): 161–162.

25. Edward Vul, Christine Harris, Piotr Winkielman, and Harold Pashler, "Puzzlingly High Correlations in fMRI Studies of Emotion, Personality, and Social Cognition," *Perspectives on Psychological Science* 4 (2009): 274–290.

26. Physicist, interview with author, Grenoble, June 2017. Interview recordings and transcripts are available upon request to the author.

27. Quadrupole dips are reductions in the proton spin-lattice relaxation time at NMR frequencies which correspond to the nuclear quadrupole transitions. The effect has been known since the 1980s, and quadrupole dips can be measured in hydrated proteins and biological samples. See David Lurie, "Quadrupole-Dip Measurement in Humans by Whole-Body Field-Cycling NMR Relaxometry and Imaging," *29th Ampere–13th ISMAR Conference*, vol. 1 (Berlin, 1998).

28. Leonelli, *Data-Centric Biology*, 69.

29. Gitelman, *Raw Data*. In her book, Gitelman discusses case studies that prove how data are cultural artifacts that need to be generated and interpreted.

30. Physicist, interview with author, Olsztyn, April 2018.

31. Regula Valérie Burri, Anna Maria Carusi, Aikaterini Aspradaki "Personalised Medicine: Visions and Visualisations," *Technoscienza. Italian Journal of Science and Technology Studies* 5, no. 1 (2014): 173.

32. Burri et al., 173.

33. Physicist, interview with author, Olsztyn, April 2018.

34. The slope of the curve is a number which is used to indicate the steepness of a curve at a particular point. The slope of a curve at a point is defined to be the slope of the tangent line.

35. Leonelli, *Data-Centric Biology*, 1–2.

36. Laboratory fieldwork, physicist to author, Aberdeen, September 2018. This and all the other dialogues reported below are faithful transcriptions of the exchanges that occurred during the fieldwork and based on notes taken by the author.

37. Peter Galison, *How Experiments End* (Chicago: University of Chicago Press, 1987).

38. Lars G. Hanson, "Is Quantum Mechanics Necessary for Understanding Magnetic Resonance?" *Concepts in Magnetic Resonance Part A* 32, no. 5 (2008): 329–340.

39. In the atomic realm, quantum mechanics rejected any deterministic thinking in relation to matter and energy. Objects no longer fit into comprehensible categories: light was not exactly a wave, an electron was not altogether a particle, each was both a wave and a particle at the same time and could act as one or the other. Physicists found that the specific characteristics of particles, or even whole atoms and molecules, were unknowable until the instant they were measured—the so-called "observer effect" described by physicist Niels Bohr. For a popular, though still scientifically reliable, account see Brian Cox and Jeff Forshaw, *The Quantum Universe: Everything That Can Happen Does Happen* (Cambridge, MA: Da Capo Press, 2011); for a historical treatment of the topic see, Jim Baggott, *The Quantum Story: A History in 40 Moments* (Oxford: Oxford University Press, 2011); and for a more rigorous treatment, see Roger Penrose, *The Road to Reality: A Complete Guide to the Laws of the Universe* (New York: Alfred Knopf, 2004).

40. Ian Hacking, *The Taming of Chance* (Cambridge: Cambridge University Press, 1990).

41. Joyce, *Magnetic Appeal*, 159.

42. See Giorgio Agamben, *Homo Sacer: Sovereign Power and Bare Life* (Palo Alto, CA: Stanford University Press, 1998).

43. On Agamben's paradigmatic method, see Giorgio Agamben, *The Signature of All Things: On Method*, trans. Luca D'Isanto with Kevin Attell (Brooklyn, NY: Zone Books, 2009); and Leland de la Durantaye, *Giorgio Agamben: A Critical Introduction* (Stanford, CA: Stanford University Press, 2009), 200–243.

44. Christian McCrea, "Giorgio Agamben," in *Film, Theory, and Philosophy: The Key Thinkers*, ed. Felicity Colman (Montreal: McGill University Press, 2009), 350.

45. Giorgio Agamben, "What Is an Apparatus?," in *What Is an Apparatus? And Other Essays* (Stanford, CA: Stanford University Press, 2009), 14.

46. Giorgio Agamben, *Che cos'è Reale? La Scomparsa di Majorana* (Vicenza: Neri Pozza, 2016). Available in English: *What Is Real*, trans. Lorenzo Chiesa (Stanford: Stanford University Press, 2018). All the citations from Agamben's book and the passages from Majorana's article included in Agamben's book are my translations.

47. The Uncertainty Principle, formulated by Heisenberg, remains a major tenet of quantum mechanics. The light used to measure particles imparts energy, altering the momentum or location of the particles, thus changing the results by the mere act of observation. An experiment can be designed to measure either momentum or location precisely, but not both (the experimenter must choose).

48. Agamben, *Che cos'è Reale?*, 14–15.

49. Majorana's article is reported in the appendix to Agamben's text. See the original article in Ettore Majorana, "Il Valore delle Leggi Statistiche nella Fisica e nelle Scienze Sociali," *Scientia* 36 (1942): 58–66. For the article's English translation, see Ettore Majorana and Rosario N. Mantegna, "The Value of Statistical Laws in Physics and Social Sciences," in *Ettore Majorana Scientific Papers*, ed. Giuseppe Franco Bassani and the Council of the Italian Physical Society (Berlin: Springer, 2006), 237–260.

50. The journal *Scientia* was funded as a monthly publication by Federigo Enriques and Eugenio Rignano in 1907 under the title *Rivista di Scienza*. Among its contributors there were Wilhelm Ostwald, Émile Picard, Paul Tannery. Books by Jules-Henri Poincaré, Étienne-Émile Boutroux, Giovanni Vailati, Pierre-Maurice Duhem, Werner Sombart, Maffeo Pantaleoni, and Vilfredo Pareto were reviewed. See Edoardo Amaldi, *La Vita e l'Opera di Ettore Majorana (1906–1938)* (Roma, Accademia Nazionale dei Lincei, 1966). See also Giuseppe Franco Bassani, *Ettore Majorana: Scientific Papers on the Occasion of the Centenary of His Birth*, Società Italiana di Fisica (Berlin: Springer, 2006).

51. Agamben, *Che Cos'è Reale?*, 75.

52. Agamben, 16.

53. Nikolas Rose and Joelle Abi-Rached. *Neuro: The New Brain Sciences and the Management of the Mind* (Princeton, NJ: Princeton University Press, 1685), 14.

54. Sander Gilman, *Illness and Image: Case Studies in the Medical Humanities* (London: Routledge, 2014).

55. Although my focus is exclusively related to the laboratory, the concept of potentiality is at work in clinical practice, in social policy, and in the way in which public discourse frames biomedicine. See Karen-Sue Taussig, Klaus Hoeyer, and Stefan Helmreich, "The Anthropology of Potentiality in Biomedicine. An Introduction to Supplement 7," *Current Anthropology* 54, no. 7 (2013): 3–14.

56. See Michel Foucault, *The Birth of the Clinic: An Archaeology of Medical Perception* (London: Tavistock Publications, 1973).

57. In his *Politics of Life Itself*, Rose cites the exhibition *Spectacular Bodies* saying that it succeeded in visualizing these historical passages in how the body was conceived anew. See Martin Kemp and Marina Wallace, *Spectacular Bodies* (Hayward Gallery, London, 2000–2001). On the history of medicine, see Roger Cooter and Claudia Stein, eds., *The History of Medicine* (New York and London: Routledge, 2015).

58. European Science Foundation (ESF), "Personalised Medicine for the European Citizen—Towards More Precise Medicine for the Diagnosis, Treatment and Prevention of Disease" (Strasbourg: ESF, 2012), accessed August 2020, http://archives.esf.org/fileadmin/Public_documents/Publications/Personalised_Medicine.pdf.

59. Olga Golubnitschaja, Judita Kinkorova, and Vincenzo Costigliola, "Predictive, Preventive and Personalised Medicine as the Hardcore of 'Horizon 2020': EPMA Position Paper," *EPMA Journal* 5, no. 1 (2014): 6.

60. François Berger, "FFC-MRI: Is This the Technology Breakthrough That Patients and Neuro-Oncologists Have Been Waiting For?" Conference presentation, one-day symposium, *Fast Field-Cycling MRI—A New Imaging Modality*, Aberdeen, UK, March 16, 2018. The concept of the body and the brain as "data" and the technique of "fingerprinting" can be reconducted to the work

of the Victorian statistician Francis Galton, who was interested in using biometric statistics to try to visualize and locate/predict current and future deviant tendencies in the body. See Francis Galton, "Composite Portraits," *Journal of the Anthropological Institute of Great Britain and Ireland* 8 (1878): 132–144.

61. Brain fingerprints are measured by an electroencephalography (EEG) event-related potential.

62. Laboratory fieldwork, physicist to author, Aberdeen, June 2018.

63. Molecular imaging researcher, interview with author, Turin, April 2018.

64. Heidi Olzscha et al., "Amyloid-Like Aggregates Sequester Numerous Metastable Proteins with Essential Cellular Functions," *Cell* 144, no. 1 (2011): 67.

65. Generation Scotland is an ethically sound resource to support medical research and identify the genetic basis of common complex diseases. The aim is to create more effective treatments based on gene knowledge for the medical, social and economic benefit of Scotland and its people. For more information, see https://www.ed.ac.uk/generation-scotland/about/general-information (accessed February 2018).

66. The seemingly proactivity of "patients" is at the center of a book written by political scientist Barbara Prainsack, who unpacks the complexities of "patient-centered personalized medicine" and the new forms of participation that are required of patients in the age of personalized medicine. See Barbara Prainsack, *Personalized Medicine: Empowered Patients in the 21st Century?* (New York: New York University Press, 2017).

67. Sarah de Rijcke and Anne Beaulieu, "Networked neuroscience: brain scans and visual knowing at the intersection of atlases and databases," in *Representations in Scientific Practice Revisited*, ed. Catelijne Coopmans et al. (Cambridge, MA: MIT Press, 2014), 133.

68. Beaulieu's image comes from a probabilistic atlas from Paul Thompson et al., "Detection and Mapping of Abnormal Brain Structure with a Probabilistic Atlas of Cortical Surfaces," *Journal of Computer Assisted Tomography* 21, no. 4 (1997), 567–581.

69. Regula Valérie Burri and Joseph Dumit, eds., *Biomedicine as Culture. Instrumental Practices, Technoscientific Knowledge, and New Modes of Life* (New York and London: Routledge, 2007).

70. This is a point made, among others, by Nikolas Rose, "Personalized Medicine: Promises, Problems and Perils of a New Paradigm for Healthcare," *Procedia—Social and Behavioral Sciences* 7 (2013): 352.

71. Margaret Lock, *The Alzheimer Conundrum: Entanglements of Dementia and Aging* (Princeton, NJ: Princeton University Press, 2003), 11. In this passage on the genealogy of risk, Lock is referring to Hacking, *Taming of Chance*.

72. Marianne Boenink, Harro van Lente and Ellen Moors, *Emerging Technologies for Diagnosing Alzheimer's Disease: Innovating with Care* (London: Palgrave, 2016): 65–66.

73. Ulrich Beck, *World at Risk* (Cambridge: Polity Press, 2007). The passage is quoted in Lock, *Alzheimer Conundrum*, 12.

74. Rose, *Politics of Life Itself*, 2007.

75. The first symposium on field-cycling NMR relaxometry was held in Berlin 1998, with the purpose of bringing together all the researchers practicing FC methods with those who do not yet but are interested in applying this technique in the future.

76. The Timavo River, known in Slovenian as the *Timav*, comes to the surface in some traits, its flow is contributed by subterranean sources. Its characteristic of disappearing and reappearing was mentioned by the poet Virgil (70–19 BC).

Intermezzo

Sections of this chapter were published in Silvia Casini, "The Material Site of Abstraction: Grid-Based Data Visualisation in Brain Scans," in *The Iconology of Abstraction. Non-Figurative Images and the Modern World*, ed. Krešimir Purgar (New York: Routledge, 2020), 221–234.

1. Phillip Thurtle, *Biology in the Grid: Graphic Design and the Envisioning of Life* (Minneapolis: University of Minnesota Press, 2018).

2. Bredekamp et al., *Technical Image*, 2015.

3. Anne Friedberg, *The Virtual Window: From Alberti to Microsoft* (Cambridge, MA: MIT Press, 2009), 40.

4. Rosalind Krauss, "Grids," *October* 9 (1979): 50–64.

5. James Elkins, *Six Stories from the End of Representation* (Stanford, CA: Stanford University Press, 2008), 66.

6. The idea of this system was developed in 1637 by Descartes. In part two of his *Discourse on Method*, Descartes introduces the idea of specifying the position of a point or object on a surface by using two intersecting axes as measuring guides. René Descartes, *Discourse on Method, Optics, Geometry, and Meteorology* (Indianapolis, IN: Hackett, 2001).

7. On photo-stereo-synthesis, see Lisa Cartwright and Brian Goldfarb, "Radiography, Cinematography, and the Decline of the Lens," in *Incorporations*, ed. Jonathan Crary and Sanford Kwinter (New York: Zone Books, 1992), 190–201.

8. On the passage from the anatomical to the atomized body, see Max Liljefors, Susan S. Lundin, and Andrea Wiszmeg, eds., *The Atomized Body: The Cultural Life of Stem Cells, Genes and Neurons* (Lund: Nordic Academic Press, 2012).

9. Jacob Beutel, Harold Kundel, and Richard L. Van Metter, *Handbook of Medical Imaging, Volume 1. Physics and Psychophysics* (Bellingham, WA: SPIE Press, 2000).

10. Prasad, "Making Images/Making Bodies," 291–316.

11. Prasad, 292.

12. Katherine N. Hayles, *Unthought: The Power of the Cognitive Nonconscious* (Chicago: Chicago University Press, 2017), 141.

13. Jonathan Sawday, *The Body Emblazoned: Dissection and the Human Body in Renaissance Culture* (London: Routledge, 1996).

14. Marta Braun, *Picturing Time: The Work of Etienne-Jules Marey* (Chicago: University of Chicago Press, 1992).

15. Krauss, "Grids," 52.

16. Cornelius Borck, "Vital Brains: On the Entanglement of Media, Minds, and Models," in *Vital Models. The Making and Use of Models in the Brain Sciences*, Progress in Brain Research 233, ed. Tara Mahfoud et al. (Cambridge: Academic Press, 2017), 3.

17. Anne Beaulieu, "A Space for Measuring Mind and Brain: Interdisciplinarity and Digital Tools in the Development of Brain Mapping and Functional Imaging, 1980–1990," *Brain and Cognition* 49 (2002): 13–33.

18. William J. Mitchell, *The Reconfigured Eye: Visual Truth in the Post-photographic Era* (Cambridge, MA: MIT Press, 1992).

19. Galit Shmueli, "To Explain or to Predict?" *Statistical Science* 25, no. 3 (2010): 291.

20. Nate Silver, *The Signal and the Noise. The Art and Science of Prediction* (London: Penguin, 2013), 241.

21. Amoore, *Politics of Possibility*, 7.

22. Amoore, 9.

23. Amoore, 50.

24. Babette Regierer et al., "Future of Medicine: Models in Predictive Diagnostics and Personalized Medicine," in *Advances in Biochemical Engineering/Biotechnology* 133 (2013): 15–33.

25. Amoore, *The Politics of Possibility*, 139.

26. For an examination of the aesthetics and politics of the interface, see Alexander L. Galloway, *The Interface Effect* (London: Polity Press, 2012). On the ubiquity of the logic of the algorithm, see William Uricchio, "The Algorithmic Turn: Photosynth, Augmented Reality and the Changing Implications of the Image," *Visual Studies* 26, no. 1 (2011): 25–35.

27. On the pervasiveness of the grid in Western visual culture, see Hannah B. Higgins, *The Grid Book* (Cambridge MA: MIT Press, 2009). On a reassessment of Descartes's grid as a system that can address affective relationships between thought and the body, see Anna Munster, *Materializing New Media: Embodiment in Information Aesthetics* (Hanover, NH: Dartmouth College Press, 2006).

Chapter 5

Sections of this chapter were published in Silvia Casini, "Beyond the Neuro-Realism Fallacy: From John R. Mallard's Hand-Painted MRI Image of a Mouse to BioArt Scenarios," *Nuncius. Journal of the Material and Visual History of Science* 32, no. 2 (2017): 440–471.

Epigraph: https://www.marcdidou.com/biographie/ (accessed December 2019).

1. Aristotle, *Parts of Animals. Movement of Animals. Progression of Animals*, trans. A. L. Peck and E. S. Forster (Cambridge, MA: Harvard University Press, 1937).

2. Throughout the Middle Ages human dissection was restricted, so the main tool for studying and representing the brain was diagrammatic drawing rather than direct observation. From the Renaissance onward, the study of the brain thrived, thanks to dissections of cadavers in anatomical theaters, demonstrated, for example, by the atlas *De Humani Corporis Fabrica*, which was produced in 1543 by the Flemish anatomist Andreas Vesalius. On the culture of dissection, see Sawday, *Body Emblazoned*, 1995.

3. de Chadarevian and Hopwood, *Models*. On the history of the different models and metaphors used to represent and investigate the brain, see Cornelius Borck, "Toys Are Us: Models and Metaphors in Brain Research," in *Critical Neuroscience: A Handbook of the Social and Cultural Contexts of Neuroscience*, ed. Suparna Choudhury and Jan Slaby (London: Blackwell, 2011), 111–133.

4. See Bart Lutters and Peter J. Koehler, "Brainwaves in Concert: The 20th Century Sonification of the Electroencephalogram," *Brain* 139, no. 10 (2016): 2809–2814. On the conceptual and historical role of sound as an art medium and on data sonification, see Peter Weibel, ed., *Sound Art: Sound as a Medium of Art* (Cambridge, MA: MIT Press, 2019).

5. Borck, "Vital Brains," 5. See also Borck, *Brainwaves*, on his work on the cultural history of electroencephalography.

6. Joseph Dumit, *Picturing Personhood: Brain Scans and Biomedical Identity* (Princeton, NJ: Princeton University Press, 2004), 141.

7. Giovanni Frazzetto and Suzanne Anker, "Neuroculture," *Nature Reviews Neuroscience* 10 (2009): 815–821. On neurocultures, see also Francisco Ortega and Fernando Vidal, eds., *Neurocultures: Glimpses into an Expanding Universe* (Frankfurt: Peter Lang, 2011).

8. Fernando Vidal, "Brainhood, Anthropological Figure of Modernity," *History of the Human Sciences* 22, no. 1 (2009): 6.

9. On the neurologization of subjectivity, see Jan De Vos, *The Metamorphoses of the Brain—Neurologisation and Its Discontents* (London: Palgrave, 2016).

10. For a critique of the neuro-turn from a history of science perspective, see Roger Cooter, "Neural Veils and the Will to Historical Critique: Why Historians of Science Need to Take the Neuro-Turn Seriously," *Isis* 105, no. 1 (2014): 145–154.

11. Dumit, "How (Not) to Do Things," 291–313.

12. See, for example, Cornelius Borck, "Recording the Brain at Work: The Visible, the Readable, and the Invisible in Electroencephalography," *Journal of the History of the Neurosciences* 17 (2008): 367–379.

13. Dumit, "How (Not) to Do Things," 297.

14. Dumit, 291–313.

15. Mallard, "Radionuclide Imaging Process," 6–7.

16. Dumit, "How (Not) to Do Things," 304. Other scholars pointed out at the flaws in functional neuroimaging. See, for example, Edward Vul and Harold Pashler, "Voodoo and Circularity Errors," *NeuroImage* 62, no. 2 (2012): 945–948; Cornelius Borck, "How to Do Voodoo with Functional Neuroimaging," *EspacesTemps.net*, accessed October 1, 2018, http://www.espacestemps.net/articles/neuroimaging/.

17. Sellars, "Philosophy," 1–40.

18. For a critical reading of Sellars's myth of the given, see Willem A. deVries and Timm Triplett, *Knowledge, Mind, and the Given: Reading Wilfrid Sellars's "Empiricism and the Philosophy of Mind"* (Indianapolis: Hackett, 2000).

19. Ortega and Vidal, *Neurocultures*, 8.

20. Eric Racine et al., "Contemporary Neuroscience in the Media," *Social Science and Medicine Journal* 71, no. 4 (2010): 725–733.

21. For example, the Portuguese artist Marta de Menezes, who has a long record of collaborative art–science projects, developed a series of artworks called *Functional Portraits* (2002) with the neuroscientist Patricia Figueiredo at the University of Oxford. See Martin Kemp, *Seen / Unseen:*

Art, Science and Intuition from Leonardo to the Hubble Telescope (New York: Oxford University Press, 2006), 319–321.

22. For a discussion of Marc Didou's work in relation to other artists' practices with MRI, see Silvia Casini, "Magnetic Resonance Imaging (MRI) as Mirror and Portrait: MRI Configurations between Science and the Arts," *Configurations* 19, no. 1 (2011): 73–99.

23. Artist, interview with author, online, September 2019. Interview recordings and transcripts are available upon request to the author. In quality of head of the media board, Lintermann contributes to the activities of the foundation Das Gehirn, accessed November 2019, https://www.dasgehirn.info.

24. See https://marileneoliver.com/home and https://www.dyscorpia.com/ (accessed December 2019).

25. Marilène Oliver, *TEDMED Talk*, accessed January 2020, https://www.youtube.com/watch?v=GfqhUO1_u28.

26. Artist, interview with author, online, December 2018.

27. For a contextualization of Carnie's installation within the broader visual culture of the neuron, see Richard Wingate and Marius Kwint, "Imagining the Brain Cell: The Neuron in Visual Culture," *Nature Reviews* 7 (2006): 746.

28. Marius Kwint, "Animated Meditations on Mortality: The Work of Andrew Carnie," in *Time Will Tell* (Winchester Gallery Publisher, 2008), 2.

29. Artist, interview with author, Winchester, December 2017.

30. Artist, interview with author, Winchester, December 2017.

31. The final film of the series *Stereoscope*, to which *WEIGHING… and WANTING* belongs, suggests the possibility of a stereoscopic vision. See Tom Gunning, "Doubled Vision: Peering through Kentridge's 'Stereoscope,'" *Parkett* 63 (2001), 66–81, accessed November 2019, http://www.parkettart.com/books/63-volume.html.

32. Dan Cameron, Carolyn Christov-Bakargiev, and John M. Coetzee, *William Kentridge* (London: Phaidon Press, 1999).

33. Borck, "Vital Brains," 2.

34. Heinz von Foerster, ed., *Cybernetics. Circular Causal, and Feedback Mechanisms in Biological and Social Systems*. Transactions of the Sixth Conference March 24–25, 1949 (New York: Josiah Macy Jr. Foundation, 1950): 9–10.

35. See Lohmeyer and Halpern, "Cinema/Cybernetics/Visuality," 3207.

36. Peter Galison, "The Ontology of the Enemy: Norbert Wiener and the Cybernetic Vision," *Critical Inquiry* 21, no. 1 (1994): 228–266.

37. Ed Finn, *What Algorithms Want: Imagination in the Age of Computing* (Cambridge, MA: MIT Press, 2017), 27. Finn's reflections are based on Norbert Wiener, *The Human Use of Human Beings: Cybernetics and Society* (Cambridge, MA: Da Capo Press, 1950[1988]), 7–9.

38. Andrew Pickering and Keith Guzik, eds., *The Mangle in Practice: Science, Society, and Becoming* (Durham, NC: Duke University Press, 2008), 13.

39. Andrew Pickering, *The Cybernetic Brain: Sketches of Another Future* (Chicago: Chicago University Press, 2010), 59. Pickering is analyzing, in particular, post–World War II British cybernetics.

40. Neuroscience (as distinct from neurophysiology and neuroanatomy as subdisciplines of physiology and anatomy) was established only in 1962 with the founding of the Neurosciences Research Program (NRP) at MIT by Francis O. Schmitt and a variety of scientists interested in the neural basis of behavior and mind. Recent advances in the neurosciences has shifted the debate on the brain from localization of brain activity to systems of active networks.

41. Hayles identifies a third wave of cybernetics in which systems show an emergent behavior capable of making the system itself evolve into new directions. Katherine Hayles, *How We Became Posthuman: Virtual Bodies in Cybernetics, Literature, and Informatics* (Chicago: University of Chicago Press, 1999).

42. See http://bcl.ece.illinois.edu/ (accessed November 2019).

43. Albert Müller, "A Brief History of the BCL. Heinz von Foerster and the Biological Computer Laboratory," in *An Unfinished Revolution? Heinz von Foerster and the Biological Computer Laboratory, BCL, 1958–1976,* ed. Albert Müller and Karl H. Müller (Vienna: Edition Echoraum, 2007), 287.

44. See Jan Müggenburg, *Lebhafte Artefakte: Heinz von Foerster und die Maschinen des Biological Computer Laboratory* (Konstanz, Germany: Konstanz University Press, 2018).

45. Lohmeyer and Halpern, "Cinema/Cybernetics/Visuality." For a rich study on the origins of computer art at the Bell Laboratories, see Zabet Patterson, *Peripheral Vision: Bell Labs, the S-C 4020, and the Origins of Computer Art* (Cambridge, MA: MIT Press, 2015).

46. Andrew Pickering, "Art, Science and Experiment," *MaHKUscript. Journal of Fine Art Research* 1, no. 1 (2016): 2.

47. Francisco Varela and Humberto Maturana, *Autopoiesis and Cognition: The Realization of the Living* (Dordrecht: Reidel, 1980).

48. "Bionics" covered attempts to analyze biological processes, to formalize them, and to implement them on computers and it was considered an alternative to artificial intelligence.

49. Varela and Maturana, *Autopoiesis.*

50. See Ronald R. Kline, *The Cybernetics Moment or Why We Call Our Age the Information Age* (Baltimore: Johns Hopkins University Press, 2015).

51. Bernard Scott, "Second-Order Cybernetics: An Historical Introduction," *Kybernetes* 33, no. 9/10 (2004): 1376.

52. See Jens Hauser, "Observations on an Art of Growing Interest: Toward a Phenomenological Approach to Art Involving Biotechnology," in *Tactical Biopolitics—Art, Activism, and Technoscience,* ed. Beatriz da Costa and Kavita Philip (Cambridge, MA: MIT Press, 2008), 83–104.

53. For an introduction to bio art, see Robert E. Mitchell, *Bioart and the Vitality of Media* (Seattle: University of Washington Press, 2010).

54. On the contentious relationship between ethics and bio art, see Nora S. Vaage, "What Ethics for Bioart?" *Nanoethics* 10 (2016): 87–104.

55. On the possibility of using the concept of biological individuality and an immunological perspective to challenge the notion of the self, see, for example, Thomas Pradeu, *The Limits of the Self: Immunology and Biological Identity* (Oxford: Oxford University Press, 2012).

56. Donna Haraway, *Simians, Cyborgs, Women: The Reinvention of Nature* (London: Free, 1991), 163.

57. Luciano Floridi, "The Informational Nature of Personal Identity," *Minds and Machines* 21, no. 4 (2011): 561–562.

58. See the artist's website, http://guybenary.com/work/cellf/ (accessed December 2019).

59. Edwin Hutchins, *Cognition in the Wild* (Cambridge, MA: MIT Press, 1995).

60. Leonardo Bich and Luisa Damiano, "Order in the Nothing: Autopoiesis and the Organizational Characterization of the Living," in *Physics of Emergence and Organization*, ed. Ignazio Licata and Ammar Sikaji (Singapore: World Scientific, 2008), 339.

61. On the concept of emergent behavior in different types of systems (organisms, robots, software), see Salter, *Alien Agency*, 138–141.

62. See Joseph Dumit, "The Fragile Unity of Neuroscience," in *Neuroscience and Critique: Exploring the Limits of the Neurological Turn*, ed. Jan De Vos and Ed Pluth (New York: Routledge, 2015), 223–229.

Chapter 6

1. Jim Hutchison, VB 2549 Personal Notebook (Special Collections of the Sir Duncan Rice Library, University of Aberdeen). The notebooks are organized in numerical (i.e., date) order. The series is not complete—it starts somewhere in the mid-1940s, but quite few of the early books are missing. The series ends in the 2000s and several of the later books are missing too.

2. Sawday, *Body Emblazoned*, 12.

3. Liz Orton, ed., "Becoming Image: An Introduction," in *Becoming Image: Medicine and the Algorithmic Gaze* (London: Digital Insides, 2018), 6.

4. The archival exhibition was then exposed in the Sir Ian Wood Building on the Garthdee Campus of Robert Gordon University in Aberdeen during the Tech Festival (October 24 through September 6, 2019).

5. See the commission opportunity launched on the website of the Suttie Arts Space, http://www.ghat-art.org.uk/the-suttie-arts-space-ffc-mri-commission-opportunity/ (accessed August 2019).

6. Felicity Callard, Des Fitzgerald, and Angela Woods, "Interdisciplinary Collaboration in Action: Tracking the Signal, Tracing the Noise," *Palgrave Communications* 1 (2015): 3.

7. Laboratory fieldwork, physicist to author, Aberdeen, September 2019. This and all the other dialogues reported below are faithful transcriptions of the exchanges that occurred during the fieldwork and are based on notes taken by the author.

8. David Lurie, "Introduction," in *Immobile Choreography* (Aberdeen: Grampian Hospitals Art Trust, 2019), 9. Exhibition catalog.

9. Lurie, 9.

10. On the concept and role of the attached observer, see the work of the social anthropologist James Leach, "Extending Contexts, Making Possibilities: An Introduction to Evaluating the Projects," *Leonardo* 39, no. 5 (2006): 447–451. On how facts are produced in the laboratory, see Bruno Latour and Steve Woolgar, *Laboratory Life: The Construction of Scientific Facts* (Princeton, NJ: Princeton University Press, 1979).

11. Ginsberg et al., *Synthetic Aesthetics.*

12. Tim Ingold, *Making: Anthropology, Archaeology, Art and Architecture* (London: Routledge, 2013): 8.

13. Erik Fisher and Roop L. Mahajan, "Embedding the Humanities in Engineering: Art, Dialogue, and a Laboratory," in *Trading Zones and Interactional Expertise: Creating New Kinds of Collaboration* ed. Michael E. Gorman (Cambridge, MA: MIT Press, 2010), 209–230.

14. Haraway takes the expression "modest witness" from the 1985 book by Shapin and Shaffer, *Leviathan and the Air-Pump.*

15. Haraway, *Modest_Witness@Second_Millennium.* Joseph Schneider, *Donna Haraway: Live Theory* (New York: Continuum, 2005).

16. Schneider, *Donna Haraway*, 91.

17. The wealth of material that Meg Foster donated to the Special Collections of the University of Aberdeen consists of following: the various medals which Jim was awarded by organizations such as the Royal Society; the photographic material held by Eleanor Hutcheon, who is the current photographer of the department and was, back then, the wife of Raymond Hutcheon, the previous photographer; photographic material held by Meg Foster; and Jim Hutchison's laboratory notebooks and personal notebooks (called the VB books, originally held by Meg and then donated to the Special Collections of the University of Aberdeen).

18. Donna J. Haraway, "Modest Witness: Feminist Diffractions in Science Studies" in *The Disunity of Science: Boundaries, Contexts, and Power*, ed. Peter Galison and David J. Stump (Stanford, CA: Stanford University Press, 1996), 432.

19. The concept of embodied techno-interfaces has been coined by contemporary art historian Mondloch in her work on new media installation art and technoscience. See Kate Mondloch, *A Capsule Aesthetic: Feminist Materialisms in New Media Art* (Minneapolis: University of Minnesota Press, 2018).

20. See https://eidolonblog.wordpress.com/ (accessed September 2019).

21. See chapters 5 and 7 for a discussion of other artists' work with MRI, neuroscientific data, and its visual imaginary.

22. Laboratory fieldwork, artist and physicist, Aberdeen, October 2018.

23. Beverley Hood, transcription of her presentation during the roundtable discussion, Friday, May 24, 2019, the Suttie Arts Space, Aberdeen Royal Infirmary. The transcription is available upon request.

24. Beverley Hood, "Being Still," in *Immobile Choreography* (Aberdeen: Grampian Hospitals Art Trust, 2019), 13. Exhibition catalog.

25. Hood, 14.

26. Hood, 22.

27. Hood, 24.

28. Bennett, *Vibrant Matter*, 2010.

29. On the feminism question in science, see Evelyn Fox Keller and Helen E. Longino, *Feminism and Science: Oxford Readings in Feminism* (Oxford: Oxford University Press, 1996); Sandra Harding, *The Science Question in Feminism* (Ithaca, NY: Cornell University Press, 1986). On the relationship

between machine learning and gender, see Clementine Collett and Sarah Dillon, *AI and Gender: Four Proposals for Future Research* (Cambridge: The Leverhulme Centre for the Future of Intelligence, 2019).

30. Laboratory fieldwork, artist to author, Aberdeen, December 2018.

31. Laboratory fieldwork, physicist to author, Aberdeen, October 2019.

32. Laboratory fieldwork, physicist to author, Aberdeen, November 2018.

33. Laboratory fieldwork, physicist to author, Aberdeen, October 2019.

34. Physicist, interview with author, Aberdeen, September 2019. Interview recordings and transcripts are available upon request to the author.

35. Feedback from patient given through Twitter, May 1, 2019.

36. Beverley Hood, transcription of her presentation during the roundtable discussion, Friday, May 24, 2019, the Suttie Arts Space, Aberdeen Royal Infirmary (edited for clarity).

37. Jennifer Burwell, *Quantum Language and the Migration of Scientific Concepts* (Cambridge, MA: MIT Press, 2018). Exploring the connections between the arts and physics, Gavin Parkinson studied how surrealism drew on the language of relativity and quantum mechanics in order to validate and authorize its artistic ambitions. See Gavin Parkinson, *Surrealism, Art and Modern Science: Relativity, Quantum Mechanics, Epistemology* (New Haven, CT: Yale University Press, 2008), 177–181.

38. Burwell discusses, for example, Samuel Coale's use of quantum entanglement in his critical reading of De Lillo's novels.

39. Burwell, *Quantum Language*, 11.

40. Burwell, 263.

41. Sean Cubitt, "Glitch," *Cultural Politics* 13, no. 1 (2017): 20.

42. See, for example, Rosa Menkman's website, http://rosa-menkman.blogspot.com/ (accessed August 2019).

43. See the approach on live performance practice, dance, and digital technologies in Susan Kozel, *Closer, Performance, Technologies, Phenomenology* (Cambridge, MA: MIT Press, 2008).

44. Beverley Hood, transcription of her presentation during the roundtable discussion, Friday, May 24, 2019, the Suttie Arts Space, Aberdeen Royal Infirmary.

45. Mondloch, *A Capsule Aesthetic*; see also Salter, *Alien Agency*.

46. Karen Barad, "Living in a Posthumanist Material World. Lessons from Schrödinger's Cat," in *Bits of Life. Feminism at the Intersections of Media, Bioscience, and Technology*, ed. Anneke Smelik and Nina Lykke (Seattle: University of Washington Press, 2008), 171.

47. Meg Foster, interview with author, Westhill, Aberdeenshire, April 2019.

48. Frederic L. Holmes, Jürgen Renn, and Hans-Jörg Rheinberger, "Introduction" in *Reworking the Bench: Research Notebooks in the History of Science* (New York: Kluwer Academic, 2003), viii.

49. See the recent exhibition projects *Immobile Choreography* and *From Where Do We See?* http://www.ghat-art.org.uk/immobile-choreography-publication-launch-and-talk/; https://www.ghat-art.org.uk/from-where-do-we-see-curated-dr-silvia-casini/.

50. Vilém Flusser, "The Gesture of Writing," in *Flusser Studies*, 9, accessed November 2019, http://www.flusserstudies.net/sites/www.flusserstudies.net/files/media/attachments/the-gesture-of-writing.pdf. The essay was originally published in Vilém Flusser, *Gesten: Versuch einer Phänomenologie* (Düsseldorf: Bollmann Verlag, 1991).

51. Jim Hutchison, VB 2553 journal, June 1972–November 1973. Hutchison discusses Thomson's work in the pages dated December 16, 1972.

52. For a nonspecialist introduction to Shannon's thought and life, see Jimmy Soni and Rob Goodman, *A Mind at Play: How Claude Shannon Invented the Information Age* (London: Simon & Schuster, 2017).

53. See the film on the mouse Theseus from the Bell Laboratories, https://www.youtube.com/watch?v=nS0luYZd4fs (accessed September 2019).

54. Jim Hutchison, VB 2553 journal, June 1972–November 1973. The pages dedicated to Shannon are dated December 16, 1972.

55. Jim Hutchison, VB 2553 journal, June 1972–November 1973.

56. Glenn Gould, "The Prospects of Recording," *High Fidelity* 16, no. 4 (1966): 46–63.

57. In Scotland, for example, the only university able to continue a funded research program on AI was the University of Edinburgh. The strong program of AI was held back by the lack of computers powerful enough to process large volumes of data.

58. Jim Hutchison, VB 2553 journal, December 16, 1972.

59. Roman Frigg, "Fiction and Science," in *Fictions and Models*, ed. John Woods (Munich: Philosophia Verlag, 2010): 248.

60. Frigg, 257.

61. See The Thomas A. Edison Papers Project, a research center at Rutgers School of Arts and Sciences, http://edison.rutgers.edu/NamesSearch/SingleDoc.php?DocId=NM003015 (accessed January 2020). On Edison and his visual thinking method, see Ian Wills, "Scientific Failure: Etheric Force" in *Thomas Edison: Success and Innovation through Failure*, Studies in History and Philosophy of Science 52 (Cham, Switzerland: Springer, 2019), 141–168.

62. According to Meg Foster, the Asahi engineers worked closely with the Aberdonian team. They managed to construct another imager and called it Mark J (for Japan). Asahi was then incorporated by Siemens.

63. Prasad, *Imperial Technoscience*, 52–53.

64. Latour, "Visualization and Cognition."

65. Latour and Woolgar, *Laboratory Life*, 1979. Quoted in Latour, "Visualization and Cognition."

66. Jacob, *Of Flies, Mice and Men*, 158.

67. See Joyce, *Magnetic Appeal*, 2008; and Dawson, *Paul Lauterbur*, 2013.

68. Other similar images of the MRI-scanned lemon are available in the MRI archive at Nottingham University. *Nature*, December 1977, highlights Dr. Paul Bottomley and colleagues' groundbreaking work in "zeugmatography," later known as MRI. See Bottomley, "On the Origins of Localized NMR."

69. Dawson, *Paul Lauterbur*, 128.

70. Meg Foster, interview with author, Westhill, Aberdeenshire, April 2019.

71. Floridi, *Philosophy of Information*, 86–87.

72. Joyce, "From Numbers to Pictures," 1–22.

73. Hans-Jörg Rheinberger, "Experimental Systems: Historiality, Narration, and Deconstruction," *Science in Context* 7, no. 1 (1994): 65–81, particularly 77–78.

74. Rheinberger, 78.

Chapter 7

1. On the implications of the shift from drawing to image making, see John May, *Signal. Image. Architecture* (New York: Columbia University Press, 2019).

2. Manfred Wolff-Plottegg, *Plottegg—Architecture beyond Inclusion and Identity Is Exclusion and Difference from Art* (Basel: Birkhäuser, 2015). See also https://zkm.de/en/exhibition/2017/10/open-codes/catalog/neuronaler-architektur-generator (accessed December 2019).

3. See http://www.neuwritewest.org/blog/2015/1/3/ask-a-neuroscientist-whats-a-spike-train (accessed October 2019).

4. Garrett B. Stanley, "Reading and writing the neural code," *Nature Neuroscience* 16 (2013): 259–263.

5. For a detailed description of the installation, see http://plottegg.tuwien.ac.at/neuro_arch_proc.htm (accessed November 2019).

6. Manuel Lima, *Visual Complexity: Mapping Patterns of Information* (New York: Princeton Architectural Press, 2011).

7. Operational images have become paradigmatic for the field of new media because they are based on the logic of the interface and database. See Lev Manovich, *The Language of New Media* (Cambridge, MA: MIT Press, 2001).

8. Harun Farocki, "Phantom Images," *Public*, no. 29 (2004): 17. He derives the concept of operational images from the notion of "technical images" elaborated by Vilém Flusser.

9. Tim Ingold, "From Science to Art and Back Again: The Pendulum of an Anthropologist," *ANUAC* 5 no. 1 (2016): 9.

10. See http://digitalinsides.org/ (accessed October 2019).

11. Orton, interview with author, London, September 2019. Interview recordings and transcripts are available upon request to the author.

12. This is an excerpt from a more extended edited conversation between Orton and John Hipwell, computational medical imaging scientist (July 2017 to March 2018). See http://digitalinsides.org/visualdialogues/7-john-hipwell/ (accessed February 2020).

13. Email correspondence with Liz Orton, February 2020. The visual dialogue with Ida Levine can be accessed here: http://digitalinsides.org/visualdialogues/lenny-levine/?images (accessed February 2020).

14. Orton, interview with author, London, September 2019.

15. Jonathon Tomlison, "The Pain of Others," in *Becoming Image: Medicine and the Algorithmic Gaze*, ed. Liz Orton (London: Digital Insides, 2018), 78. For further reading, see Louise Amoore, "Doubt and the Algorithm: On the Partial Accounts of Machine Learning," *Theory, Culture & Society* 36, no. 6 (2019): 147–169.

16. See Pratik Shah et al., "Artificial Intelligence and Machine Learning in Clinical Development: A Translational Perspective," *Npj Digital Medicine 2*, no. 69 (2019): 1–5. See also Editorial, "Ascent of Machine Learning in Medicine," *Nature Materials* 18 (May 2019): 407, April 18, https://www.nature.com/articles/s41563-019-0360-1.pdf.

17. Anne Trafton, "Doctors Rely On More Than Just Data for Medical Decision Making," *MIT News*, 2018, accessed November 2019, http://news.mit.edu/2018/doctors-rely-gut-feelings-decision-making-0720.

18. For the Foucauldian understanding of biopower, see Michel Foucault, *A History of Sexuality*, vol. 1, *An Introduction* (New York: Vintage, 1980). For Michel Foucault, power and the human body are intertwined. Biopower is not just a repressive force exercised upon the body, for it is literally embodied. Foucault identified a politics that centers on the body defining and measuring the health of the individual body (the "*anatomo-politics of the human body*") and another that classifies and manages human populations for matters of life and death relying on statistics ("*a biopolitics of the population*") (139, emphasis in original).

19. Nikolas Rose, *Politics of Life*, 2007.

20. Roger Cooter, "The Turn of the Body: History and the Politics of the Corporeal," *ARBOR Ciencia, Pensamiento y Cultura CLXXXVI* 743 (2010): 401. See also Roger Cooter, "The End? History-Writing in the Age of Biomedicine (and Before)," in *Writing History in the Age of Biomedicine*, ed. Roger Cooter and Claudia Stein (New Haven, CT: Yale University Press, 2013), 1–40.

21. Barry F. Saunders, *CT Suite. The Work of Diagnosis in the Age of Noninvasive Cutting* (Durham and London: Duke University Press, 2008).

22. Saunders, *CT Suite*, 3.

23. Designed by engineer Owen Williams, in 1935 this center was hailed by Walter Gropius, the architect and founder of the Bauhaus School, as Britain's best new building.

24. Innes H. Pearse and Lucy H. Crocker, *The Peckham Experiment* (New York: Routledge, 2009).

25. The original passage is taken from Pearse and Crocker, *The Peckham Experiment*, 27.

26. Ilona Sagar, *Correspondence O*, transcript.

27. Sagar, *Correspondence O*, transcript.

28. On the aesthetics and politics of structural films which comprises works by, among others, Michael Snow and Hollis Frampton, see Paul Adams Sitney, *Visionary Film: The American Avant-Garde 1943–1978* (Oxford: Oxford University Press, 1979); and Peter Gidal, *Materialist Film* (New York: Routledge, 1989).

29. George Scott Williamson and Innes Hope Pearse, *The Case for Action: A Survey of Everyday Life Under Modern Industrial Conditions, with Special Reference to the Question of Health* (Edinburgh: Scottish Academic Press, 1982).

30. Sagar, *Correspondence O*, transcript.

31. LiDAR uses a laser to bounce lights from objects and collect measurements that can then be used to create 3D models and maps of objects and environments.

32. Beatriz Colomina, *X-Ray Architecture* (Baden, Germany: Lars Müller, 2019), 16.

33. Michael Sappol, *Body Modern: Fritz Kahn, Scientific Illustration, and the Homuncular Subject* (Minneapolis: University of Minnesota Press, 2017), 165.

34. Eloise Hawser has recently been exploring the connection between the liquid flow within the body and below the city. Like Sagar, Hawser too uses archival material and cutting-edge medical technology (in her case phantoms used to calibrate medical equipment) to explore the correlation between the medical measurement of a bodily phenomenon such as the circulation of fluid and the models used to study the river Thames in its urban environment. See https://www.somersethouse.org.uk/whats-on/eloise-hawser-deep-mark (accessed November 2019).

35. Sagar, interview with author, London, December 2019. The archival material is accessible at the Wellcome Trust.

36. Sagar, *Correspondence O*, transcript.

37. Sagar, interview with author, London, December 2019.

38. Tom Gunning, "To Scan a Ghost: The Ontology of Mediated Vision," *Grey Room* 26 (2007): 94–127.

39. Aristotle, "On the Soul (De Anima)," in *The Basic Works of Aristotle*, ed. Richard McKeon (New York: Random House, 1966), 595 (432a).

40. Gunning, "To Scan a Ghost," 115–116.

41. Rose, *Politics of Life Itself*, 2009.

42. Kathryn Lloyd, "No Measure of Health: Ilona Sagar Scans the Politics of Wellbeing," *MoMus*, 2018, accessed September 2019, https://momus.ca/no-measure-health-ilona-sagar-scans-politics-wellbeing/.

43. Thomas Häusle, "Poetics of Cannibalism." Thomas Häusle in conversation with Thomas Feuerstein, n.d., 131, accessed November 2019, https://www.thomasfeuerstein.net/20_BIBLIOGRAPHY/30_TEXTS_&_ARTICLES/Haeusle-Feuerstein_en.pdf.

44. See https://www.thomasfeuerstein.net/50_WORKS/70_NETART/70_BORGY_BES_01 (accessed November 2019).

45. John D. Kelleher and Brendan Tierney, *Data Science* (Cambridge MA: MIT Press, 2018), 121–124.

46. Lily E. Kay, "From Logical Neurons to Poetic Embodiments of Mind: Warren S. McCulloch's Project in Neuroscience," *Science in Context* 14, no. 4 (2001): 597.

47. Thomas Feuerstein, "Metabolic Machines & Demons of Life," presented at Kunst und Künstliche Intelligenz, May 2019, accessed October 2019, https://www.youtube.com/watch?v=MzZhZYLliac&vl=en. On the metabolic subject, Deleuze stated how "the speed or slowness of metabolisms, perceptions, actions and reactions link together to constitute a particular individual in the world." See Gilles Deleuze, "Ethology: Spinoza and Us," in *Incorporations*, ed. Jonathan Crary and Sanford Kwinter (New York: Zone Books, 1992), 624–633, 628.

48. Elizabeth Wilson, "Gut Feminism," *Differences: A Journal of Feminist Cultural Studies* 15, no. 3 (2004): 70.

49. Wilson, 14 and 6, respectively.

50. Wilson, 5.

51. Bernhard J. Dotzler, "Demons-Magic-Cybernetics: On the Introduction to Natural Magic as Told by Heinz von Foerster," *Systems Research* 13, no. 3 (1996): 249. Dotzler cites from Heinz von Foerster, *KybernEthik* (Berlin: Merve, 1993). See also Heinz von Foerster et al., "Cybernetics Computer Science Computer Art: The Beginnings of an Epistemology of Responsibility," in *Beyond Art: A Third Culture. A Comparative Study in Cultures, Art and Science in 20th Century Austria and Hungary*, ed. Peter Weibel (Vienna: Springer-Verlag, 2005), 294–367.

52. Häusle, "Poetics of Cannibalism," 135–136, citing von Foerster 1993.

53. Pickering, *Cybernetic Brain*, 6.

54. The Greek idea of demon first appeared in ancient Greece through the works of Plato.

55. See Thomas Feuerstein in Hartmut Böhme "Demons of Art. Hartmut Böhme in Conversation with Thomas Feuerstein," August 2012, accessed November 2019, https://daimon.myzel.net/Demons_of_Art.

56. The label of "new realism" is first motivated by the fact that Feuerstein works only with real-world data; second, his installations are not representing subject matters in a naturalistic manner, almost photographic quality, as it was the case with the mid-nineteenth-century artistic movement of Realism.

57. Thomas Elsaesser, "The Future of 'Art' and 'Work' in the Age of Vision Machines: Harun Farocki," in *After the Avant-garde: Contemporary German and Austrian Experimental Film*, ed. Randall Halle and Reinhild Steingröver (Rochester, NY: Camden House, 2008), 31–49.

58. Feuerstein, interview with author, online, October 2019.

59. On the concept of "life forms," see Michael M. J. Fischer, *Emergent Forms of Life and the Anthropological Voice* (Durham, NC: Duke University Press, 2003).

60. Lisa Gitelman and Virginia Jackson, "Introduction," in *Raw Data Is an Oxymoron*, ed. Lisa Gitelman (Cambridge, MA: MIT Press, 2013), 1–14.

61. Bachelard 1949, 133, quoted in Hans-Jörg Rheinberger, *On Historicizing Epistemology: An Essay*, trans. David Fernbach (Stanford, CA: Stanford University Press, 2010).

62. Joseph Dumit, "Afterward," in *The Neuroscientific Turn: Transdisciplinarity in the Age of the Brain*, ed. J. Johnson and M. M. Littlefield (Ann Harbor: University of Michigan Press, 2012), 235.

Bibliography

Agamben, Giorgio. *Che cos'è Reale? La Scomparsa di Majorana*. Vicenza: Neri Pozza, 2016.

Agamben, Giorgio. *Homo Sacer: Sovereign Power and Bare Life*. Palo Alto, CA: Stanford University Press, 1998.

Agamben, Giorgio. *The Signature of All Things: On Method*. Translated by Luca D'Isanto with Kevin Attell. Brooklyn, NY: Zone Books, 2009.

Agamben, Giorgio. *What Is an Apparatus? And Other Essays*. Stanford, CA: Stanford University Press, 2009.

Alač, Morana. *Handling Digital Brains: A Laboratory Study of Multimodal Semiotic Interaction in the Age of Computers*. Cambridge, MA: MIT Press, 2011.

Amaldi, Edoardo. *La Vita e l'Opera Di Ettore Majorana (1906–1938)*. Rome: Accademia Nazionale dei Lincei, 1966.

Amoore, Louise. "Doubt and the Algorithm: On the Partial Accounts of Machine Learning." *Theory, Culture and Society* 36, no. 6 (2019): 147–169.

Amoore, Louise. *The Politics of Possibility: Risk and Security beyond Probability*. Durham, NC: Duke University Press, 2013.

Aristotle. "On the Soul (De Anima)." In *The Basic Works of Aristotle*, edited by Richard McKeon. New York: Random House, 1966.

Aristotle. *Parts of Animals. Movement of Animals. Progression of Animals*. Translated by A. L. Peck and E. S. Forster. Cambridge, MA: Harvard University Press, 1937.

Arnheim, Rudolf. *Art and Visual Perception: A Psychology of the Creative Eye*. Berkeley: University of California Press, 1954.

Arnheim, Rudolf. *Visual Thinking*. Berkeley: University of California Press, 1969.

Bachelard, Gaston. *Le Rationalisme Appliqué*. Paris: Presses Universitaires de France, 1949.

Baggott, Jim. *The Quantum Story: A History in 40 Moments*. Oxford: Oxford University Press, 2011.

Baltrušaitis, Jurgis. *Aberrations: An Essay on the Legend of Forms*. Cambridge, MA: MIT Press, 1989.

Barad, Karen. "Living in a Posthumanist Material World. Lessons from Schrödinger's Cat." In *Bits of Life: Feminism at the Intersections of Media, Bioscience, and Technology*, edited by Anneke Smelik and Nina Lykke, 165–176. Seattle: University of Washington Press, 2008.

Barad, Karen. *Meeting the Universe Halfway: Quantum Physics and the Entanglement of Matter and Meaning*. Durham, NC: Duke University Press, 2007.

Bassani, Giuseppe Franco. *Ettore Majorana: Scientific Papers on the Occasion of the Centenary of His Birth*. Società Italiana di Fisica. Berlin: Springer, 2006.

Bateson, Nora. "Warm Data: Contextual Research and the Evolution of Science." N.p.: The International Bateson Institute, April 10, 2017, web edition.

Beaulieu, Anne. "A Space for Measuring Mind and Brain: Interdisciplinarity and Digital Tools in the Development of Brain Mapping and Functional Imaging, 1980–1990." *Brain and Cognition* 49, no. 1 (2002): 13–33.

Beck, Ulrich. *World at Risk*. Cambridge: Polity Press, 2007.

Benjamin, Walter. *The Arcades Project*. Cambridge, MA: Harvard University Press, 1999.

Benjamin, Walter. "Little History of Photography." In *Walter Benjamin: Selected Writings*, edited by Michael W. Jennings, Howard Eiland, and Gary Smith, vol. 2, pt. 2, *1931–1934*, 507–530. Cambridge, MA: Belknap Press of Harvard University Press, 2005.

Benjamin, Walter. *One Way Street*. London: Verso, 1999.

Bennett, Jane. *Vibrant Matter: A Political Ecology of Things*. Durham, NC: Duke University Press, 2010.

Berger, François. "FFC-MRI: Is This the Technology Breakthrough That Patients and Neuro-Oncologists Have Been Waiting For?" Talk presented at the one-day symposium, *Fast Field-Cycling MRI—A New Imaging Modality*, University of Aberdeen, March 2018.

Biagioli, Mario. "Postdisciplinary Liaisons: Science Studies and the Humanities." *Critical Inquiry* 35, no. 4 (2009): 816–832.

Bich, Leonardo, and Luisa Damiano. "Order in the Nothing: Autopoiesis and the Organizational Characterization of the Living." In *Physics of Emergence and Organization*, edited by Ignazio Licata and Ammar Sakaji, 339–369. Singapore: World Scientific, 2008.

Blackman, Lisa. *Haunted Data: Affect, Transmedia, Weird Science*. London: Bloomsbury Academic, 2019.

Blok, Anders, Ignacio Farias, and Celia Roberts, eds. *The Routledge Companion to Actor-Network Theory*. New York: Routledge, 2020.

Boehm, Gottfried. *Was Ist Ein Bild*. Munich: Fink Verlag, 1994.

Boenink, Marianne, Harro van Lente, and Ellen Moors. *Emerging Technologies for Diagnosing Alzheimer's Disease: Innovating with Care*. London: Palgrave Macmillan, 2016.

Böhme, Hartmut. "Demons of Art. Hartmut Böhme in Conversation with Thomas Feuerstein," August 2012. https://daimon.myzel.net/Demons_of_Art.

Borck, Cornelius. *Brainwaves: A Cultural History of Electroencephalography*. New York: Routledge, 2018.

Borck, Cornelius. "How to Do Voodoo with Functional Neuroimaging," *EspacesTemps.Net*, n.d., http://www.espacestemps.net/articles/neuroimaging/.

Borck, Cornelius. "How We May Think: Imaging and Writing Technologies across the History of the Neurosciences." *Studies in History and Philosophy of Biological and Biomedical Sciences* 57 (2016): 112–120.

Borck, Cornelius. "Recording the Brain at Work: The Visible, the Readable, and the Invisible in Electroencephalography." *Journal of the History of the Neurosciences* 17, no. 3 (2008): 367–379.

Borck, Cornelius. "Toys Are Us: Models and Metaphors in Brain Research." In *Critical Neuroscience: A Handbook of the Social and Cultural Contexts of Neuroscience*, edited by Suparna Choudhury and Jan Slaby, 111–133. London: Blackwell, 2011.

Borck, Cornelius. "Vital Brains: On the Entanglement of Media, Minds, and Models." In *Vital Models: The Making and Use of Models in the Brain Sciences*, Progress in Brain Research 233, edited by Tara Mahfoud, Sam McLean, and Nikolas Rose, 1–24. Cambridge: Academic Press, 2017.

Bottomley, Paul A. "On the Origins of Localized NMR: View from an Accomplice." In *The Development of Magnetic Resonance Imaging and Spectroscopy*, edited by G. Mark Bydder, Ian R. Young, and Martyn Paley, 1–56. MRIS History vol. 1. 2019. https://mrishistory.org.uk/paul-bottomley.

Boyle, Robert. *The Sceptical Chymist*. London: Cadwell, 1661.

Braun, Marta. *Picturing Time: The Work of Etienne-Jules Marey*. Chicago: University of Chicago Press, 1992.

Breaker, Jeanine. "The Complexion of Two Bodies. Part One: Nuance Drawn Out." *Leonardo* 46, no. 5 (2013): 425–431.

Bredekamp, Horst, Vera Dankel, and Birgit Schneider. *The Technical Image: A History of Styles in Scientific Imagery*. Chicago: University of Chicago Press, 2015.

Breen, Benjamin. "The Alchemy of Madness: Understanding a Seventeenth-Century 'Brain Scan.'" *Res Obscura: A Catalogue of Obscure Things* (blog), December 17, 2015. https://resobscura.blogspot.com/2015/12/the-alchemy-of-madness.html.

Broche, Lionel M., P. James Ross, Gareth R. Davies, Mary-Joan MacLeod, and David J. Lurie. "A Whole-Body Fast Field-Cycling Scanner for Clinical Molecular Imaging Studies." *Scientific Reports* 9, no. 10402 (2019): 1–11.

Bruno, Giuliana. *Atlas of Emotion: Journeys in Art, Architecture and Film*. London: Verso, 2007.

Buck-Morss, Susan. *The Dialectics of Seeing: Walter Benjamin and the Arcades Project*. Cambridge, MA: MIT Press, 1991.

Buiani, Roberta. "Squatting for SciArt." *Antennae: The Journal of Nature in Visual Culture* no. 47 (2019): 27–47.

Burri, Regula Valérie. "Pictures, Practices, Paradoxes: Medical Imaging and Modernity." *Tecnoscienza. Italian Journal of Science & Technology Studies* 5, no. 1 (2014): 165–171.

Burri, Regula Valérie. "Sociotechnical Anatomy. Technology, Space and Body in the MRI Unit." In *Biomedicine as Culture: Instrumental Practices, Technoscientific Knowledge, and New Modes of Life*, edited by Regula Valérie Burri and Joseph Dumit, 109–121. New York: Routledge, 2007.

Burri, Regula Valérie. "Visual Rationalities: Towards a Sociology of Images." *Current Sociology* 60, no. 1 (2012): 45–60.

Burri, Regula Valérie, Annamaria Carusi, and Aikaterini A. Aspradaki. "Personalised Medicine: Visions and Visualisations." *Technoscienza. Italian Journal of Science and Technology Studies* 5, no. 1 (2014): 165–189.

Burri, Regula Valérie, Annamaria Carusi, and Aikaterini A. Aspradaki. "Visualising Bodies within and beyond Laboratories and Clinics." *Tecnoscienza. Italian Journal of Science and Technology Studies* 5, no. 1 (2014): 165–189.

Burri, Regula Valérie, and Joseph Dumit, eds. *Biomedicine as Culture: Instrumental Practices, Technoscientific Knowledge, and New Modes of Life*. New York: Routledge, 2010.

Burri, Regula Valérie, and Joseph Dumit. "Social Studies of Scientific Imaging and Visualization." In *The Handbook of Science and Technology Studies*, edited by Edward J. Hackett et al., 297–317. Cambridge, MA: MIT Press, 2008.

Burwell, Jennifer. *Quantum Language and the Migration of Scientific Concepts*. Cambridge, MA: MIT Press, 2018.

Cajal, Santiago Ramón y. *Recollections of My Life*. Cambridge, MA: MIT Press, 1989.

Callard, Felicity, Des Fitzgerald, and Angela Woods. "Interdisciplinary Collaboration in Action: Tracking the Signal, Tracing the Noise." *Palgrave Communications* 1 (2015): 1–7.

Callon, Michel. "Struggles and Negotiations to Define What Is Problematic and What Is Not: The Sociology of Translation." In *The Social Process of Scientific Investigation: Sociology of the Sciences Yearbook*, edited by Karin D. Knorr et al., 197–219. Dordrecht: Reidel, 1980.

Calvert, Jane, and Pablo Schyfter. "What Can Science and Technology Studies Learn from Art and Design? Reflections on Synthetic Aesthetics." *Social Studies of Science* 47, no. 2 (2017): 195–215.

Cameron, Dan, Carolyn Christov-Bakargiev, John M. Coetzee, and William Kentridge. *William Kentridge*. London: Phaidon Press, 1999. Reprinted in 2010.

Cartwright, Lisa. *Screening the Body: Tracing Medicine's Visual Culture*. Minneapolis: University of Minnesota Press, 1995.

Cartwright, Lisa, and Brian Goldfarb. "Radiography, Cinematography, and the Decline of the Lens." In *Incorporations*, edited by Jonathan Crary and Sanford Kwinter, 190–201. New York: Zone Books, MIT, 1992.

Carusi, Annamaria, Aud Sissel Hoel, Timothy Webmoor, and Steve Woolgar, eds. *Visualization in the Age of Computerization*. New York: Routledge, 2015.

Casini, Silvia. "Beyond the Neuro-Realism Fallacy. From John R. Mallard's Hand-Painted MRI Image of a Mouse to BioArt Scenarios." *Nuncius. Journal of the Material and Visual History of Science* 32, no. 2 (2017): 440–471.

Casini, Silvia. "Magnetic Attractions: Sculpture, Magnetic Resonance Imaging and Cinema." In *Marc Didou*, edited by Silvia Casini, 4–18. Belfast: Queen's University Editions, 2008. Exhibition catalog.

Casini, Silvia. "Magnetic Resonance Imaging (MRI) as Mirror and Portrait: MRI Configurations between Science and the Arts." *Configurations* 19, no. 1 (2011): 73–99.

Casini, Silvia. "The Material Site of Abstraction: Grid-Based Data Visualisation in Brain Scans." In *The Iconology of Abstraction: Non-Figurative Images and the Modern World*, edited by Krešimir Purgar. New York: Routledge, 2020.

Cetina, Karin Knorr. *Epistemic Cultures: How the Sciences Make Knowledge*. Cambridge, MA: Harvard University Press, 1999.

Cetina, Karin Knorr. "Laboratory Studies: The Cultural Approach to the Study of Science." In *Handbook of Science and Technology Studies*, edited by Sheila Jasanoff, Gerald E. Markle, James C. Peterson, and Trevor Pinch, 140–167. London: SAGE, 1995.

Chen, Min, and Luciano Floridi. "An Analysis of Information in Visualization." *Synthese* 190, no. 16 (2013): 3421–3438.

Clair, Jean. "Le Farfalle Dell'anima." *Museologia Scientifica Memorie* 15 (2016): 13–18.

Collett, Clementine, and Sarah Dillon. *AI and Gender: Four Proposals for Future Research*. Cambridge: The Leverhulme Centre for the Future of Intelligence, 2019.

Colomina, Beatriz. *X-Ray Architecture*. Baden, Germany: Lars Müller, 2019.

Coopmans, Catelijne, Janet Vertesi, Michael E. Lynch, and Steve Woolgar, eds. *Representation in Scientific Practice Revisited*. Cambridge, MA: MIT Press, 2014.

Cooter, Roger. "The End? History-Writing in the Age of Biomedicine (and Before)." In *Writing History in the Age of Biomedicine*, edited by Roger Cooter and Claudia Stein, 1–40. New Haven, CT: Yale University Press, 2013.

Cooter, Roger. "Neural Veils and the Will to Historical Critique: Why Historians of Science Need to Take the Neuro-Turn Seriously." *Isis* 105, no. 1 (2014): 145–154.

Cooter, Roger. "The Turn of the Body: History and the Politics of the Corporeal." *ARBOR Ciencia, Pensamiento y Cultura CLXXXVI*, no. 743 (2010): 339–340.

Cooter, Roger, and Claudia Stein, eds. *The History of Medicine*. New York: Routledge, 2015.

Coppo, Simone, Bhairav B. Mehta, Debra McGivney, Dan Ma, Yong Chen, Yun Jiang, Jesse Hamilton, et al. "Overview of Magnetic Resonance Fingerprinting." *MAGNETOM Flash* 65, no. 2 (2016): 12–21.

Cover, Thomas, and Joy Thomas. *Elements of Information Theory*. Hoboken, NJ: Wiley Interscience, 2006.

Cox, Brian, and Jeff Forshaw. *The Quantum Universe: Everything That Can Happen Does Happen*. Cambridge, MA: Da Capo Press, 2011.

Crary, Jonathan. *Techniques of the Observer: On Vision and Modernity in the Nineteenth Century*. Cambridge, MA: MIT Press, 1990.

Cubitt, Sean. "Glitch." *Cultural Politics* 13, no. 1 (2017): 19–33.

Daninos, Davide. "The Necessary." In *Intuition*, edited by Luc Derycke and Axel Vervoordt, 63–81. Gent, Belgium: AsaMER, 2017. Exhibition catalog.

Daston, Lorraine, and Peter Galison. *Objectivity*. New York: Zone Books, MIT, 2010.

Daston, Lorraine, and Elizabeth Lunbeck. *Histories of Scientific Observation*. Chicago: University of Chicago Press, 2011.

Dawson, Mary Joan. *Paul Lauterbur and the Invention of MRI*. Cambridge, MA: MIT Press, 2013.

de Chadarevian, Soraya, and Nick Hopwood. *Models: The Third Dimension of Science*. Stanford, CA: Stanford University Press, 2004.

de Chadarevian, Soraya, and Harmke Kamminga, eds. *Molecularizing Biology and Medicine: New Practices and Alliances, 1910s–1970s*. Amsterdam: Harwood, 1998.

de la Durantaye, Leland. *Giorgio Agamben: A Critical Introduction*. Stanford, CA: Stanford University Press, 2009.

de la Verpillière, Leclerc. "Visceral Creativity: Digestion, Earthly Melancholy, and Materiality in the Graphic Arts of Early Modern France and the German-Speaking Lands (c. 1530–1675)." PhD thesis, University of Cambridge, 2019. https://doi.org/10.17863/CAM.35715.

Deleuze, Gilles. "Ethology: Spinoza and Us." In *Incorporations*, edited by Jonathan Crary and Sanford Kwinter, 624–633. New York: Zone Books, 1992.

Del Giudice, Daniele. *Atlante Occidentale*. Turin, Italy: Einaudi, 1985.

Dennett, Daniel. "Ontology, Science, and the Evolution of the Manifest Image." Keynote lecture, New College for the Humanities, London, March 14, 2016. https://www.nchlondon.ac.uk/videos/daniel-dennett-on-ontology-science-and-the-evolution-of-the-manifest-image/.

de Regt, Henk W. *Understanding Scientific Understanding*. Oxford: Oxford University Press, 2017.

de Rijcke, Sarah, and Anne Beaulieu. "Networked Neuroscience: Brain Scans and Visual Knowing at the Intersection of Atlases and Databases." In *Representations in Scientific Practice Revisited*, edited by Catelijne Coopmans, Mike Lynch, Janet Vertesi, and Steve Woolgar, 131–152. Cambridge, MA: MIT Press, 2014.

Descartes, René. *Discourse on Method, Optics, Geometry, and Meteorology*. Translated by Paul J. Olscamp. Indianapolis: Hackett, 2001.

De Vos, Jan. *The Metamorphoses of the Brain—Neurologisation and Its Discontents*. London: Palgrave Macmillan, 2016.

deVries, Willem A., and Timm Triplett. *Knowledge, Mind, and the Given: Reading Wilfrid Sellars's "Empiricism and the Philosophy of Mind."* Indianapolis: Hackett, 2000.

Didi-Huberman, Georges. "Glimpses. Between Appearance and Disappearance." *Zeitschrift Fuer Medien Und Kulturforschung* 7 (2016): 109–124.

Dolby, Riki G. A. *Uncertain Knowledge: An Image of Science for a Changing World*. Cambridge: Cambridge University Press, 1996.

Dotzler, Bernhard J. "Demons-Magic-Cybernetics: On the Introduction to Natural Magic as Told by Heinz von Foerster." *Systems Research* 13, no. 3 (1996): 245–250.

Dotzler, Bernhard J., and Henning Schmidgen. "Einleitung zu einer Epistemologie der Zwischenräume." In *Parasiten und Sirenen: Zwischenräume als Orte der materiellen Wissensproduktion*, edited by Bernhard J. Dotzler and Henning Schmidgen, 7–18. Bielefeld, Germany: Transcript Verlag, 2008.

Dumit, Joseph. "The Fragile Unity of Neuroscience." In *Neuroscience and Critique: Exploring the Limits of the Neurological Turn*, edited by Jan De Vos and Ed Pluth, 223–229. New York: Routledge, 2015.

Dumit, Joseph. "How (Not) to Do Things with Brain Images." In *Representation in Scientific Practice Revisited*, edited by Michael E. Lynch and Steve Woolgar, 291–313. Cambridge, MA: MIT Press, 2014.

Dumit, Joseph. *Picturing Personhood: Brain Scans and Biomedical Identity*. Princeton, NJ: Princeton University Press, 2004.

Ede, Siân. *Art & Science*. London: Tauris, 2005.

Ede, Siân. *Strange and Charmed: Science and the Contemporary Visual Arts*. London: Calouste Gulbenkian Foundation, 2010.

Edelstein, William. "An American Physicist in Aberdeen: Good Enough Engineering." In *MRI25*, edited by P. Antell, R. Jobson, and D. Woods, 56–65. London: Faircount, 2006.

Edelstein, William, James M. S. Hutchison, George Johnson, and Thomas Redpath. "Spin Warp NMR Imaging and Applications to Human Whole-Body Imaging." *Physics in Medicine & Biology* 25, no. 4 (1980): 751–756.

Editorial. "Ascent of Machine Learning in Medicine." *Nature Materials* 18 (May 2019): 407. April 18. https://www.nature.com/articles/s41563-019-0360-1.pdf.

Edwards, David. *Artscience: Creativity in the Post-Google Generation*. Cambridge, MA: Harvard University Press, 2009.

Elkins, James. "Aesthetics and the Two Cultures: Why Art and Science Should Be Allowed to Go Their Separate Ways." In *Rediscovering Aesthetics: Transdisciplinary Voices from Art History, Philosophy, and Art Practice*, edited by Francis Halsall, Julia Alejandra Jansen, and Tony O'Connor, 34–50. Stanford, CA: Stanford University Press, 2009.

Elkins, James. *Six Stories from the End of Representation*. Stanford, CA: Stanford University Press, 2008.

Elsaesser, Thomas. "The Future of 'Art' and 'Work' in the Age of Vision Machines: Harun Farocki." In *After the Avant-Garde: Contemporary German and Austrian Experimental Film*, edited by Randall Halle and Reinhild Steingröver, 31–49. Rochester, NY: Camden House, 2008.

Elster, Allen D., and Jonathan H. Burdette. *Questions and Answers in Magnetic Resonance Imaging*. Chicago: Mosby, 2000.

Farocki, Harun. "Phantom Images." *Public* 29 (2004): 12–22.

Felipe, Javier De. *Cajal's Butterflies of the Soul: Science and Art*. Oxford: Oxford University Press, 2010.

Ferran, Bronac. "Creating a Program of Support for Art and Science Collaborations." *Leonardo Journal* 39, no. 5 (2006): 442–445.

Ferrante, Gianni, and Stanislav Sykora. "Technical Aspects of Fast Field Cycling." In *Advances in Inorganic Chemistry Volume 57: Relaxometry of Water-Metal Ion Interactions*, edited by Rudi Van Eldik, 405–470. Amsterdam: Elsevier, 2004.

Feuerstein, Thomas. "Metabolic Machines & Demons of Life." Presented at the Kunst und Künstliche Intelligenz, May 2019. https://www.youtube.com/watch?v=MzZhZYLliac&vl=en.

Finn, Ed. *What Algorithms Want: Imagination in the Age of Computing*. Cambridge, MA: MIT Press, 2017.

Fischer, Michael M. J. *Emergent Forms of Life and the Anthropological Voice*. Durham, NC: Duke University Press, 2003.

Fisher, Erik, and Roop L. Mahajan. "Embedding the Humanities in Engineering: Art, Dialogue, and a Laboratory." In *Trading Zones and Interactional Expertise: Creating New Kinds of Collaboration*, edited by Michael E. Gorman, 209–230. Cambridge, MA: MIT Press, 2010.

Floridi, Luciano. "The Informational Nature of Personal Identity." *Minds and Machines* 21, no. 4 (2011): 549–566.

Floridi, Luciano. *The Philosophy of Information*. Oxford: Oxford University Press, 2011.

Flusser, Vilém. *Gesten: Versuch Einer Phänomenologie*. Düsseldorf: Bollmann Verlag, 1991.

Flusser, Vilém. "The Gesture of Writing." In *Flusser Studies*, 1–18, n.d. http://www.flusserstudies.net/sites/www.flusserstudies.net/files/media/attachments/the-gesture-of-writing.pdf.

Foucault, Michel. *The Birth of the Clinic: An Archaeology of Medical Perception*. London: Tavistock Publications, 1973.

Foucault, Michel. *A History of Sexuality*. Vol. 1, *An Introduction*. New York: Vintage, 1980.

Frampton, Michael. *Embodiments of Will: Anatomical and Physiological Theories of Voluntary Animal Motion from Greek Antiquity to the Latin Middle Ages, 400 B.C.–A.D. 1300*. Berlin: VDM Verlag, 2008.

Frazzetto, Giovanni, and Suzanne Anker. "Neuroculture." *Nature Reviews Neuroscience* 10 (2009): 815–821.

Friedberg, Anne. *The Virtual Window: From Alberti to Microsoft*. Cambridge, MA: MIT Press, 2009.

Frigg, Roman. "Fiction and Science." In *Fictions and Models*, edited by John Woods. Munich: Philosophia Verlag, 2010.

Galison, Peter. *How Experiments End*. Chicago: Chicago University Press, 1987.

Galison, Peter. *Image and Logic: Material Culture of Microphysics*. Chicago: University of Chicago Press, 1997.

Galison, Peter. "The Ontology of the Enemy: Norbert Wiener and the Cybernetic Vision." *Critical Inquiry* 21, no. 1 (1994): 228–266.

Galison, Peter. "Trading with the Enemy." In *Trading Zones and Interactional Expertise: Creating New Kinds of Collaboration*, edited by Michael E. Gorman, 25–52. Cambridge, MA: MIT Press, 2010.

Galloway, Alexander. "Are Some Things Unrepresentable?" *Theory, Culture and Society* 28, no. 7–8 (2011): 85–102.

Galloway, Alexander. *The Interface Effect*. London: Polity Press, 2012.

Galton, Francis. "Composite Portraits." *Journal of the Anthropological Institute of Great Britain and Ireland* 8 (1878): 132–144.

Gidal, Peter. *Materialist Film*. New York: Routledge, 1989.

Gilman, Sander. "Representing Health and Illness: Thoughts for the Twenty-First Century." *Medical History* 55, no. 3 (2011): 295–300.

Gilman, Sander. *Seeing the Insane: A Visual and Cultural History of Our Attitudes toward the Mentally Ill*. Brattleboro, VT: Echo Point Books and Media, 1982.

Gilman, Sander L. *Illness and Image: Case Studies in the Medical Humanities*. London: Routledge, 2014.

Ginsberg, Alexandra Daisy, Jane Calvert, Pablo Schyfter, Alistair Elfick, and Drew Endy. *Synthetic Aesthetics: Investigating Synthetic Biology's Designs on Nature*. Cambridge, MA: MIT Press, 2014.

Ginzburg, Carlo. *The Cheese and the Worms: The Cosmos of a Sixteenth Century Miller*. Baltimore: Johns Hopkins University Press, 1980.

Ginzburg, Carlo. "Microhistory: Two or Three Things That I Know about It." *Critical Inquiry* 20, no. 1 (1993): 10–35.

Gitelman, Lisa. *"Raw Data" Is an Oxymoron*. Cambridge, MA: MIT Press, 2013.

Glinkowski, Paul, and Anne Bamford. *Insight and Exchange: An Evaluation of the Wellcome Trust's SciArt Programme*. London: Wellcome Trust, 2009. https://wellcome.ac.uk/sites/default/files/wtx057228_0.pdf.

Golubnitschaja, Olga, Judita Kinkorova, and Vincenzo Costigliola. "Predictive, Preventive and Personalised Medicine as the Hardcore of 'Horizon 2020': EPMA Position Paper." *EPMA Journal* 5, no. 1 (2014): 6.

Goodchild, Michael F. "Reimagining the History of GIS." *Annals of GIS* 24, no. 1 (2018): 1–8.

Goodman, Nelson. *Ways of Worldmaking*. Indianapolis: Hackett, 1978.

Goodman, Nelson. "Words, Works, Worlds." *Erkenntnis* 9, no. 1 (1975): 57–73.

Gould, Glenn. "The Prospects of Recording." *High Fidelity* 16, no. 4 (1966): 46–63.

Graham, Scott. "Object-Oriented Ontology's Binary Duplication and the Promise of Thing-Oriented Ontologies." In *Rhetoric, through Everyday Things*, edited by Scot Barnett and Casey Boyle, 108–122. Tuscaloosa: University of Alabama Press, 2016.

Grau, Oliver, and Thomas Veigl, eds. *Imagery in the 21st Century*. Cambridge, MA: MIT Press, 2011.

Gunning, Tom. "Doubled Vision: Peering through Kentridge's 'Stereoscope.'" *Parkett* 63 (2001): 68–81.

Gunning, Tom. "To Scan a Ghost: The Ontology of Mediated Vision." *Grey Room* 26 (2007): 94–127.

Hacking, Ian. *Representing and Intervening: Introductory Topics in the Philosophy of Natural Science*. Cambridge: Cambridge University Press, 1983.

Hacking, Ian. *The Taming of Chance*. Cambridge: Cambridge University Press, 1990.

Halpern, Orit. *Beautiful Data: A History of Vision and Reason since 1945*. Durham, NC: Duke University Press, 2015.

Hansen, Mark. *New Philosophy for New Media*. Cambridge, MA: MIT Press, 2004.

Hanson, Lars G. "Is Quantum Mechanics Necessary for Understanding Magnetic Resonance?" *Concepts in Magnetic Resonance Part A* 32, no. 5 (2008): 329–340.

Haraway, Donna. "Modest Witness: Feminist Diffractions in Science Studies." In *The Disunity of Science: Boundaries, Contexts, and Power*, edited by Peter Galison and David J. Stump. Stanford, CA: Stanford University Press, 1996.

Haraway, Donna. *Modest_Witness@Second_Millennium.FemaleMan_Meets_OncoMouse: Feminism and Technoscience*. New York: Routledge, 1997.

Haraway, Donna. *Simians, Cyborgs, Women: The Reinvention of Nature*. London: Free, 1991.

Haraway, Donna. *When Species Meet*. Minneapolis: University of Minnesota Press, 2008.

Harding, Sandra. *The Science Question in Feminism*. Ithaca, NY: Cornell University Press, 1986.

Harding, Sandra. *Sciences from Below: Feminisms, Postcolonialities, and Modernities*. Durham, NC: Duke University Press, 2008.

Hauser, Jens. "Observations on an Art of Growing Interest: Toward a Phenomenological Approach to Art Involving Biotechnology." In *Tactical Biopolitics—Art, Activism, and Technoscience*, edited by Beatriz da Costa and Kavita Philip, 83–104. Cambridge, MA: MIT Press, 2008.

Häusle, Thomas. "Poetics of Cannibalism." Thomas Häusle in conversation with Thomas Feuerstein n.d., 130–141. https://www.thomasfeuerstein.net/20_BIBLIOGRAPHY/30_TEXTS_&_ARTICLES/Haeusle-Feuerstein_en.pdf.

Hayles, Katherine. *How We Became Posthuman: Virtual Bodies in Cybernetics, Literature, and Informatics*. Chicago: Chicago University Press, 1999.

Hayles, Katherine N. *Unthought: The Power of the Cognitive Nonconscious*. Chicago: Chicago University Press, 2017.

Henriksen, Danah. "Full STEAM Ahead: Creativity in Excellent STEM Teaching Practices." *The STEAM Journal* 1, no. 2 (2014): 1–7.

Hentschel, Klaus. *Visual Cultures in Science and Technology: A Comparative History*. Oxford: Oxford University Press, 2014.

Higgins, Hannah B. *The Grid Book*. Cambridge, MA: MIT Press, 2009.

Holmes, Frederic L., Jürgen Renn, and Hans-Jörg Rheinberger. "Introduction." In *Reworking the Bench: Research Notebooks in the History of Science*, vi–xiii. New York: Kluwer Academic, 2003.

Hood, Beverley. "Being Still." In *Immobile Choreography*, 11–30. Aberdeen: Grampian Hospitals Art Trust, 2019. Exhibition catalog.

Hutchins, Edwin. *Cognition in the Wild*. Cambridge, MA: MIT Press, 1995.

Hutchison, James M. S. "Imaging by Nuclear Magnetic Resonance." In *Medical Imaging Techniques*, edited by B. William Watson, 79–93. London: Peter Peregrinus, 1979.

Hutchison, James M. S., William Edelstein, and Glyn Johnson. "A Whole-Body NMR Imaging Machine." *Journal of Physics E: Scientific Instruments* 13, no. 9 (1980): 947.

Hutchison, James M. S., John R. Mallard, and G. C. Goll. "In-Vivo Imaging of Body Structures Using Proton Resonance." In *Proceedings, 18th Ampere Congress*, edited by P. S. Allen et al., 283–284. Nottingham: University of Nottingham, 1974.

Hytten, Kathy, and Kurt Stemhagen. "When STEM and STEAM Really Mean ABC: A Democratic Critique of 'Anything but Civics' Schools." *Educational Studies* 56, no. 1 (2020): 18–36.

Ingold, Tim. "Beyond Art and Technology: The Anthropology of Skill." In *Anthropological Perspectives on Technology*, edited by Michael Brian Schiffer, 17–31. Albuquerque: University of New Mexico Press, 2001.

Ingold, Tim. "Bringing Things to Life: Creative Entanglements in a World of Materials." National Centre for Research Methods Working Paper Series no. 15. 2010. http://eprints.ncrm.ac.uk/1306/1/0510_creative_entanglements.pdf. Original version (April 2008) presented at Vital Signs: Researching Real Life, 9 September 9, 2008, University of Manchester.

Ingold, Tim. *Essays on Movement, Knowledge and Description*. London: Routledge, 2011.

Ingold, Tim. "From Science to Art and Back Again: The Pendulum of an Anthropologist." *ANUAC* 5, no. 1 (2016): 5–23.

Jacob, François. *Of Flies, Mice and Men*. Cambridge, MA: Harvard University Press, 1998.

Jasanoff, Sheila. "Future Imperfect: Science, Technology and the Imaginations of Modernity." In *Dreamscapes of Modernity: Sociotechnical Imaginaries and the Fabrication of Power*, edited by Sheila Jasanoff and Sang-Hyun Kim, 1–33. Chicago: University of Chicago Press, 2015.

Jevtić, Iva. "Between Word and Image: Walter Benjamin's Images as a Species of Space." *Inter-Disciplinary.Net* 3 (2008). http://citeseerx.ist.psu.edu/viewdoc/download?doi=10.1.1.522.5174&rep=rep1&type=pdf.

Johnston, Sean F. "Technological Parables and Iconic Illustrations: American Technocracy and the Rhetoric of the Technological Fix." *History and Technology* 33, no. 2 (2017): 196–219.

Jones, Caroline A., and Peter Galison, eds. *Picturing Science, Producing Art*. New York: Routledge, 1998.

Joyce, Kelly A. "From Numbers to Pictures: The Development of Magnetic Resonance Imaging and the Visual Turn in Medicine." *Science as Culture* 15, no. 1 (2006): 1–22.

Joyce, Kelly A. *Magnetic Appeal: MRI and the Myth of Transparency*. Ithaca: Cornell University Press, 2008.

Kac, Eduardo. *Signs of Life: Bio Art and Beyond*. Cambridge, MA: MIT Press, 2007.

Karnes, Michelle. *Imagination, Meditation, and Cognition in the Middle Ages*. Chicago: Chicago University Press, 2011.

Kay, Lily E. "From Logical Neurons to Poetic Embodiments of Mind: Warren S. McCulloch's Project in Neuroscience." *Science in Context* 14, no. 4 (2001): 591–614.

Kay, Lily E. *The Molecular Vision of Life: Caltech, the Rockefeller Foundation, and the Rise of the New Biology*. Oxford: Oxford University Press, 1993.

Keating, Peter, and Alberto Cambrosio. *Biomedical Platforms: Realigning the Normal and the Pathological in Late-Twentieth-Century Medicine*. Cambridge, MA: MIT Press, 2003.

Keller, Evelyn Fox, and Helen E. Longino. *Feminism and Science: Oxford Readings in Feminism*. Oxford: Oxford University Press, 1996.

Kemp, Martin. *Leonardo*. Oxford: Oxford University Press, 2005.

Kemp, Martin. *Seen | Unseen: Art, Science, and Intuition from Leonardo to the Hubble Telescope*. New York: Oxford University Press, 2006.

Kemp, Martin, and Marina Wallace. *Spectacular Bodies*. London: Hayward Gallery, 2001. Exhibition catalog.

Kevles, Bettyann. *Naked to the Bone: Medical Imaging in the Twentieth Century*. Reading, MA: Addison-Wesley, 1998.

Kimmich, Rainer. "Field Cycling NMR Relaxometry." *Bulletin Magnetic Resonance* 1, no. 4 (1980): 195.

Kline, Ronald R. *The Cybernetics Moment or Why We Call Our Age the Information Age*. Baltimore: Johns Hopkins University Press, 2015.

Knorr-Cetina, Karin. *The Manufacture of Knowledge: An Essay on the Constructivist and Contextual Nature of Science*. Oxford: Pergamon Press, 1981.

Koek, Ariane. "In/Visible: The inside Story of the Making of Arts at CERN." *Interdisciplinary Science Reviews* 42, no. 4 (2017): 345–358.

Koenig, Seymour H., and Rodney D. Brown. "Relaxometry of Tissue." *Progress in NMR Spectroscopy* 22 (1990): 487.

Kozel, Susan. *Closer, Performance, Technologies, Phenomenology*. Cambridge, MA: MIT Press, 2008.

Krauss, Rosalind. "Grids." *October* 9 (1979): 50–64.

Kuhn, Thomas S. *The Trouble with the Historical Philosophy of Science*. Cambridge, MA: Dept. of the History of Science, Harvard University, 1992.

Kwint, Marius. "Animated Meditations on Mortality: The Work of Andrew Carnie." In *Time Will Tell*, 1–4. Winchester Gallery Publisher, 2008.

Latour, Bruno. *Pandora's Hope: Essays on the Reality of Science Studies*. Cambridge, MA: Harvard University Press, 1999.

Latour, Bruno. *Reassembling the Social: An Introduction to Actor-Network-Theory*. Oxford: Oxford University Press, 2005.

Latour, Bruno. *Science in Action: How to Follow Scientists and Engineers through Society*. Milton Keynes: Open University Press, 1987.

Latour, Bruno. "Visualization and Cognition: Thinking with Eyes and Hands." In *Knowledge and Society: Studies in the Sociology of Culture Past and Present*, vol. 6, 1–40. Greenwich, CT: JAI Press, 1986.

Latour, Bruno. "What Is Iconoclash? Or Is There a World beyond the Image Wars?" In *Iconoclash, Beyond the Image-Wars in Science, Religion and Art*, edited by Peter Weibel and Bruno Latour, 14–37. Cambridge, MA: ZKM and MIT Press, 2002.

Latour, Bruno, and Steve Woolgar. *Laboratory Life: The Construction of Scientific Facts*. Princeton, NJ: Princeton University Press, 1979.

Lauterbur, Paul. "Cancer Detection by Nuclear Magnetic Resonance Zeugmatographic Imaging." *Cancer* 57 (1986): 1899–1904.

Lauterbur, Paul. "MRI: A New Way of Seeing." *Nature* 242 (1973): 190–191.

Law, John. "Actor Network Theory and Material Semiotics," April 25, 2007. http://www.heterogeneities.net/publications/Law2007ANTandMaterialSemiotics.pdf.

Leach, James. "Extending Contexts, Making Possibilities: An Introduction to Evaluating the Projects." *Leonardo Journal* 39, no. 5 (2006): 447–451.

Leder, Drew. *The Body in Medical Thought and Practice*. Dordrecht: Kluwer Academic, 1992.

Leonelli, Sabina. *Data-Centric Biology: A Philosophical Study*. Chicago: University of Chicago Press, 2016.

Leonelli, Sabina. "Lakatos Award Lecture." Lecture, London School of Economics, October 2018.

Leonelli, Sabina, and Niccolò Tempini, eds. *Data Journeys in the Sciences*. Cham, Switzerland: Springer Nature, 2020.

Lévi-Strauss, Claude. *The Savage Mind*. Chicago: Chicago University Press, 1966.

Liljefors, Max, Susan S. Lundin, and Andrea Wiszmeg, eds. *The Atomized Body: The Cultural Life of Stem Cells, Genes and Neurons*. Lund, Sweden: Nordic Academic Press, 2012.

Lima, Manuel. *Visual Complexity: Mapping Patterns of Information*. New York: Princeton Architectural Press, 2011.

Lippit, Akira Mizuta. *Atomic Light Shadow Optics*. Minneapolis: University of Minnesota Press, 2005.

Lloyd, Kathryn. "No Measure of Health: Ilona Sagar Scans the Politics of Wellbeing." *MoMus*, 2018. https://momus.ca/no-measure-health-ilona-sagar-scans-politics-wellbeing/.

Lock, Margaret. *The Alzheimer Conundrum: Entanglements of Dementia and Aging*. Princeton, NJ: Princeton University Press, 2003.

Lohmeyer, Eddie, and Orit Halpern. "Cinema/Cybernetics/Visuality: A Conversation with Orit Halpern." *International Journal of Communication* 10 (2016): 3203–3215.

Löwy, Ilana. "Historiography of Biomedicine 'Bio,' 'Medicine,' and In Between." *Isis* 102 (2011): 116–122.

Lumière, Louis. "Répresentation Photographique d'un Solide Dans l'espace. Photo-Stéreo-Synthèse." *Comptes Rendus Hebdomadaires des Séances de l'académie Des Sciences* 171 (1920): 891–896.

Lurie, David J. "Introduction." In *Immobile Choreography*, 9. Aberdeen: Grampian Hospitals Art Trust, 2019. Exhibition catalog.

Lurie, David J. "Quadrupole-Dip Measurement in Humans by Whole-Body Field-Cycling NMR Relaxometry and Imaging." In *29th Ampere–13th ISMAR Conference*, vol. 1. Berlin, 1998.

Lurie, David J., Silvio Aime, Simona Baroni, Nuala A. Booth, Lionel M. Broche, Chang-Hoon Choi, Gareth R. Davies, Saadiya Ismail, and Dara Ó hÓgáin. "Fast Field-Cycling Magnetic Resonance Imaging." *Comptes Rendus Physique* 11, no. 2 (2010): 136–148.

Lurie, David J., David M. Bussell, Lawrence H. Bell, and John R. Mallard. "Proton-Electron Double Magnetic Resonance Imaging of Free Radical Solutions." *Journal of Magnetic Resonance* 76 (1988): 366–370.

Lurie, David J., James M. S. Hutchison, Lawrence H. Bell, David M. Bussell, and John R. Mallard. "Field-Cycled Proton-Electron Double-Resonance Imaging of Free Radicals in Large Aqueous Samples." *Journal of Magnetic Resonance* 84 (1989): 431–437.

Lutters, Bart, and Peter J. Koehler. "Brainwaves in Concert: The 20th Century Sonification of the Electroencephalogram." *Brain* 139, no. 10 (2016): 2809–2814.

Lynch, Michael. "Discipline and the Material Form of Images: An Analysis of Scientific Visibility." *Social Studies of Science* 15, no. 1 (1985): 37–66.

Lynch, Michael. "The Externalized Retina: Selection and Mathematization in the Visual Documentation of Objects in the Life Sciences." *Human Studies* 11, no. 2/3 (1988): 201–234.

Lynch, Michael. "Laboratory Space and the Technological Complex: An Investigation of Topical Contextures." *Science in Context* 4, no. 1 (1991): 51–78.

Lynch, Michael. *Scientific Practice and Ordinary Action: Ethnomethodology and Social Studies of Science*. Cambridge: Cambridge University Press, 1993.

Lynch, Michael, and Steve Woolgar. *Representation in Scientific Practice*. Cambridge, MA: MIT Press, 1990.

Ma, Dan, Vikas Gulani, Nicole Seiberlich, Kecheng Liu, Jeffrey L. Sunshine, Jeffrey L. Duerk, and Mark A. Griswold. "Magnetic Resonance Fingerprinting." *Nature* 14, no. 495 (2013): 187–192.

Ma, Dan, Vikas Gulani, Nicole Seiberlich, Kecheng Liu, Jeffrey L. Sunshine, Jeffrey L. Duerk, and Mark A. Griswold. "Music-Based Magnetic Resonance Fingerprinting to Improve Patient Comfort during MRI Examinations." *Magnetic Resonance in Medicine* 75, no. 6 (2016): 2303–2314.

Majorana, Ettore. "Il Valore delle Leggi Statistiche nella Fisica e nelle Scienze Sociali." *Scientia* 36 (1942): 58–66.

Majorana, Ettore, and Rosario N. Mantegna. "The Value of Statistical Laws in Physics and Social Sciences." In *Ettore Majorana Scientific Papers*, edited by Giuseppe Franco Bassani and the Council of the Italian Physical Society, 237–260. Berlin: Springer, 2006.

Mallard, John R. "Contributions from Aberdeen to the Emergence of Worldwide, Clinically Diagnostic, MRI." *Encyclopedia of Magnetic Resonance*. 2010. https://onlinelibrary.wiley.com/doi/abs/10.1002/9780470034590.emrhp1073.

Mallard, John R. "The Evolution of Medical Imaging: From Geiger Counters to MRI—A Personal Saga." *Perspectives in Biology and Medicine* 46, no. 3 (2003): 349–370.

Mallard, John R. "Hevesy Memorial Medal Lecture 1985 (September 4th, 1985). Some Call It Laziness: I Call It Deep Thought (with Apologies to Garfield)." *Nuclear Medicine Communications* 8, no. 9 (1987): 691–710.

Mallard, John R. "Magnetic Resonance Imaging—The Aberdeen Perspective on Developments in the Early Years." *History of Medical Biology* 51 (2006): 45–60.

Mallard, John R. "The New Bacon-Slicing Machine—A Non-Invasive Gadget for Human Beings." *Health Care Equipment and Technology* 4 (1978): 7–13. GB 0231 University of Aberdeen, Special Collections, Ref. No MS 3819/1/123.

Mallard, John R. "Nuclear Imaging." In *Electronic Imaging*, edited by T. P. McLean and P. Schagen, 419–459. London: Academic Press, 1979.

Mallard, John R. "Nuclear Imaging." *Journal of Medical Progress through Technology* 7 (1980): 87–110. Printed in the *Proceedings of the International Symposium Electronic Imaging at the Royal Society, London, September 1978* (London: Academic Press, 1978): 419–459.

Mallard, John R. "Principles of Scanning and Current Physical Problems." In *Radioactive Isotopes in the Localization of Tumours*, 1–6. London: William Heinemann Medical Books, 1969.

Mallard, John R. "Radioisotope Imaging—The End of the Beginning." *Separata Do Arquivo de Patologia* 46, no. 1 (1974): 3–26.

Mallard, John R. "The Radionuclide Imaging Process and Factors Influencing the Choice of an Instrument for Brain Scanning." *Progress in Nuclear Medicine* 1 (1972): 1–114.

Mallard, John R., James M. S. Hutchison, William Edelstein, Richard Ling, and Margaret Foster. "Imaging by Nuclear Magnetic Resonance and Its Bio-Medical Implications." *Journal of Biomedical Engineering* 1, no. 3 (1979): 153–160.

Mallard, John, James M. S. Hutchison, William A. Edelstein, Charles R. Ling, Margaret A. Foster, Glyn Johnson, Stephen F. J. Cox, et al. "In Vivo N.M.R. Imaging in Medicine: The Aberdeen Approach, Both Physical and Biological [and Discussion]." *Philosophical Transactions of the Royal Society of London: Series B, Biological Sciences* 289, no. 1037 (1980): 519–530.

Mallard, John R., and M. J. Myers. "The Performance of a Gamma Camera for the Visualization of Radioactive Isotopes in Vivo." *Physics in Medicine & Biology* 8, no. 2 (1963): 165.

Manovich, Lev. *The Language of New Media*. Cambridge, MA: MIT Press, 2001.

Mansfield, Peter. Letter from Peter Mansfield to Allen Garroway, April 6, 1976. Peter Mansfield Collection, PPM/11/1/5, US Naval Research Laboratory, Washington, DC.

Mansfield, Peter. "Multi-Planar Imaging Formation Using NMR Spin-Echo." *Journal of Physics C: Solid State Physics* 10, no. 3 (1977): 55–58.

Mansfield, Peter, and Andrew A. Maudsley. "Medical Imaging by NMR." *British Journal of Radiology* 50, no. 591 (1977): 188–194.

Massey, Lyle. *Picturing Space, Displacing Bodies: Anamorphosis in Early Modern Theories of Perspective*. University Park, PA: Pennsylvania University Press, 2008.

May, John. *Signal. Image. Architecture*. New York: Columbia University Press, 2019.

McCrea, Christian. "Giorgio Agamben." In *Film, Theory, and Philosophy: The Key Thinkers*, edited by Felicity Colman, 349–357. Montreal, Canada: McGill University Press, 2009.

McRobbie, Donald W., Elisabeth A. Moore, Martin J. Graves, and Martin R. Prince. *MRI: From Picture to Proton*. Cambridge: Cambridge University Press, 2003.

Michael, Mike, and Marsha Rosengarten. "Medicine: Experimentation, Politics, Emergent Bodies." *Body & Society* 18, no. 3/4 (2012): 1–17.

Miller, Arthur I. *Colliding Worlds: How Cutting-Edge Science Is Redefining Contemporary Art*. London: W. W. Norton, 2014.

Mitchell, Robert E. *Bioart and the Vitality of Media*. Seattle: University of Washington Press, 2010.

Mitchell, Robert, and Phillip Thurtle. *Data Made Flesh: Embodying Information*. New York: Routledge, 2004.

Mitchell, William J. T. *Picture Theory: Essays on Verbal and Visual Representation*. Chicago: University of Chicago Press, 1994.

Mitchell, William J. *The Reconfigured Eye: Visual Truth in the Post-Photographic Era*. Cambridge, MA: MIT Press, 1992.

Mitchell, W. J. T. *What Do Pictures Want? The Lives and Loves of Images*. Chicago: University of Chicago Press, 2006.

Mody, Cyrus C. M. "The Sounds of Science: Listening to Laboratory Practice." *Science, Technology, & Human Values* 30, no. 2 (2005): 175–198.

Mol, Annemarie. "Actor-Network Theory: Sensitive Terms and Enduring Tensions." *Kölner Zeitschrift Für Soziologie Und Sozialpsychologie. Sonderhefte* 50 (2010): 253–269.

Mol, Annemarie. *The Body Multiple: Ontology in Medical Practice*. Durham, NC: Duke University Press, 2002.

Mondloch, Kate. *A Capsule Aesthetic: Feminist Materialisms in New Media Art*. Minneapolis: University of Minnesota Press, 2018.

Müggenburg, Jan. *Lebhafte Artefakte: Heinz von Foerster und die Maschinen des Biological Computer Laboratory*. Konstanz, Germany: Konstanz University Press, 2018.

Müller, Albert. "A Brief History of the BCL: Heinz von Foerster and the Biological Computer Laboratory." In *An Unfinished Revolution? Heinz von Foerster and the Biological Computer Laboratory, BCL, 1958–1976*, edited by Albert Müller and Karl H. Müller, 277–302. Vienna: Edition Echoraum, 2007.

Munster, Anna. *Materializing New Media: Embodiment in Information Aesthetics*. Hanover, NH: Dartmouth College Press, 2006.

Myers, Natasha. *Rendering Life Molecular: Models, Modelers, and Excitable Matter*. Durham, NC: Duke University Press Books, 2015.

Noack, Frank. "NMR Field Cycling Spectroscopy: Principles and Applications." *Progress in NMR Spectroscopy* 18 (1986): 171–176.

Noë, Alva. *Strange Tools: Art and Human Nature*. New York: Hill & Wang, 2015.

Olzscha, Heidi, Sonya M. Schermann, Andreas C. Woerner, Stefan Pinkert, Michael H. Hecht, Gian G. Tartaglia, Michele Vendruscolo, Manajit Hayer-Hartl, F. Ulrich Hartl, and R. Martin Vabulas. "Amyloid-like Aggregates Sequester Numerous Metastable Proteins with Essential Cellular Functions." *Cell* 144, no. 1 (2011): 67–78.

Ortega, Francisco, and Fernando Vidal, eds. *Neurocultures: Glimpses into an Expanding Universe*. Frankfurt: Peter Lang, 2011.

Orton, Liz, ed. *Becoming Image: Medicine and the Algorithmic Gaze*. London: Digital Insides, 2018.

Parikka, Jussi. "Machine Learned Futures." *JussiParikka* (blog), September 2018. https://jussiparikka.net/2018/09/06/machine-learned-futures/.

Parkinson, Gavin. *Surrealism, Art and Modern Science: Relativity, Quantum Mechanics, Epistemology*. New Haven, CT: Yale University Press, 2008.

Patterson, Zabet. *Peripheral Vision. Bell Labs, the S-C 4020, and the Origins of Computer Art*. Cambridge, MA: MIT Press, 2015.

Pearse, Innes H., and Lucy H. Crocker. *The Peckham Experiment*. New York: Routledge, 2009.

Penrose, Roger. *The Road to Reality: A Complete Guide to the Laws of the Universe*. New York: Alfred Knopf, 2004.

Perini, Laura. "The Truth in Pictures." *Philosophy of Science* 72 (2005): 262–285.

Pickering, Andrew. "Art, Science and Experiment." *MaHKUscript. Journal of Fine Art Research* 1, no. 1 (2016): 1–6.

Pickering, Andrew. *The Cybernetic Brain: Sketches of Another Future*. Chicago: Chicago University Press, 2010.

Pickering, Andrew. *The Mangle of Practice: Time, Agency, and Science*. Chicago: University of Chicago Press, 1995.

Pickering, Andrew, ed. *Science as Practice and Culture*. Chicago: Chicago University Press, 1992.

Pickering, Andrew, and Keith Guzik. *The Mangle in Practice: Science, Society, and Becoming*. Durham, NC: Duke University Press, 2008.

Pradeu, Thomas. *The Limits of the Self: Immunology and Biological Identity*. Oxford: Oxford University Press, 2016.

Prainsack, Barbara. *Personalized Medicine: Empowered Patients in the 21st Century?* New York: New York University Press, 2017.

Prasad, Amit. *Imperial Technoscience: Transnational Histories of MRI in the United States, Britain, and India*. Cambridge, MA: MIT Press, 2014.

Prasad, Amit. "Making Images/Making Bodies: Visibilizing and Disciplining through Magnetic Resonance Imaging (MRI)." *Science, Technology, & Human Values* 30, no. 2 (2005): 291–316.

Prasad, Amit. "Scientific Culture in the 'Other' Theatre of 'Modern Science': An Analysis of the Culture of Magnetic Resonance Imaging (MRI) Research in India." *Social Studies of Science* 30, no. 3 (2005): 463–489.

Rabinow, Paul. *Making PCR: A Story of Biotechnology*. Chicago: Chicago University Press, 1997.

Racine, Eric, Sarah Waldman, Jarrett Rosenberg, and Judy Illes. "Contemporary Neuroscience in the Media." *Social Science and Medicine Journal* 71, no. 4 (2010): 725–733.

Rancière, Jacques. *The Future of the Image*. London: Verso, 2007.

Regierer, Babette, Valeria Zazzu, Ralph Sudbrak, Alexander Kühn, and Hans Lehrach. "Future of Medicine: Models in Predictive Diagnostics and Personalized Medicine." *Advances in Biochemical Engineering/Biotechnology* 133 (2013): 15–33.

Reinsborough, Michael. "Art-Science Collaboration in an EPSRC/BBSRC-Funded Synthetic Biology UK Research Centre." *NanoEthics* 14 (2020): 93–111.

Rheinberger, Hans-Jörg. "Afterword: Instruments as Media, Media as Instruments." *Studies in History and Philosophy of Biological and Biomedical Sciences* 57 (2016): 161–162.

Rheinberger, Hans-Jörg. "Difference Machines: Time in Experimental Systems." *Configurations* 23, no. 2 (2015): 165–176. https://doi.org/10.1353/con.2015.0013.

Rheinberger, Hans-Jörg. *An Epistemology of the Concrete: Twentieth-Century Histories of Life*. Durham, NC: Duke University Press, 2010.

Rheinberger, Hans-Jörg. "Experimental Systems: Historiality, Narration, and Deconstruction." *Science in Context* 7, no. 1 (1994): 65–81.

Rheinberger, Hans-Jörg. "From Microsomes to Ribosomes: 'Strategies' of 'Representation.'" *Journal of the History of Biology* 28, no. 1 (1995): 49–89.

Rheinberger, Hans-Jörg. "Gaston Bachelard and the Notion of 'Phenomenotechnique.'" *Perspectives on Science* 13, no. 3 (2005): 313–328.

Rheinberger, Hans-Jörg. "Infra-Experimentality: From Traces to Data, from Data to Patterning Facts." *History of Science* 49, no. 3 (2011): 337–348.

Rheinberger, Hans-Jörg. "Making Visible. Visualization in the Sciences—and in Exhibitions?" In *The Exhibition as Product and Generator of Scholarship*, 9–23. Berlin: Max Planck Institute for the History of Science, pre-print, 2010. https://www.mpiwg-berlin.mpg.de/sites/default/files/Preprints/P399.pdf.

Rheinberger, Hans-Jörg. *On Historicizing Epistemology: An Essay*. Translated by David Fernbach. Stanford, CA: Stanford University Press, 2010.

Rheinberger, Hans-Jörg. "On the Possible Transformation and Vanishment of Epistemic Objects." *Theory of Science* 38, no. 3 (2016): 269–278.

Rheinberger, Hans-Jörg. "Scripts and Scribbles." *MLN* 118, no. 3 (2003): 622–636.

Rheinberger, Hans-Jörg. *Toward a History of Epistemic Things: Synthesizing Proteins in the Test Tube*. Stanford, CA: Stanford University Press, 1997.

Rock, Jenny, and Sierra Adler. "From 'SciArt' to 'Art Science.'" *Antennae: The Journal of Nature in Visual Culture* 47, no. 14 (2019): 14–26.

Rohdie, Sam. *Promised Lands: Cinema, Geography, Modernism*. London: BFI, 2001.

Rose, Nikolas. "Genomic Susceptibility as an Emergent Form of Life? Genetic Testing, Identity, and the Remit of Medicine." In *Biomedicine as Culture: Instrumental Practices, Technoscientific Knowledge, and New Modes of Life*, edited by Regula Valérie Burri and Joseph Dumit, 141–150. New York: Routledge, 2010.

Rose, Nikolas. "The Human Sciences in a Biological Age." ICS Occasional Paper Series 3, no. 1. Edited by David Rowee and Reena Dobson. 2012.

Rose, Nikolas. "Personalized Medicine: Promises, Problems and Perils of a New Paradigm for Healthcare." *Procedia—Social and Behavioral Sciences* 7 (2013): 341–352.

Rose, Nikolas. *The Politics of Life Itself: Biomedicine, Power, and Subjectivity in the Twentieth-First Century*. Princeton, NJ: Princeton University Press, 2007.

Rose, Nikolas, and Joelle M. Abi-Rached. *Neuro: The New Brain Sciences and the Management of the Mind*. Princeton, NJ: Princeton University Press, 1685.

Rosenberg, Nathan. *Studies on Science and the Innovation Process*. London: World Scientific, 2010.

Røstvik, Camilla M. "At the Edge of Their Universe: Artists, Scientists and Outsiders at CERN." Unpublished PhD thesis, University of Manchester, 2016. https://www.research.manchester.ac.uk/portal/en/theses/at-the-edge-of-their-universe-artists-scientists-and-outsiders-at-cern(1a75c456-967e-4c71-a88e-3632f4b9745a).html.

Rudwick, Martin J. S. "The Emergence of a Visual Language for Geological Science 1760–1840." *History of Science* 14, no. 3 (1976): 149–195.

Salter, Chris. *Alien Agency: Experimental Encounters with Art in the Making*. Cambridge, MA: MIT Press, 2015.

Sappol, Michael. *Body Modern: Fritz Kahn, Scientific Illustration, and the Homuncular Subject*. Minneapolis: University of Minnesota Press, 2017.

Saunders, Barry F. *CT Suite: The Work of Diagnosis in the Age of Noninvasive Cutting*. Durham, NC: Duke University Press, 2008.

Sawday, Jonathan. *The Body Emblazoned: Dissection and the Human Body in Renaissance Culture*. London: Routledge, 1996.

Schneider, Joseph. *Donna Haraway: Live Theory*. New York: Continuum, 2005.

Schnugg, Claudia. *Creating Art Science Collaboration: Bringing Value to Organizations*. New York: Palgrave Macmillan, 2019.

Schuppli, Susan. "Atmospheric Correction." In *Imaging beyond Representation*, edited by Daniel Rubinstein et al., 16–32. Birmingham, UK: Birmingham Article Press, 2013.

Schwab, Michael, ed. *Experimental Systems: Future Knowledge in Artistic Research*. Adapted edition. Leuven, Belgium: Leuven University Press, 2015.

Scott, Bernard. "Second-Order Cybernetics: An Historical Introduction." *Kybernetes* 33, no. 9/10 (2004): 1365–1378.

Sejnowski, Terrence. "The Brain as Circuit." In *Portraits of the Mind: Visualizing the Brain from Antiquity to the 21st Century*, edited by Carl E. Schoonover, 168–172. New York: Abrams, 2010.

Selin, Cynthia. "Merging Art and Design in Foresight: Making Sense of Emerge." *Futures* 70 (2015): 24–35.

Sellars, Wilfrid. "Philosophy and the Scientific Image of Man." In *Science, Perception and Reality*, edited by Robert Colodny, 35–78. New York: Humanities Press, 1963.

Shah, Pratik, Francis Kendall, Sean Khozin, Ryaan Goosen, Jianying Hu, Jason Laramie, Michael Ringel, and Nicholas Schork. "Artificial Intelligence and Machine Learning in Clinical Development: A Translational Perspective." *Npj Digital Medicine* 2, no. 69 (2019): 1–5.

Shapin, Stephen, and Simon Shaffer. *Leviathan and the Air-Pump: Hobbes, Boyle and the Experimental Life*. Princeton, NJ: Princeton University Press, 1985.

Sherrington, Charles Scott. "Santiago Ramón y Cajal, 1852–1934." *Obituary Notices of Fellows of the Royal Society* 1, no. 4 (December 1935): 430.

Shmueli, Galit. "To Explain or to Predict?" *Statistical Science* 25, no. 3 (2010): 289–310.

Silver, Nate. *The Signal and the Noise: The Art and Science of Prediction*. London: Penguin, 2013.

Sitney, Paul Adams. *Visionary Film: The American Avant-Garde 1943–1978*. Oxford: Oxford University Press, 1979.

Smelik, Anneke, and Nina Lykke. *Bits of Life: Feminism at the Intersections of Media, Bioscience, and Technology*. Seattle: University of Washington Press, 2008.

Smith, Barry. *Foundations of Gestalt Theory*. Munich: Philosophia Verlag, 1988.

Smith, Francis, John Mallard, James Hutchison, A. Reid, Glyth Johnson, Thomas Redpath, and Robert Selbie. "Clinical Application of Nuclear Magnetic Resonance." *The Lancet* 1, no. 8211 (1981): 78–79.

Smith, Pamela H. *The Body of the Artisan: Art and Experience in the Scientific Revolution*. Chicago: Chicago University Press, 2004.

Smith, Scott. "From Nobel Ideas to Industrial Success—Bill Edelstein's Legacy." June 13, 2014. https://web.archive.org/web/20170031110622/http://www.geglobalresearch.com/blog/translating-nobel-beginnings-industrial-success-bill-edelsteins-legacy.

Smith, Shawn Michelle, and Sharon Sliwinski, eds. *Photography and the Optical Unconscious*. Durham, NC: Duke University Press, 2017.

Snow, Charles P. *The Two Cultures and the Scientific Revolution*. Cambridge: Cambridge University Press, 2011.

Soni, Jimmy, and Rob Goodman. *A Mind at Play: How Claude Shannon Invented the Information Age*. London: Simon & Schuster, 2017.

Sormani, Philippe, Guelfo Carbone, and Priska Gisler, eds. *Practicing Art/Science: Experiments in an Emerging Field*. New York: Routledge, 2018.

Stanley, Garrett B. "Reading and Writing the Neural Code." *Nature Neuroscience* 16 (2013): 259–263.

Star, Susan L. "This Is Not a Boundary Object: Reflections of the Origin of a Concept." *Science, Technology, & Human Values* 35, no. 5 (2010): 601–617.

Star, Susan Leigh, and James Griesemer. "Institutional Ecology, 'Translations' and Boundary Objects: Amateurs and Professionals in Berkeley's Museum of Vertebrate Zoology, 1907–39." *Social Studies of Science* 19, no. 3 (1989): 387–420.

Stengers, Isabelle. *Another Science Is Possible: A Manifesto for Slow Science*. Cambridge: Polity Press, 2018.

Stengers, Isabelle. *Cosmopolitics II*. Stanford, CA: Stanford University Press, 2011.

Taussig, Karen-Sue, Klaus Hoeyer, and Stefan Helmreich. "The Anthropology of Potentiality in Biomedicine. An Introduction to Supplement 7." *Current Anthropology* 54, no. 7 (2013): 3–14.

Thompson, Paul, David MacDonald, Michael Mega, Colin Holmes, Alan Evans, and Arthur Toga. "Detection and Mapping of Abnormal Brain Structure with a Probabilistic Atlas of Cortical Surfaces." *Journal of Computer Assisted Tomography* 21, no. 4 (1997): 567–581.

Thurtle, Phillip. *Biology in the Grid: Graphic Design and the Envisioning of Life*. Minneapolis: University of Minnesota Press, 2018.

Toga, Arthur W., and John C. Mazziotta. *Brain Mapping: The Methods*. San Diego, CA: Academic Press, 1996.

Toga, Arthur W., and John C. Mazziotta. *Brain Mapping: The Systems*. San Diego, CA: Academic Press, 2000.

Tomlison, Jonathon. "The Pain of Others." In *Becoming Image: Medicine and the Algorithmic Gaze*, edited by Liz Orton, 76–83. London: Digital Insides, 2018.

Trafton, Anne. "Doctors Rely On More Than Just Data for Medical Decision Making." *MIT News* (blog), 2018. http://news.mit.edu/2018/doctors-rely-gut-feelings-decision-making-0720.

Triscott, Nicola. "Art and Intervention in the Stewardship of the Planetary Commons: Towards a Curatorial Model of Co-Inquiry." PhD thesis, University of Westminster, 2017.

Tucker, Jennifer. "The Historian, the Picture, and the Archive." *Isis* 97, no. 1 (2006): 111–120.

Tufte, Edward. *The Visual Display of Quantitative Information*. Cheshire, CT: Graphics Press, 2001.

Turkle, Sherry. *Evocative Objects: Things We Think With*. Cambridge, MA: MIT Press, 2007.

Uricchio, William. "The Algorithmic Turn: Photosynth, Augmented Reality and the Changing Implications of the Image." *Visual Studies* 26, no. 1 (2011): 25–35.

Vaage, Nora S. "What Ethics for Bioart?" *Nanoethics* 10 (2016): 87–104.

van Dijck, José. "Memory Matters in the Digital Age." *Configurations* 12, no. 3 (2004): 349–373.

van Dijck, José. *The Transparent Body: A Cultural Analysis of Medical Imaging*. Seattle: University of Washington Press, 2005.

Varela, Francisco, and Humberto Maturana. *Autopoiesis and Cognition: The Realization of the Living*. Dordrecht: Reidel, 1980.

Vertesi, Janet. *Seeing Like a Rover: How Robots, Teams, and Images Craft Knowledge of Mars*. Chicago: University of Chicago Press, 2015.

Vidal, Fernando. "Brainhood, Anthropological Figure of Modernity." *History of the Human Sciences* 22, no. 1 (2009): 5–36.

von Foerster, Heinz, ed. *Cybernetics: Circular Causal, and Feedback Mechanisms in Biological and Social Systems*. Transactions of the Sixth Conference, March 24–25, 1949. New York: Josiah Macy Jr. Foundation, 1950.

von Foerster, Heinz. *KybernEthik*. Berlin: Merve, 1993.

von Foerster, Heinz. *Memory without Record: Essays on Cybernetics and Cognition*. New York: Springer, 2003.

von Foerster, Heinz, Ernst von Glasersfeld, Győző Kovács, Peter Weibel, Tihamér Nemes, Nicolas Schöffer, Heinz Zemanek, et al. "Cybernetics Computer Science Computer Art: The Beginnings of an Epistemology of Responsibility." In *Beyond Art: A Third Culture. A Comparative Study in Cultures, Art and Science in 20th Century Austria and Hungary*, edited by Peter Weibel, 294–367. Vienna: Springer-Verlag, 2005.

Vons, Jacqueline. "Le Medecin Guarissant Phantasie: Purgeant Aussi Par Drogues la Folie." *Histoire Des Sciences Médicales* 44, no. 2 (2010): 121–129.

von Schomberg, René. "Prospects for Technology Assessment in a Framework of Responsible Research and Innovation." In *Technikfolgen Abschätzen Lehren: Bildungspotenziale Transdisziplinärer Methoden*, edited by Marc Dusseldorp and Richard Beechcroft, 39–61. Wiesbaden, Germany: Springer-Verlag, 2012.

Vul, Edward, Christine Harris, Piotr Winkielman, and Harold Pashler. "Puzzlingly High Correlations in FMRI Studies of Emotion, Personality, and Social Cognition." *Perspectives on Psychological Science* 4 (2009): 274–290.

Vul, Edward, and Harold Pashler. "Voodoo and Circularity Errors." *NeuroImage* 62, no. 2 (2012): 945–948.

Waldby, Catherine. *The Visible Human Project: Informatic Bodies and Posthuman Medicine*. London: Routledge, 2000.

Webster, Stephen. "Science and Society: Art and Science Collaborations in the United Kingdom." *Nature Reviews Immunology* 5 (2005): 965–969.

Weibel, Peter, ed. *Sound Art: Sound as a Medium of Art*. Cambridge, MA: MIT Press, 2019.

Wiener, Norbert. *Cybernetics, or, Control and Communication in the Animal and the Machine*. Cambridge, MA: MIT Press, 1948.

Wiener, Norbert. *The Human Use of Human Beings: Cybernetics and Society*. Cambridge, MA: Da Capo Press, 1950.

Williamson, George Scott, and Innes Hope Pearse. *The Case for Action: A Survey of Everyday Life Under Modern Industrial Conditions, with Special Reference to the Question of Health*. Edinburgh: Scottish Academic Press, 1982.

Wills, Ian. "Scientific Failure: Etheric Force." In *Thomas Edison: Success and Innovation through Failure*, 141–168. Studies in History and Philosophy of Science 52. Cham, Switzerland: Springer, 2019.

Wilson, Elizabeth. "Gut Feminism." *Differences: A Journal of Feminist Cultural Studies* 15, no. 3 (2004): 66–94.

Wilson, Elizabeth A. *Affect and Artificial Intelligence*. Seattle: University of Washington Press, 2010.

Wilson, Stephen. *Art+Science Now*. London: Thames and Hudson, 2010.

Wingate, Richard, and Marius Kwint. "Imagining the Brain Cell: The Neuron in Visual Culture." *Nature Reviews* 7 (2006): 745–752.

Winner, Langdon. "Upon Opening the Black Box and Finding It Empty: Social Constructivism and the Philosophy of Technology." *Science, Technology, & Human Values* 18, no. 3 (1993): 365–368.

Wise, Norton. "Making Visible." *Isis* 97, no. 1 (2006): 75–82.

Wolff-Plottegg, Manfred. *Plottegg—Architecture beyond Inclusion and Identity Is Exclusion and Difference from Art*. Basel, Switzerland: Birkhäuser, 2015.

Index

Page numbers in italics refer to figures.